Managing Motherhood, Managing Risk

Managing Motherhood, Managing Risk

Fertility and Danger in
West Central Tanzania

Denise Roth Allen

Ann Arbor

THE UNIVERSITY OF MICHIGAN PRESS

Copyright © by the University of Michigan 2002
All rights reserved
Published in the United States of America by
The University of Michigan Press
Manufactured in the United States of America
♾ Printed on acid-free paper

2005   2004   2003   2002   4   3   2   1

A CIP catalog record for this book is available from the British Library.

Library of Congress Cataloging-in-Publication Data

Allen, Denise Roth, 1959–
    Managing motherhood, managing risk : fertility and danger in West
Central Tanzania / Denise Roth Allen.
        p.   cm.
    Includes bibliographical references and index.
    ISBN 0-472-11284-8 (cloth : alk. paper)
    1. Childbirth—Tanzania.   2. Pregnancy—Tanzania.   3. Mothers—
Tanzania—Mortality.   4. Maternal and infant welfare—Tanzania.
5. Maternal health services—Tanzania.   I. Title.

GN659.T3   A45   2002
304.6'32'09678—dc21   2002000564

*To the women of "Bulangwa," some of whose stories
can be found in the following pages,
and to the memory of Mama Tumaini and Simon Masasi*

Contents

Tables

Preface

> It is quite plausible, in terms of meaning, to say that multiple meanings
> may co-exist in a culture—even in a single room or a single head. But a
> definition is much less democratic. It sets limits, determines
> boundaries, outlines. Unlike meanings, which are bound up in what
> people think and have in their minds and intend, definitions claim to
> state what is. A definition is a meaning that has become "official" and
> thereby appears to tell us how things are in the real world.
> —Paula Treichler, "What Definitions Do: Childbirth,
> Cultural Crisis, and the Challenge to Medical Discourse"

My decision to structure this book on motherhood and risk in the way that
I have has its genesis in an incident that occurred during my first visit to
Tanzania in the summer of 1990. I was a doctoral student in anthropology
at the time and had traveled to Tanzania to explore the possibility of conducting an ethnographic study of maternal health there at some point in
the future.

While visiting a large government hospital in Dar es Salaam, the capital city, I was given a tour of the maternity ward by one of the Tanzanian
nurses on duty. At one point during my visit, she brought me to the bed-
side of a sixteen-year-old girl. The girl's father, the nurse told me, had
brought his daughter into the city from a village, five days after the onset
of labor. Due to the trauma of that prolonged labor, the young girl had
suffered extensive vaginal and rectal tears, as well as nerve damage in her
upper legs that left her temporarily paralyzed. The baby had not survived
the ordeal.

According to the nurse showing me around that day, the delay in the
girl's arrival at the hospital was a result of the father's "ignorance." The
nurse seemed quite certain that before finally deciding to bring his daughter to the hospital, he had first made the rounds of traditional healers in his
community, who most likely had declared sorcery to be the cause of the
birth complications. According to some of the maternal health literature

produced by the World Health Organization that I had read prior to my arrival in Tanzania, however, a variety of factors contributed to such delays, including distance to the hospital, poverty, and women's diminished status in society (Royston and Armstrong 1989; WHO 1986).

Despite the above explanations, I found myself wondering about the ordeal from the point of view of the young girl and her father, two perspectives that neither the nurse showing me around that day nor the maternal health literature offered much insight into. If those two people had been asked to recount their versions of the events that led to their delayed arrival at the hospital, what would we have learned?

At the end of that summer I returned to the States, unable to shake from my mind the image of the young girl lying on that hospital bed; the unanswered questions surrounding her story continued to occupy my thoughts over the next year of my studies. What actually happened from the time her labor began in the village to her eventual arrival at the hospital in the capital city five days later? If, as the nurse suggested, the father had made the round of healers in his community before finally bringing his daughter to the hospital, *why* had he done so? Or if, as the maternal health literature I had read suggested, poverty and women's status in society had a bearing on the outcome of that young girl's pregnancy, *how* did they do so?

In the following pages, I take the unanswered questions surrounding this young girl's story as a starting point from which to explore the cultural construction of maternal health risk in a different Tanzanian setting: a small, rural community in the Shinyanga Region of west central Tanzania. I will suggest that there are official and unofficial definitions of maternal health risk, and that although both address the similar domains of motherhood, fertility, and health, their respective definitions of what constitutes risk are oftentimes strikingly different. Kaufert and O'Neil's (1993) notion of "different languages of risk," the idea that "different definitions of risk stem from different versions of reality" (Lindenbaum and Lock 1993:4), is especially useful here. In terms of this specific study, those "versions of reality" reflect a contrast between international, national, and local languages of maternal health risk, differences in biomedical and local cultural approaches to health and healing, as well as the diversity of experience present within a small, rural community—a community shaped by various factors, including history, ethnicity, and notions of identity.

Although my fieldwork in west central Tanzania began in September 1992, my initial exposure to the management of pregnancy and childbirth began nine months earlier in El Paso, Texas, where I took part in a six-month course in lay midwifery offered through one of the two existing lay midwifery clinics in that town. My hands-on training in lay midwifery created many expectations on my part as to what constituted appropriate care for pregnant women. How those expectations influenced in positive as well as negative ways my own perceptions and responses to the pregnancy and birth complications I encountered while in Tanzania will be addressed at various points throughout this book.

Both my preliminary training in El Paso and my fieldwork experience in Tanzania were for very different reasons emotionally intense. Never before had I been involved at such a personal level with the joys of birth and the sorrows of death for such an extended period of time, with much of that involvement occurring on a daily basis. In El Paso, my role was an active one in the sense that I was actually "catching babies" (as the process of assisted birth was referred to at the clinic) as well as conducting prenatal and postpartum exams and nutritional counseling for the clinic's predominantly Mexican clientele who crossed the border from Juárez. In Tanzania, although my position was less active in that I was observing how births were managed rather than catching babies myself, I gradually took on a more active role in a different way as people in the community became familiar with me and what I was studying. In the latter context, I often found myself in two very different roles. In one sense, I became a kind of ambulance driver, in that I was often asked to drive people to the hospital when emergency transportation was needed. But once at the hospital, my role changed into one of negotiator/mediator between the families of the person I had transported and the hospital personnel. I had a certain amount of power as a mediator in that sometimes I would insist that the person receive immediate treatment, and I usually prevailed. But the source and effects of that power are themselves debatable issues and will be addressed in more detail in some of the case studies presented in the second half of this book.

My position as participant/observer at births in El Paso and Tanzania also enabled me to understand more clearly how the positioning of the various actors within the birth drama (the birthing woman, her family and friends, hospital and clinic personnel, local healers, myself as the midwifery trainee and anthropologist) and the value and aspirations each brings to the experience are all important in identifying and defining the context of maternal health risk. It was through my participation at births in both locales that I became acutely aware of how various ideologies play out within that context.

My study in Tanzania incorporates data from a variety of historical and contemporary sources, including colonial archives, international and national documents, informal interviews with many people, observations in the community, and semistructured interviews with a sample of 154 women about their pregnancy-related experiences and concerns. Throughout I was interested in particular kinds of information: perceptions of normal versus abnormal pregnancy, labor, and childbirth, and cultural norms surrounding the proper behavior of women and men during those periods. I was also interested in the perspective of practitioners working within the biomedical and nonbiomedical systems of health care. The former included doctors, nurses, and medical assistants in the maternity wards of hospitals and rural clinics; the latter included healers, diviners, spirit mediums, midwives, and vendors of herbal and spiritual medicines. I was particularly interested in how people working within these two different systems of health care defined "at risk" mothers, maternal health problems, and pregnancy and childbirth complications.

My study also included observations of births within hospital and village settings. In the hospital setting, I paid a lot of attention to the interactions between hospital staff and their clients and how emergencies were handled in each case. I also spent much time observing births in the village setting, at the home of a local midwife who was also well known as a healer and specialist in a variety of reproductive health problems, including infertility. Many pregnant women came from far away to birth with her, or to receive treatment during pregnancy.

Ginsburg and Rapp (1995:1) have suggested that reproduction can be used as an entry point into the analysis of social life. It is by doing so, they argue, that one can begin to understand not only how global processes have an impact on reproductive experiences at the local level, but how local culture is produced *and* contested. This book, with its attention to the interplay of colonial, international, national, and local debates surrounding the management of motherhood and risk, is an effort to highlight those processes in a rural Tanzanian setting.

Most of the local terms that appear throughout this book are in Kiswahili, the official national language of Tanzania. When I use Kisukuma terms, I make that distinction in the text.

Acknowledgments

This book, which is a revision of my dissertation thesis, has had a long gestation. The list of people and institutions who helped in the process and to whom I owe many thanks is also long. The initial research on which this book is based was funded by a grant from the Joint Committee on African Studies of the Social Science Research Council and the American Council of Learned Societies with funds provided by the Rockefeller Foundation and by a Fulbright-Hays Doctoral Dissertation Research Training Grant. Summer grants from the Center for African Studies and the Department of Anthropology at the University of Illinois at Urbana-Champaign provided funds for my preliminary trip to Tanzania in the summer of 1990. The revision of my thesis into book form was funded by a Mellon Foundation Postdoctoral Fellowship in Anthropological Demography offered through the Office of Population Research at Princeton University from January 1999 to December 2000.

In Tanzania, I am indebted to many people, only a few of whom I mention here formally by name. I thank the Tanzania Commission for Science and Technology for permission to undertake research in the United Republic of Tanzania from 1992 through 1994, in particular Mr. Nguli who helped facilitate the research clearance process. The Institute of Development Studies at the University of Dar es Salaam kindly accorded me research affiliation, and Dr. A. D. Kiwara served as a resourceful contact person. I also thank Dr. Ali A. Mzige at the Ministry of Health for allowing me to observe the first National Safe Motherhood Conference in Tanzania in the summer of 1990.

Many thanks are also in order for the various government officials and health-care personnel who helped facilitate my research in the Shinyanga Region. Many of the latter were quite patient with my endless questions during the period I observed their work. I hope my descriptions of how some health-care workers interacted with their pregnant clients will be understood in the spirit they are meant: not as a critique of individuals—who are themselves working in less than ideal conditions—but, rather, as illustrations of the complex and often unacknowledged ways global processes have an impact on people living at the local level. I am also deeply and forever indebted to my Tanzanian friends and neighbors in the community of "Bulangwa" and its surrounding villages, especially to the women who shared their stories with me and without whom this research would not have been possible. Although many miles now separate us in terms of physical distance, they are always in my thoughts. It is to them that I dedicate this book.

Many thanks are also due to the many mentors, colleagues, and friends in the United States I have encountered along the way. First and foremost are the members of my original dissertation committee: Alma Gottlieb, Clark Cunningham, Bill Kelleher, and Paula Treichler at the University of Illinois at Urbana-Champaign; and Bill Arens from the Department of Anthropology at SUNY who served as an outside reader. Their insightful and critical comments were especially helpful; I have learned much from all of them. I am particularly indebted to Alma Gottlieb, my thesis adviser and committee chair, whose role in this process can be compared to that of a midwife during birth, in that her encouragement through the various stages of this project—proposal writing, fieldwork, the writing of the dissertation, and words of wisdom during the revision phase—helped in bringing this book to completion. I am also indebted to Clark Cunningham, who, during the course of one conversation we had soon after I returned from the field, assured me that there was, indeed, a thesis buried deep within the seemingly amorphous mass of data I had collected over two years, and that it revolved around the notion of risk. I would also like to mention the crucial role played by the late Demitri Shimkin, who first encouraged me to work in Tanzania, and who provided the initial contacts with Tanzanian officials working within the health sector. The late Albert Scheven, who worked for many years in Tanzania, also provided help on many fronts. In addition to teaching me the basics of the Sukuma language, he generously shared with me all kinds of wonderful documents pertaining to Sukuma culture, including a copy of proverbs collected by Fr. George Cotter and unpublished works by missionaries and scholars who have worked among the Sukuma over the years. I also benefited immensely from discussions I had with fellow graduate students, many of whom provided comments and shared pertinent articles and books: Carolee Berg, Stacie Colwell, Sandra Hamid, Richard Howard, Michelle Johnson, her husband and fellow anthropologist Ned

Searles, Caroline Princehouse, Nancy Sikes, Maria Tapias, and Tesfaye Wolde-Medhin. Sheryl McCurdy and Corinne Whitaker shared their insights into research methodology and questionnaire design during the course of our respective research projects in Tanzania.

Many thanks are also due to the Population Fellows Program at the University of Michigan. As a result of their generous support, I was able to attend the 1997 Technical Consultation on Safe Motherhood in Colombo, Sri Lanka, during my tenure as a Michigan Population Fellow at WHO from 1996 through 1998.

Many people generously offered comments and suggestions during the revision phase of this book. I am particularly grateful to Robbie Davis-Floyd and Carolyn Sargent who provided detailed and insightful comments on the first draft. I also thank Ties Boerma, Zaida Mgalla, Elisha Renne, Hania Sholkamy, Etienne van de Walle, and Susan Watkins for their comments on earlier versions of chapters or articles I submitted elsewhere for publication. Ulla Larsen offered invaluable insight into the demography of secondary infertility in Tanzania.

I am also indebted to colleagues and friends at the Office of Population Research at Princeton University for their willingness to read and comment on different parts of the manuscript, in particular Sigal Alon, Marcy Carlson, Sara Curran, Patricia Fernandez-Kelly, Linda Potter, and Juerg Utzinger. Parts of this manuscript were also presented as talks at seminars in the Department of Anthropology, the Office of Population Research, and the Shelby Cullom Davis Center for Historical Studies at Princeton, forums in which I received many helpful comments from members of the audience. Many thanks are also due to Wayne Appleton, Maryann Belanger, Joyce Lopuh, Kathy Niebo, Debbie Stark, and Judith Tilton, all of whom provided the necessary logistical and/or computer support during my tenure as a postdoctoral fellow. The assistance I received from Tsering Wangyal Shawa, the Geographic Information System librarian, is also very much appreciated. I thank Kata Chillag, Patricia Hammer, and Deborah Swartz for their close readings of different sections of the book, and Terry Njoroge for her correction of my Swahili.

Grateful acknowledgment is made to the World Health Organization for permission to reprint the figures "Mrs. X" and the "Road to Maternal Death" from the publication *Foundation Module: The Midwife in the Community,* copyright 1996. I also thank the World Bank for permission to reprint a revised version of the table "Selected Measures of Maternal and Perinatal Mortality by Region and Subregion" from the World Bank Discussion Paper no. 202, *Making Motherhood Safe,* copyright 1993. Grateful acknowledgment is also made to the Women's Global Network of Reproductive Rights for permission to reprint a revised version of the table "Maternal Mortality Rates for Selected Countries," from their publication *Maternal Mortality. Special Issue. International Day of Action for Women's Health, 28 May 1988,* copyright 1988. Part of chapter 8 is revised from an article originally published in *Africa Today,* volume 47, numbers 3/4 (2000) and is reprinted with permission from Indiana University Press. Parts of chapter 8 also appear as a chapter in the edited volume *Women and Infertility in Sub-Saharan Africa: A Multi-Disciplinary Perspective* (2001) and are reprinted with permission of Kit Publishers.

These acknowledgments would not be complete without thanking my family for their support throughout my seemingly endless years in school, in particular my sister and brother-in-law Lisa and Stanley Maloy. Last, but certainly not least, I thank my husband, Bill Allen, whose support and encouragement during the final stage of the revision process helped me see it through calmly to the end.

Abbreviations

MCH	Maternal and child health
TBA	Traditional birth attendant
TSH	Tanzanian shilling
UNDP	United Nations Development Programme
UNFPA	United Nations Population Fund (formerly United Nations Fund for Population Activities)
UNICEF	United Nations Children's Fund
WHO	World Health Organization

A Note on the Buying Power of the Tanzanian Shilling

When I began my fieldwork in July 1992, one U.S. dollar was equivalent to 385 Tanzanian shillings. By the end of my fieldwork two years later in July 1994, one U.S. dollar bought 500 Tanzanian shillings. The official government minimum wage in 1992 was 5,000 TSH per month. In the last six months of my fieldwork, this minimum wage was doubled to 10,000 TSH.

To give a sense of how some of the health-care costs listed throughout this book translate into local economic terms, below I provide a list of the approximate costs of some basic food and nonfood items. Prices of some of the food items fluctuated from 1992 through 1994 according to their availability and quality.

Kilo of meat	350–400 TSH
Kilo of beans	150–200 TSH
One chicken	300–600 TSH
Kilo of peanuts	200–300 TSH
Kilo of corn or millet flour	150–200 TSH
Kilo of rice	200–300 TSH
Meal at local food establishment	200–400 TSH

Liter of milk	50–100 TSH
Bottled beer	300–400 TSH
Bottled soft drink	150–200 TSH
Liter of kerosine	150–200 TSH
Liter of gasoline	190–320 TSH
Bus fare of one-hour trip	400–500 TSH
Bicycle	25,000–30,000 TSH

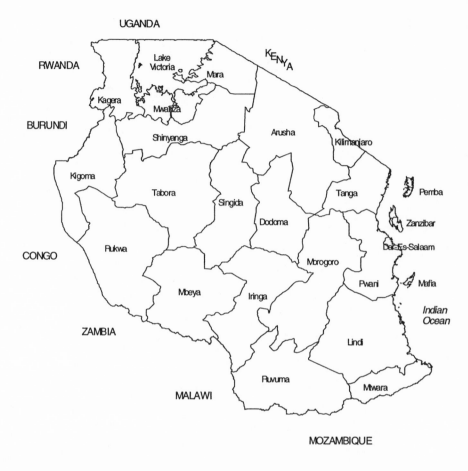

Fig. 1.   Map of Tanzania. (From UNEP/GRID. Map created by Tsering Wangyal Shawa.)

CHAPTER 1

Motherhood as a Category of Risk

Mrs. X died in the hospital during labor. The attending physician certified that the death was from hemorrhage due to placenta previa. The consulting obstetrician said that the hemorrhage might not have been fatal if Mrs. X had not been anemic owing to parasitic infection and malnutrition. There was also concern because Mrs. X had only received 500 ml of whole blood, and because she died on the operating table while a caesarean section was being performed by a physician undergoing specialist training. The hospital administrator noted that Mrs. X had not arrived at the hospital until four hours after the onset of severe bleeding, and that she had several episodes of bleeding during the last month for which she did not seek medical attention. The sociologist observed that Mrs. X was 39 years old, with seven previous pregnancies and five living children. She had never used contraceptives and the last pregnancy was unwanted. In addition, she was poor, illiterate and lived in a rural area.

—World Health Organization,
"Helping Women off the Road to Death"

The questions start with how people explain misfortune. For example, a woman dies; the mourners ask: why did she die? After observing a number of instances, the anthropologist notices that for any misfortune there is a fixed repertoire of possible causes among which a plausible explanation is chosen, and a fixed repertoire of obligatory actions follow on the choice. Communities tend to be organized on one or another dominant form of explanation.

—Mary Douglas, *Risk and Blame*

I first heard the story of Mrs. X in February 1988 during an afternoon talk in the School of Public Health at the University of California, Los Angeles. The guest speaker, a senior medical officer from the World Health Organization (WHO), had come to speak to graduate students about the recently launched Safe Motherhood Initiative, an international effort to address the problem of maternal mortality in the "developing" world.[1] "From the very beginning, even before labor began," the speaker told us,

"Mrs. X was on the road to death." The challenge, as he put it that day, was getting her off that road. Projected onto the large overhead screen before us was a hand-drawn image of a downhill road. At the bottom of the road were two stick figures holding a stretcher on which lay a stick figure corpse, Mrs. X. And handwritten at several intervals along this downhill road were the various key dramatic points of the story: "placenta previa"; "anemia"; "several episodes of bleeding during pregnancy"; "39 years old"; "unwanted pregnancy"; "illiterate"; and so on. We were then asked as a group to determine the cause of Mrs. X's death.

Eight months later I again came across the story of Mrs. X as I was browsing through a WHO publication (1986). I had just begun doctoral studies in anthropology and was researching a paper for a class on health problems in Africa. Remembering the story of Mrs. X, I decided to focus my paper on maternal mortality.

I encountered Mrs. X a third time, three years later in June 1991, at the Eighteenth Annual National Council for International Health Conference in Arlington, Virginia. The theme of the conference was "Women's Health: The Action Agenda for the 90's," and Mrs. X was once again in the limelight. After presenting Mrs. X's medical and social history to the audience, the keynote speaker thoughtfully posed the following question: "Why did Mrs. X die?"

Mrs. X achieved a certain amount of notoriety during the first decade of the Safe Motherhood Initiative (1987–97). Versions of her story were recounted in international journals and conference keynote speeches, developed as the central theme in advocacy videos and classroom lectures, and used in training workshops to sensitize health-care workers to the multiple causes of preventable maternal deaths (see fig. 2). Although we were not told what country she actually came from, certain key phrases— "poor, illiterate, and lived in a rural area," "anemic owing to parasitic infection and malnutrition," "seven previous pregnancies and five living children"—were hints to the audience that she didn't reside in any Western industrialized nation. She was a "developing country" woman, and through her story we came to understand the experiences of all pregnant women labeled as such.

The "road to maternal death" was another concept widely invoked during the first decade of the Safe Motherhood Initiative (see fig. 3). Often shown in conjunction with the story of Mrs. X, the road served as a visual summary of the causes of and solutions to maternal mortality. Signposts along the road reminded the audience of the four main factors that con-

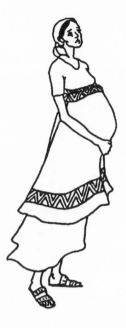

Fig. 2.   Mrs. X. (Reprinted by permission of the World Health Organization, from WHO 1996:17.)

tributed to Mrs. X's death: life-threatening complications, excessive fertility, high-risk pregnancy, and poor socioeconomic development. Another set of signposts along the road indicated the policies and programs that would have enabled Mrs. X to exit that road. Those exits included curative and preventive measures such as first-referral-level obstetric service, community-based maternity services, family planning, and the implementation of social policies to raise the status of women.

Without question, Mrs. X's death is a tragic one; I still remember how deeply her story moved me the first time I heard it in 1988. But since completing my own research on women's pregnancy-related experiences in a rural community of west central Tanzania, I have come to see the short account of her death in a different light: as a story that shapes and then freezes this unfortunate woman's experiences—and thus, by extrapolation, the experiences of all women she is supposed to represent—into a particular representation of facts. It is, ultimately, a story that conceals more than it reveals.

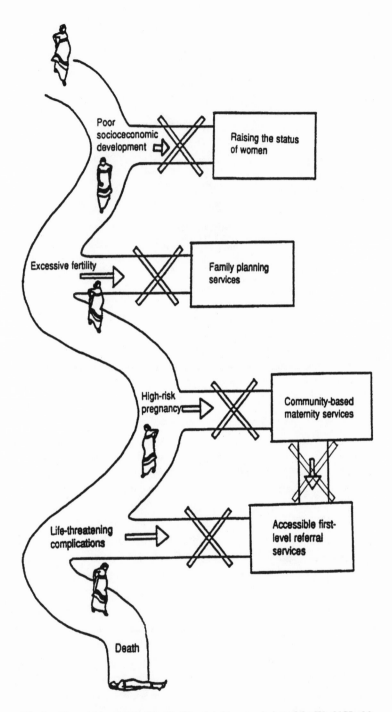

Fig. 3. The road to maternal death. (Reprinted by permission of the World Health Organization, from WHO 1996:30.)

For example, although we are told that the social and demographic characteristics of Mrs. X's life—her unwanted pregnancy, her illiteracy, her poverty, her rural address—contributed to her demise, we are not offered much insight into how they did so. Nor are we told anything about the context in which decisions that affected her survival were made. Instead, we are presented with a partial telling of the events that led to her death, one that seems crafted to suggest that the "real" solutions to the problem are, for the most part, biomedical.

But what if we asked different kinds of questions about Mrs. X's death; would it change our perception of the problem? For example, by the title she is given—Mrs. X—we can assume this woman was married. What about unmarried women? Are their health issues different from or similar to those of the married Mrs. X? We also learn that Mrs. X was "illiterate." If we limit our questions to what happened once she arrived at the hospital, had she been able to read, would she have gotten better care? Mrs. X's story reveals that she came to the hospital four hours after the onset of bleeding. What was the cause of that specific delay? Her story notes that she hadn't sought medical attention for the bleeding during her pregnancy. Why hadn't she? Was her "illiteracy" the reason she had not sought medical care, or had she gone to her local clinic but been turned away by nurses? We learn that Mrs. X never used contraceptives. Do we know why? Could it be that she had tried several times, but the only method available at her local clinic always made her sick? We are told that this last pregnancy of hers was unwanted. How do we know that? We have already been told that she arrived at the hospital in serious condition and died on the operating table. When did anyone have time to ask her if she had wanted to be pregnant at all?

What if we learn that Mrs. X was actually from a rural part of northern India; would our understanding of the factors that contributed to her death begin to change? Or if we learn that she came from southern Sudan? From an urban setting in postwar Liberia? From a village in Tanzania? Would the causes of her death and thus the solutions to "the problem" be the same? What if we learn that she was actually from rural Kentucky, couldn't afford medical insurance, and that the "physician undergoing specialist training" was a resident working at the county hospital who had been working nonstop for the past thirty-two hours? Would the definition of the problem and thus the proposed solutions change?

In *Writing Women's Worlds,* Lila Abu-Lughod (1993:7) cautions against a homogenization of women's experiences, what she calls a "trafficking in generalizations." A language that abounds in generalizations, she notes, forms "part of a professional discourse of objectivity and expertise, [and thus] it is inevitably a language of power. It is the language of those who seem to stand apart from and outside of what they are describing" (8). Drawing from Dorothy Smith's (1987) critique of sociological discourse, Abu-Lughod continues:

> This seemingly detached mode of reflecting on social life is actually located: it represents the perspective of those involved in professional, managerial, and administrative structures, and its origins lie in the management of internal social groups like workers, women, blacks, the poor, or prisoners. It is thus part of what [Smith] calls "the ruling apparatus of this society." (1993:8)

Others have called attention to the use of trauma stories in the popular media and development literature (Kleinman and Kleinman 1996). Kleinman and Kleinman point out that such stories, although usually based on real-life events, homogenize human experience, reducing the complexity of people's everyday experiences to "a core cultural image of victimization," an image that is then used to "rewrite social experience in medical terms" (1996:10; Scheper-Hughes and Lock 1987).

Within the international health and development literature specifically, "third world" or "developing country" women as a category are often depicted as thinking, feeling, believing, and responding in similar ways (Kabeer 1994; Mohanty 1991; Parpart 1993; Sen and Grown 1987). This homogenization of experience also has practical consequences: it can lead to the development of generic policies and programs in the belief that what works in one third world locale will surely work in another.

The Safe Motherhood Initiative: Unfulfilled Expectations

Maternal mortality reemerged as an issue of international public health concern in the mid-1980s with the publication of the article "Maternal Mortality—A Neglected Tragedy: Where Is the M in MCH" (Rosenfield and Maine 1985).[2] In that article, maternal health advocates Allan Rosenfield and Deborah Maine from the Center of Population and Family Health at Columbia University called health professionals, policymakers, and politicians to task for neglecting mothers in maternal and child health programming:

> It is difficult to understand why maternal mortality receives so little serious attention from health professionals, policy makers, and politicians. The world's obstetricians are particularly neglectful of their duty in this regard. Instead of drawing attention to the problem and lobbying for major programmes and changes in priorities, most obstetricians concentrate on subspecialities that puts [*sic*] emphasis on high technology. By reviewing the issue here we hope to stimulate those concerned with international health and doctors and policy makers in developing countries to make reduction of maternal mortality one of their priorities. (Rosenfield and Maine 1985:83)

In November 1985, four months after the publication of Rosenfield and Maine's article, WHO hosted the Interregional Meeting on the Prevention of Maternal Mortality at WHO headquarters in Geneva, Switzerland. The meeting brought maternal health professionals, researchers, and policymakers from twenty-six countries and agencies together to review factors that contribute to maternal mortality in developing country settings (WHO 1986). From the perspective of the various experts attending the meeting, risks to maternal health were defined in terms of the medical, reproductive, and socioeconomic factors that contribute to the high rates of maternal mortality in many of the world's poorer countries. They noted that a woman's age, her physical health, the number of her previous pregnancies, her socioeconomic status, and her desire to be pregnant all had a bearing on whether or not she would survive a given pregnancy. The physical distance from a woman's home to a health center or hospital was also identified as an important factor that affected whether or not she would survive a given pregnancy should complications arise.

In response to the issues raised at the 1985 meeting, WHO, in collaboration with the World Bank and the United Nations Population Fund (UNFPA), formulated a set of curative and preventive measures to help ensure that motherhood became a safe aspect of women's lives.[3] Billed as the "Safe Motherhood Initiative" and launched at an international conference in Nairobi in February 1987, this joint international effort set out to reduce by half by the year 2000 the then estimated 500,000 annual maternal deaths associated with complications during pregnancy, childbirth, and the postpartum period (Starrs 1987). As noted already above, a standard set of preventive and curative interventions were seen as key to achieving this goal. These included, but were not limited to, the establishment of emergency obstetric and community maternal health services, the promotion of family planning, and the implementation of social policies to raise the status of women.

Despite the Initiative's efforts, revised global estimates of maternal mortality reveal that the number of annual maternal deaths is now estimated at 585,000, an upward revision of 85,000 deaths per year since the Initiative was first launched in 1987 (WHO and UNICEF 1996).[4] In terms of the impact of maternal health interventions during the first decade of the Initiative in Africa specifically, a recent article notes that sub-Saharan Africa is the only region in the developing world where maternal health standards have actually declined (Harrison 1997). Clearly, something is not working as intended.

This book offers insight into why efforts to "make motherhood safe" have not always worked as intended in "Bulangwa," the pseudonym for a small, rural community in the Shinyanga Region of west central Tanzania.[5] Drawing upon twenty-two months of ethnographic research that explored women's pregnancy-related concerns, my intention is to examine the processes by which a set of seemingly well-intentioned international recommendations go awry when they are implemented at the local level. My analysis of some of the Initiative's effects in this small, rural setting is focused on a particular period of time: from July 1992, when my fieldwork in Tanzania began, up until July 1994 when my research in Bulangwa came to an end. My discussion of the Safe Motherhood Initiative is also limited to a particular period of time: from the mid-1980s when the issue of maternal mortality began receiving more international attention, until the late 1990s when the first decade of the Initiative drew to a close.

Post–first decade assessments of the Safe Motherhood Initiative acknowledge that some of the recommended strategies to reduce maternal mortality were not as effective as originally hoped (Nowak 1995; Maine and Rosenfield 1999; Starrs 1998). According to an article that appeared in a 1995 issue of the journal *Science,* the failure of the Initiative to reach the goal of reducing maternal mortality by half by the year 2000 is now seen as a result of some of the recommended strategies themselves, "especially those selected initially by key organizations such as WHO, UNFPA, and UNICEF" (Nowak 1995:781). Despite such acknowledgments, many of the post–first decade assessments of the Initiative's impact on maternal health outcomes still provide very limited insight into the context in which such failures occurred.

This book provides that context. Central to my analysis is the notion of official and unofficial definitions of maternal health risk. I define as *official* the various factors that have been identified by international and national policymakers as posing risks to women's survival during pregnancy and childbirth. I define as *unofficial* those risks that, although valid for community members at the local level, did not become part of any official policy. I argue more specifically that official definitions of risk do not always accurately reflect the realities of women's experiences of pregnancy and childbirth; that these incomplete or inaccurate definitions of risk have sometimes led to the development of inadequate solutions for reducing maternal mortality in Tanzania; and that some of the solutions proposed as a result of relying exclusively on official definitions are, in turn, perceived as risks themselves by local community members.

Situating Motherhood and Risk

The Fieldwork Setting

Although the Shinyanga Region is located in a part of Tanzania that is often referred to as the home of the Sukuma people, the cultural and ethnic diversity that characterized the community of Bulangwa belies this generalization. Whereas the Sukuma people constituted the largest ethnic group in the community, people from a variety of other ethnicities also counted among its members. The result was a fluidity in social interactions, a fluidity that often transcended specific ethnic, cultural, or religious boundaries (Abrahams 1981).[6] When placed within the historical context of the Shinyanga Region, this aspect of the community's social relations is hardly surprising. From the Bantu migrations into this area several centuries ago, to the nineteenth-century trade caravans that passed through neighboring areas with their cargoes of slaves and ivory, to the movement of Arab traders into the interior in the 1850s, to the impact of colonial rule, west central Tanzania has long been a site for a coming together of different peoples, for a fluidity in social and cultural interactions, for incorporation and assimilation, but for resilience as well (Abrahams 1967; Alpers 1968; Bennett 1968; Holmes and Austen 1972; Roberts 1968a, 1970; Koponen 1988).

Social interactions related to the management of maternal health risk in the contemporary setting were also notable for their fluidity. For example, many of the Muslim women living in the community, both Arab and African, tended to speak about risks during pregnancy, childbirth, and the postpartum period in relation to Islam (Good 1980), while spiritual ties to ancestors and perceived threats of sorcery were some of the key risk factors for maternal health mentioned by non-Muslim women (Sargent 1982, 1989). But these distinctions themselves were often blurred. Some Muslim women in the community consulted non-Islamic healers for medicines to safeguard against sorcery or for herbal remedies to prevent miscarriage, while non-Muslim women might use Islamic medicine to prevent miscarriage or "cure" their infertility. In addition, most of the women who sought care from local healers also visited the local government prenatal clinic when pregnant. A closer look at the reasons why reveals that these two very different systems of maternal health care, the biomedical and the nonbiomedical, were addressing and responding to two very different perspectives on maternal risk: risks *of* motherhood (as articulated in the government's Safe Motherhood strategy) and risks *to* motherhood (as articulated through the healing strategies adopted by women in the community).

Given these two different framings of motherhood and risk, how are some of the concepts and assumptions of the Safe Motherhood Initiative perceived and interpreted by women at the local level? To what extent were people in the community even aware of these latter definitions of risk, and if they were aware of them, to what extent did they acknowledge them as risks? Over the course of my fieldwork I learned that while some women may have heard about the biomedical risk factors associated with pregnancy through health education lessons at government prenatal clinics and hospitals, there was oftentimes a radically different perception of what the actual dangers might be, or even how they were prioritized in the community.

For example, in contrast to the Initiative's emphasis on the risks of "excessive fertility" (a risk *of* motherhood), many of the women I spoke with seemed much more concerned with the risk of "unsuccessful fertility" (a risk *to* motherhood). As a result, many had used local herbal or spiritual remedies at some point in their lives, either to become pregnant or ensure that their pregnancies would be carried to term (Feldman-Savelsberg 1999; Inhorn 1994a). Similarly, most of the women I interviewed were not using any family planning methods, and when I asked them why not, it soon became clear that concerns about the harmful side effects of birth control methods expressed by women in many Western countries mirror some of those raised by women living in Bulangwa. Irregular periods, fears of getting *kansa* (cancer), and threats to their future fertility were some of the reasons women gave for either deciding to discontinue use of a chosen birth control method or for avoiding the use of family planning methods altogether.

In addition to the physical risks women associated with pregnancy and childbirth, they also acknowledged a spiritual set of risk factors, such as ancestral displeasures or sorcery practiced by family members or neighbors. As a result of these perceived spiritual risks, local healers' advice on the prevention of spiritual risks was often followed more closely than the advice handed out by health personnel in hospitals and clinics.

Even the seemingly straightforward issue of access to maternal health care takes on new meaning when looked at from the perspective of women living in Bulangwa. In addition to physical distance, one must also consider the concept of "social distance." In other words, who are the women who actually make it to the hospital on time, and, once there, who are the women who receive immediate, competent treatment? In some cases, a lack of essential supplies resulted in a delay in treatment, but at other times the delay was a result of negative interaction between the woman, her family members, and hospital or clinic personnel. Although some of the maternal health literature dating from the early 1990s makes the point that *how* women are treated by health personnel within biomedical institutions has a bearing on their access to care, this crucial aspect of care was not alluded to in Mrs. X's story, nor was it stressed at the time the Initiative was launched in 1987 (Fonn et al. 1998; Okafor and Rizzuto 1994; Sargent and Rawlins 1991; Sundari 1992; Thaddeus and Maine 1990).[7]

The Literature

Contrasting Perspectives on Risk
One of the defining differences between expert and lay perceptions of risk, according to Mary Douglas, can be found in their respective approaches to the individual subject (1992:11). The expert, she notes, has a commitment to methodological individualism: "To start with the individual and to stay with the individual to the bitter end, is their chosen escape route to objectivity" (11). The problem with the objective approach of the expert, Douglas suggests, is that it says nothing at all about subjectivities, nor about the influence of a person's social support network. Nor does the

expert acknowledge that "anger, hope and fear are part of most risky situations" and that a decision that involves cost also involves consultations with neighbors, family, and work friends (12).

The distinction Douglas makes between expert and lay perceptions of risk is similar in many ways to how biomedical and nonbiomedical approaches to health and healing have been characterized in the medical anthropological literature.[8] It has been noted, for example, that within the biomedical context, sickness and ill health are seen in terms of how disease affects the individual person, and as a result, the focus of treatment is on the individual (Good 1995; DiGiacomo 1987; Lock and Gordon 1988). Some have suggested that this approach reflects the values of Western, industrialized countries, wherein individualism and an emphasis on high-tech treatment figure significantly (Davis-Floyd 1987, 1992; Martin 1987; Scheper-Hughes and Lock 1987). Nonbiomedical approaches to ill health, in contrast, often include a focus on the social and symbolic aspects of sickness and ill health and, in doing so, call into play a wider set of relationships external to the individual (Hepburn 1988:62; Young 1982).[9] As we will see at various points throughout this book, differences between expert and lay perspectives on risk and biomedical and nonbiomedical approaches to health and healing matter in the context of women's fertility-related experiences in Bulangwa as well.

The Context of Risk: Past and Present Considerations
Appadurai's (1996) reflections on the production and meaning of locality in an increasingly globalized world offer some useful ways of thinking about how past and present social relations both within and outside of Tanzania have shaped the management of motherhood and risk in the contemporary setting of Bulangwa. For Appadurai, locality has a phenomenological, albeit inherently fragile, quality. He describes it as a "structure of feeling" that is actively produced and carefully maintained "against various kinds of odds" (179). He is careful to point out, however, that this structure of feeling is related to actual settings or "neighborhoods," noting at the same time that there is a historical and dialectical relationship between how local subjects and local neighborhoods are "produced, named, and empowered to act socially" (181).

As Appadurai's work suggests, and as Ginsburg and Rapp (1995) have noted elsewhere, global processes can have an impact on everyday experiences at the local level, affecting how local culture is both produced and contested. These authors' observations are important to keep in mind as we explore the cultural context of maternal health risk in Bulangwa. In what ways has the history of social relations in west central Tanzania shaped women's pregnancy-related experiences in the ethnographic present? To what extent is the "structure of feeling" that surrounds the management of maternal health risk in contemporary Bulangwa a reflection of how motherhood and risk were managed during Tanzania's colonial past? And in what ways, if any, do the discourses and practices related to the management of motherhood and risk continue to be actively produced and carefully maintained at the international, national, and local levels today?

Discourses of Development
Critical assessments of the impact of colonial and contemporary development interventions in African, Latin American, and Asian settings focus attention on how the languages and practices associated with development produce particular kinds of truths about societies or groups of people and on the power relations and unintended consequences related to the production of that knowledge (Escobar 1985, 1995; Ferguson 1990; Pigg 1993, 1995; Vaughan 1991; Wood 1985).[10] Recent analyses of colonial maternal health policies, for example, note that the maternal body often served as the starting point from which British colonial interventions to modernize and transform native populations were launched (Jolly 1998a; Manderson 1998; Sargent and Rawlins 1992; Vaughan 1991). These "interventions in mothering," as the anthropologist Margaret Jolly refers to them (1998a:5), were articulated through policies and practices that involved the surveillance and supervision of pregnant and birthing women, mothers, and wives.[11]

The historian Megan Vaughan's analysis of colonial biomedical discourse in eastern and southern Africa is also important in this regard. Her aim is to treat biomedicine as an "exotic system of healing" (not unlike past analyses of indigenous healing systems, she notes) and in doing so to highlight "the humiliating rituals of biomedicine in the colonial context" (1991:11; see also Comaroff 1993; Hunt 1999). She pays particular attention to how African women as a category became an object of knowledge, and thus concern, for colonial administrators and health officials. According to Vaughan, Christian missionaries saw African women as the "repository of all that was dark and evil in African culture and social practices" (1991:23), and therefore regarded with suspicion many of the local practices surrounding midwifery, initiation, and fertility cults (23). As we will see later in this book, African women in colonial Tanganyika (present-day Tanzania) were also constructed as objects in colonial and missionary discourse. Tanzanian archival documents reveal that older African women were perceived as particularly dangerous to society in that they were, in the words of one missionary doctor working in the Shinyanga District in the 1920s, "contaminated by native customs" and thus bypassed in government programs to train native midwives. Native mothers were also constituted as a distinct category of dangerous women, and, as a result, education programs geared to transforming native mothers into useful mothers were launched throughout the territory. My examination of the British colonial discourse on development in general and the role of native women in Tanganyika in particular sets the stage for my discussion of international and national approaches to managing maternal health risk in the contemporary context.

James Ferguson's analysis of the unintended effects of a World Bank-sponsored rural development project in Lesotho focuses on contemporary discourses of development and in so doing "takes as its primary object not the people to be 'developed,' but the apparatus that is to do the 'developing'" (1990:17; Justice 1986).[12] Ferguson's study illustrates what can happen when development planners hold "certain kinds of ideas" about third world countries without taking into account the specific historical, political, and cultural contexts in which a particular country's "development problem" emerged. According to Ferguson, many of the planned economic interventions in Lesotho failed precisely because they were based on ideas that had no counterpart to the reality of how Lesotho's economy was actually structured. Instead, the Lesotho project interacted with what Ferguson refers to as "unacknowledged structures," an interaction that produced, in turn, a set of "unintended outcomes" (20). It is precisely because interventions are planned and implemented on the basis of such generic definitions, he suggests, that standardized development interventions more often than not fail. Ferguson is careful to point out, however, that the failure of a project does not necessarily mean that the project did nothing at all: the failure may simply mean that the project did "something else" not quite intended by development planners (276).

Ferguson's notions of unacknowledged structures and unintended outcomes are important to keep in mind as we examine the "something elses" that emerge when generic Safe Motherhood policies were implemented in a west central Tanzanian community. Much of the international and national attention in the early years of the Initiative was focused on the direct and indirect medical causes of maternal mortality. When mention of social and cultural factors was made, very little attention was paid to how power relations between providers of health care and their clients affected women's access to care. Nor was much attention paid to how economic hardships affected the quality of care that health-care workers provided (Bassett 1997; Ruck 1996; Walraven 1996). Instead, attention to social and cultural factors was focused on eliminating "harmful cultural practices" and "traditional attitudes" that were assumed to be common to all third world country settings. As we will see later in this book, some of these assumptions about the widespread applicability of traditional practices resulted in the implementation of programs and recommendations that were not always relevant to women's pregnancy and childbearing experiences in Bulangwa.

Stacy Pigg's analysis of the discourse associated with UN-sponsored training programs for "traditional" healers in the Nepalese context explores similar issues (1995). Like Ferguson, Pigg is interested in highlighting both the intended as well as unintended consequences of development interventions, and like Ferguson and Vaughan, she grounds her analysis in Foucault's work on the relation between discourse, knowledge, and power (Foucault 1979, 1980). Pigg notes, for example, that the language used by development agencies is not neutral. This "moral discourse of saving lives," as she refers to it, presents particular versions of reality as truth and fact and, in the process, "reasserts the inevitability of institutional practices" (Pigg 1995:48). Following Foucault, Pigg suggests that studies of interventions implemented in the name of development pay attention to how particular definitions of problems "enable particular techniques for managing, organizing and disciplining people" (48). As we will see at various points throughout this book, techniques for managing, organizing, and disciplining Tanzanian mothers have been employed both within and outside of the biomedical setting. We will also see that techniques for managing rural women were present during the period of British colonial rule in Tanganyika as well.

Modernity as Discourse and Practice
That the above discussions of development programs, whether in their colonial or contemporary contexts, must be located within a broader discourse on modernity is a point that has been raised by many scholars (Comaroff and Comaroff 1993; Escobar 1995; Ong 1988). Ong, for example, problematizes what she sees as "a kind of magical thinking about

modernity," a thinking that she believes permeates much of the early Western feminist scholarly literature (1988). She sees this as problematic on at least two fronts. First, much of this literature employed what she refers to as a "traditional/modernity framework" in the analysis of women's status in many third world societies, despite the fact that a distinction between what constitutes the "traditional" and the "modern" is often blurred (83). She is also critical of how the modernity discourse, with its key theme of individual freedom, underlay many feminist analyses of gender relations in the Third World. She notes that in a large part of this literature "there is insufficient attention to nonmodern social values which do not conceptualize gender relations in those terms [of individualism]" (Ong 1988:86; Caplan 1988; Mohanty 1991; Pala 1977). Collier and Yanagisako (1989) have also problematized some social and cultural analyses that focus on the "individual," noting that these analyses "can easily lead to assuming that the 'interests' of individuals are focused on themselves" (33). These authors' cautionary notes will be important to keep in mind as we explore women's fertility-related experiences in Bulangwa. As the case studies presented in this book reveal, local perceptions of what constitutes risk during pregnancy and childbirth are not always seen in terms of the pregnant woman herself, but also in terms of the risks posed to her wider social network. We will also see how a distinction between "traditional" versus "modern" beliefs and practices in the context of maternal health is not always so clear-cut.

More recently, in his study of the modernizing state and local culture in highland Ethiopia, Tesfaye (2002) employs the concept "performing modernity" to describe the current form that modernity takes in that context. In brief, Tesfaye's notion of performing modernity captures the reality that in Ethiopia, as in much of the rest of Africa, modernity of state institutions and practices is often not much more than the performance of "modernity scripts" that serve as imitations of Western institutions. Tesfaye's concept of performing modernity is particularly relevant in some hospital and clinic settings in Tanzania where nurses, garbed in their modern attire of white uniforms and nurses' caps, attempt to perform biomedicine (i.e., modernity) in working conditions characterized by a scarcity of even the most basic essentials of biomedicine: gloves, syringes, and medicines. We will also see that the notion of performing modernity is applicable even at the village level when we encounter the healing practice of a midwife and healer who defines herself as a Christian (another symbol of modernity) and who proudly notes that women who give birth at her home usually do so in the European way (*kuzaa Kizungu*), that is, lying flat on their backs.

Outline of the Book

This book provides, in a sense, alternative tellings of Mrs. X's story. As we will see at various points throughout this book, a contextualization of women's fertility-related experiences is crucial to understanding the complexity of events that shape and affect their pregnancy outcomes. It is my hope that by highlighting rural women's experiences of pregnancy and childbirth, and by foregrounding their own analyses of the various factors that pose risks to their well-being, we will better understand not only how material conditions interact with individual or collective symbolic schemes, but how historical processes, notions of identity, and relations of power are also part of that complexity (Collier and Yanagisako 1989; Ginsburg and Rapp 1995; Greenhalgh 1995; Lindenbaum and Lock 1993).

Official Maternal Health Risks

Chapters 2 through 4 explore the cultural construction of maternal health risk in three distinct contexts or "communities": (1) Tanganyika during the period of British colonial rule; (2) the "international health development community" as it pertains to the Safe Motherhood Initiative; and (3) Tanzania at the national level, in discussions of how best to adapt the Safe Motherhood Initiative to the Tanzanian context. The problems as defined in each of these three communities—the colonial, the international, and the national—are described as official risks in the sense that it is from their identification, their naming, that problems are (were) defined, solutions proposed, and programs implemented. These three chapters set the stage for the discussion of unofficial risks that appears in later chapters.

The Context of Risk

In chapter 5, I provide a description of the Shinyanga Region from a historical perspective. This chapter is particularly crucial to my argument regarding official versus unofficial risks, in that I am trying to show that past social and cultural formations in west central Tanzania continue to play out in the contemporary fieldwork setting. It is in this chapter that I also present material that suggests some women may have held significant local positions of social and ritual power in the past. In chapter 6 I introduce the reader to Bulangwa, the site of my fieldwork from 1992 through 1994, paying attention to the cultural heterogeneity in the community and to distinctions between Muslim and non-Muslim women, and discussing some of the available biomedical and nonbiomedical sources of maternal health care.

Unofficial Maternal Health Risks

Chapters 7 through 11 explore the unofficial risks associated with motherhood and maternal health. In chapter 7 we take a closer look at risk and tradition. Chapters 8 through 11 address specific stages of pregnancy: the prenatal period, childbirth, and the postpartum period. Because my primary concern is with women's perceptions of risk factors, the prenatal period has been divided further into two separate chapters. Chapter 8 focuses on prenatal risks that take place prior to conception. It is here that I examine women's concerns with infertility and their use of herbal and ritual medicines in their efforts to ensure their fertility, and that I begin to explore the concept of spiritual as well as physical risks associated with maternal health. I pay particular attention to women's discussions of sorcery and the perceived role of ancestral and nonancestral spirits in women's experiences of infertility.

In chapter 9, I explore women's perceptions of spiritual and physical risks once conception has taken place. I include a discussion of miscarriage as well as a local condition in which pregnancies are said to "turn to the back" and women's analyses of the spiritual and physical causes of these conditions. I also explore women's experiences of attending the government prenatal clinic, an experience about which many spoke quite negatively. Chapter 10 examines the physical and spiritual risks associated with the management of birth, both in the hospital and village setting. The focus of chapter 11 is on the physical and spiritual risks associated with the postpartum period.

In chapter 12, the final chapter, we briefly revisit Mrs. X's story in light of the other stories presented throughout this book.

CHAPTER 2

The Colonial Community:
Managing Native Motherhood

Societies interested in women's welfare have been concerned about the
high rates for maternal mortality, by the great lack of education for
girls, by the lack of attention to the training of local nurses, and by the
insufficient investigation of certain social conditions which react
unfavorably upon women. . . . In talking to those engaged in medical
work in the colonies, one cannot help being impressed by the
constancy with which a great deal of the ill-health among the people is
considered to be attributable to ignorance, poverty and to harmful
social environment and customs.

—Dr. Mary Blacklock, "Certain Aspects of the
Welfare of Women and Children in the Colonies"

A comparison of colonial and contemporary documents that have
addressed motherhood and maternal health risk in the Third World
reveals similarities in the language used and solutions proposed despite the
passage of time. In 1937, for example, a reprint of the article "Certain
Aspects of the Welfare of Women and Children in the Colonies" was sent
out to colonial administrators throughout the British Empire. The author,
Dr. Mary Blacklock, wrote the article after returning from a trip to the
British colonies of Hong Kong, Malaya, and Ceylon (Blacklock 1936).[1]
The document presents her reflections on the status of maternal and child
health in the colonies and outlines a series of interrelated steps colonial
administrators should take to improve the dismal state of affairs.[2] These
included: (1) improving native women's access to the medical management
of pregnancy and childbirth, (2) eliminating cultural superstitions and traditional practices surrounding childbirth and child rearing, and (3)
increasing young girls' access to formal education.

Fifty years after Blacklock's article was sent out to colonial administrators, another set of recommendations related to motherhood and
maternal health risk appeared on the scene. Referred to as the "Safe

19

Motherhood Initiative" and launched at an international conference in Nairobi, Kenya, in 1987, the Initiative recommended a variety of interventions to improve maternal health outcomes in the developing world (Starrs 1987). These included: (1) improving community-based maternal health services and first-level-referral obstetric services, (2) changing cultural attitudes and behaviors that undermine maternal health, and (3) improving women's access to education.

But just as there are similarities in these two sets of maternal health recommendations, so, too, are there differences. Although both express a concern with high levels of maternal mortality, their conclusions with respect to how education and fertility interact to pose risks to women's well-being are very different. In the Safe Motherhood Initiative, the link between low levels of female education, high fertility, and maternal death is made quite explicit. The 1987 Safe Motherhood conference proceedings note, for example, that 25 to 50 percent of the estimated 494,000 maternal deaths occurring each year in developing countries are the result of unsafe abortion, a method sought out by women when their pregnancies are "unwanted" or "unplanned" (Starrs 1987).[3] The presentation of data in this way underscores one of the main conclusions of the Safe Motherhood Initiative: reducing high levels of fertility is key to reducing maternal mortality. The proceedings further note that the health consequences associated with unwanted fertility are linked, in turn, to the level of female education. The argument supporting this particular definition of risk is that improving women's access to education will improve their overall status in society, thus enabling women to decide (and control) the number of pregnancies they have through the use of family planning (Starrs 1987; cf. Morsy 1995).[4]

The interaction between fertility, education, and maternal death is discussed quite differently in Blacklock's 1936 article. Although she notes that maternal mortality rates in some colonial settings were as high as 30 maternal deaths for every 1,000 live births, she does not identify high levels of fertility as the source of the problem.[5] Instead, anemia due to deficiencies in a woman's diet, to hookworm, and to malaria are presented as the main factors contributing to maternal death. When she makes reference to an association between fertility and education, it is in terms of how "a low population may be and frequently is due to ignorance on the part of the mothers" (Blacklock 1936:224). In other words, low population levels were associated with the high levels of maternal and infant mortality seen in some colonies at that time (Jolly 1998b; Koponen 1996; Manderson 1998).[6] Eliminating the cultural superstitions and practices surrounding childbirth and child rearing as well as educating mothers in proper nutrition and sanitation practices were seen as key to addressing the problem.

The anthropologist Mary Douglas has suggested that definitions of what constitutes danger or risk reveal a lot about the underlying moral principles of the communities from which those definitions emerge. The argument is not so much about the reality of the dangers identified, she notes, but how those dangers are politicized and the actions that follow (1985:60). "Disasters," according to Douglas, "are often turned to political account: someone already unpopular is going to be blamed" (1992:5). Douglas's observations are important to keep in mind in this and subsequent chapters as we explore how maternal health risk has been defined and managed in four different contexts: the colonial, the international, the national, and the local.

In this chapter we examine how policies and actions surrounding motherhood and maternal health risk were defined by administrators within the colonial community in Tanganyika from the 1920s to the 1950s. By referring to it as a *community,* I do not mean to imply that it was a homogeneous one. Indeed, as other scholars have noted elsewhere, and as my discussion of archival documents in this chapter reveals, differences of opinion and even dissent were not uncommon among Europeans working within colonial administrations (Stoler 1992; Vaughan 1991).[7] I refer to it this way in order to highlight some of the overarching themes in the policies and approaches to maternal health risk during a specific period of time, and to compare it to definitions of and approaches to managing maternal health risk that emerge later in the contemporary setting.

I begin by reviewing some of the main issues raised in Dr. Blacklock's 1936 article. I then move to a discussion of how some of those issues played out in the Tanganyikan context specifically. I pay particular attention not only to how risk in the context of motherhood and maternal health in Tanganyika was defined, but also to how that definition changed over time. My examination of the colonial and missionary discourse on development in general and the role of native women in Tanganyika in particular sets the stage for the examination of the international and national Safe Motherhood recommendations that are the focus of chapters 3 and 4.

Risk and the Native Woman

The Welfare of Women and Children in the Colonies

For those interested in colonial discourses of development, Dr. Mary Blacklock's reflections on native life, her views on the proper role of native women in society, and her recommendations for setting colonized peoples on the right path to development are certainly gems (1936). Her article is particularly interesting from a public health perspective, for what it reveals about British colonial discourse surrounding motherhood and maternal health risk in the colonies at a particular point in time. Her analysis of the state of gender relations in the colonies—in particular African women's lower use of health services in relation to African men's, as well as her views on colonial administrators' patriarchal attitudes toward European women—is another theme present throughout the document.

Throughout Blacklock's article, "the natives" are portrayed as being under the care of the colonial government: native populations were undergoing a process of development through the benevolent institution of colonial rule (Beck 1981).[8] Blacklock acknowledges, however, that a "one-sided state of affairs" that gave preference to men over women was a problem in many of the colonies. As a result, native women were at a disadvantage not only in terms of education, but also in terms of their access to health care.

In the following passage she alludes to colonialism's role in creating this unequal state of affairs:

> The early activities in the development of most colonies were chiefly the concern of men; such activities, for example, as the maintenance of law and order, the development of trade, of transport and the utilization of natural resources. Men from the home countries generally originated these works, and it was the male members of the local population who assisted in developing them. As a result of this, the first schools which were built were for the education of boys, the hospitals were engaged chiefly in treating men patients, and in some cases, as in certain projects such as the construction of railways or mines, even the housing accommodation was sometimes for the use of male labour alone. (Blacklock 1936:221)

Blacklock provides insight into how local community members reacted to some colonial policies and programs, although she seems surprised that such reactions would have occurred at all. As we see in the following passage, the blame for not fully understanding and thus for resisting what she saw as the good intentions of colonial educators and healthcare workers appears to lie with the native population itself:

> In colonies where a markedly one-sided state of affairs existed it was soon seen that serious results were arising, but when efforts were made to improve matters surprising difficulties were often encountered. Difficulty sometimes arose from the timidity of the local women and from their suspicions of strange foreign customs and institutions; in countries where women lived in a more or less secluded position it was often found very difficult to get them to make use of educational or medical institutions when these were provided. Again, the type of education given in earlier days in girls' schools was often considered by the people to be neither useful nor suitable, and the women were reluctant to attend hospitals staffed by men. (1936:221–22)

Local suspicions of colonial intentions were apparently also common in Tanganyika, as we see in a letter written on March 3, 1937, by a colonial administrator in response to Blacklock's article and subsequent inquiry by the Secretary of State for the Colonies:

> In a country with a large Mahommedan population and where the non-Mahommedans also are exceedingly conservative in their ideas regarding the training of girls, a good deal of suspicion and actual opposition has been encountered and had to be overcome before girls have been permitted to attend schools in any large numbers. Not many years ago we had to be content if the native girls were brought to school one by one at long intervals, usually attended by parents who would stay to see exactly what would happen. Soon the mothers grew interested, and convinced that no danger was to be apprehended, they often requested to be allowed to join the classes themselves. (TNA 24840/1:7)

Although Blacklock's aim does not appear to be a questioning of the moral authority of the colonial governments per se, she does seem to be suggesting that certain British colonial policies worked directly or indirectly to undermine the health of the local population. Her article is filled with references to poor nutrition, to economic hardships of women whose husbands are recruited to work elsewhere, or to poor health in general. At some points, she suggests that colonial labor policies were adversely affecting the structure of local domestic life:

> When male labourers have been withdrawn from villages for labour elsewhere, have the effects on the women and children in the villages from which they go been sufficiently studied? In a number of towns of recent growth in Africa, many of the people who have come to reside there have become detribalized. Has adequate study yet been made of what social consequences these changing conditions are having on women and children? (Blacklock 1936:262; see also Beck 1977; Little 1991; Turshen 1984)[9]

At other points her words imply that the hardships suffered by the local population are inherent to all native societies. In the following passage we see that although labor policies are mentioned, the "real" problem appears to be with the local women's social role as wife and mother:

> The vast majority of women in the colonies are mainly occupied in looking after a home and a husband and in giving birth to and bringing up children. That this occupation has often to be combined with work in the farm or field, with plantation or factory labour, with street- or shop-trading is true, but it is the first mentioned factors which make their problems distinct. (Blacklock 1936:223–24)

Despite the article's focus—"The Welfare of Women and Children in the Colonies"—Blacklock's proposed solutions do not address women as a target population in and of themselves. Instead, her call for the provisions of funds for education and health services for women emphasized women's roles as mothers and wives; the problem from the colonial point of view seemed to be one of quality. Local women, in effect, needed to be taught how to be *good* mothers and wives so that order could be imposed on the unordered native communities:

> In order to keep a home and to care for a family in a healthy manner, women require a special type of education; special facilities must be provided so that they and their children may have adequate medical treatment; special arrangements must be made so that they receive education in health matters; and a special study must be made of the

social and industrial conditions which may have harmful effects on their well-being. Were these factors attended to, were the women given the knowledge and opportunity to keep a healthy home and family, the good effects would naturally be felt also by the men and so by the whole community. (1936:224)

Archival documents reveal that similar types of instruction were undertaken in west central Tanganyika during the 1920s. African women, it appears, needed to be taught how to be good mothers, based on colonial notions of what motherhood entailed:

At Tabora mothercraft and hygiene occupy a large part of the syllabus and when possible a baby is borrowed, usually from an African woman teacher, for mothercraft lessons. Other domestic subjects such as laundry work, cooking, sewing and mending form regular parts of the syllabus. (TNA 24840/1:7; see also Hunt 1990)[10]

Another important target, according to Blacklock, was the training of native women to enter the health field:

Again, in the early development of a country it would seem necessary that a relatively large proportion of medical expenditure should be devoted to the training of local [hospital] staff, of which an adequate number should be women. (1936:225)

Female health-care workers were needed, as was already mentioned above, because women were refusing to use health services if men were the health-care providers. This was less the case in mission-run hospitals, according to Blacklock, where the majority of health services were provided by European women who traveled to the colonies to work as missionaries. This reference to mission work is also relevant in the context of west central Tanzania. In the next section I examine how maternity care and the training of local women as nurses and midwives were taken up as issues in the Shinyanga District and other parts of Tanganyika during the early years of British colonial rule.

The African Inland Mission, Shinyanga District

In 1913, the Americans Dr. and Mr. Maynard traveled to southern Sukumaland to establish a Protestant mission outpost for the African Inland

Mission Society.[11] While her husband occupied himself with the mission's evangelical work, Dr. Maynard tended to the health problems of the local population, a medical practice that became known as the Kolondoto Mission Hospital and would eventually include a leprosy clinic and a maternity and child welfare center. By 1926 the number of people seeking treatment at the mission was quite significant: 360 people had been hospitalized during that year, and 26,062 outpatient visits were recorded, 6 of which were listed as Europeans, and 18 as Indians (TNA 10721:2).[12]

Initially, few women came to the mission to give birth. In one colonial document dated March 19, 1934 (TNA 10721:14), a colonial administrator notes that Dr. Maynard had told the administrator's wife that "she [Dr. Maynard] worked amongst the Sukuma for 14 years before she got one woman to enter her maternity ward." Why this reluctance? A possible explanation is provided in a letter written on September 16, 1927, by the Shinyanga district officer to the provincial commissioner of the Tabora Province:

> In this district, it is considered unlucky for a woman to be confined in a house in a village where the family had not cultivated land. It is considered an omen of ill luck and that it prevents the rain and thereby creates a famine. Such being the case natives are naturally prejudiced in coming to the Maternity Home for confinement. It is only now being overcome gradually in this district and Chief Makwaia bin Mwandu was one of the first chiefs to break away from this superstition by sending his wives to Kolondoto. I have not as yet been able to induce other Chiefs. They admit the superstition exists but deny that this is the reason. They merely state that their women prefer to be confined in their homes. (TNA 10409:25)

Despite the impression left by the above passage that women were avoiding birthing outside of their homesteads, by 1926 the number of babies born at the Kolondoto mission was deemed significant enough that the Native Authorities provided funds for the building of a maternity clinic at the mission outpost.[13] In a 1927 report written by the acting provincial commissioner of Tabora to the director of medical and sanitary services in Dar es Salaam, we learn that 176 babies were born at Kolondoto's maternity clinic in 1926. During the first six months of 1927 an additional 266 births were recorded (TNA 10721:19).[14]

Risk and the Native Midwife

Archival documents indicate that the issue of medically assisted births and the training of native midwives in Tanganyika received much attention from colonial administrators in the late 1920s. In April 1927 (ten years before the appearance of Dr. Blacklock's article), the director of medical and sanitary services in Dar es Salaam sent a letter to all the provincial commissioners and medical officers in Tanganyika requesting information about the feasibility of training native midwives in their respective provinces (TNA 10409:1). Candidates for training, he informed them, must be residents of the districts where they were to work, be able to read and write, and be able to "overcome the opposition of the grandmothers and the older members of the tribe" (1–3). According to some of the responses he received, the major obstacles to training native midwives in 1927 were the lack of suitable candidates, as well as a lack of facilities for training them.

In his reply, the acting provincial commissioner of Tabora Province suggests that the government adopt a position supporting the movement of births out of the home and into the hospital environment:

> For a considerable while we should look only to established Maternity Hospitals to attend to maternity work, and not to native women working without supervision in the villages. At such established hospitals much instruction can be disseminated not only amongst the women assistants but also amongst the native mothers who come there for confinements. (TNA 10409:8)[15]

Along with this emphasis on the superiority of medically managed births was a request for trained health personnel to assist with the anticipated increase in work load within hospital settings. The district officer for Shinyanga, for example, noted that he looked to Dr. Maynard and to Native Authorities for suggestions as to who would make suitable candidates for training. According to him, Dr. Maynard was firm in her belief that young girls (fifteen to eighteen years of age) as opposed to older women should be the ones to obtain training:

> I have discussed the matter with [Dr. Maynard] and with several of my Native Authorities and we have come to the conclusion that it is

far better to train girls, many of whom we admit may not agree to continue the work when they are married but at any rate they will become useful mothers and if we do fail to retain the services of all of them we can at any rate console ourselves with the fact that some useful and intelligent mothers have been given to the community. Older women are, as Mrs. Maynard rightly state[s]: "*deeply contaminated by native customs*" and the percentage of success is practically nil. (TNA 10409:10; emphasis in the original)

The reply sent in by the district officer in Arusha in the Northern Province, in contrast, expressed the opinion that native women were not capable of being trained:

It is difficult to believe that even in the remote future a native midwife, trained in European practices, will ever be anything but a danger at normal confinements in normal native areas. (TNA 10409:15)

Although it isn't clear how he acquired his information, he provides a description of a "native birth":

At present a native women is delivered in almost complete darkness in suffocating smoke in a foetid atmosphere in indescribable filth in a kennel or a hut. She is surrounded by cattle and sheep and goats and attended by women covered with dried sweat and dirt and clad in stenching skins. Confinement and labor in such conditions are almost unbelievable and yet in normal cases women are delivered as easily as peas are shelled. It is nothing but a miracle and any interference with conditions short of a complete revolution, *would only disturb balances which nature has struck.* Normal labor is nothing to native women and they are quite capable of looking after themselves without the assistance of midwives as we understand the term. (TNA 10409:15; emphasis added)

Other colonial officials anticipated problems with the training of native midwives on the grounds that finding a suitable location where such training could be undertaken might prove difficult. The only government institution that conducted training of health personnel at the time was located in the Asiatic Section of the European hospital in Dar es Salaam.[16] The Dar es Salaam facility was deemed an unsuitable locale for training native women because the patients at that hospital who paid fees "would certainly object if they were used for instructional purposes" (TNA 10409:4; see also TNA 12548:75).[17] In addition, "native women sent from the country to be trained as midwives should not be subjected to the temptations of a large town such as Dar es Salaam" (TNA 10409:4).

Government officials in the Shinyanga District hoped that Dr. Maynard would be able to conduct some of this training at Kolondoto Hospital, but she pleaded overwork as well as lack of funds. Nevertheless, she did informally train some of the local young women in nursing skills, and they usually stayed on to work with her at the mission hospital upon completion of their training (TNA 10409:21).[18]

Maternal Health Care as a Contentious Issue in Post–World War II Tanganyika

By the mid-1940s the anticipated increase in work load mentioned above had become a reality. African women had become quite amenable to the notion of hospital-based maternity care—so amenable, in fact, that many maternity clinics in the Territory were experiencing overcrowding.[19] It was during this time that the issue of the availability of maternity services for the African population also began to be debated in more public forums by African representatives in government. A two-part question raised during the Legislative Council meeting of March 7, 1946, by Chief Abdiel Shangali, for example, appeared to set off a series of inquiries and debates regarding government-funded maternity services, debates that lasted into the early 1950s.[20] Shangali wanted to know the number of existing maternal and welfare clinics for Africans and whether the government intended to increase their number.

In his formal reply to Shangali's inquiry, Dr. Sneath, the Director of Medical Services, responds to the first part of Shangali's question by listing the actual number of clinics in the Territory (see table 2.1). In the second part of his reply to Shangali, Sneath notes that although "the Government is anxious to improve and expand maternity, infant and child welfare services to the full extent that resources permit," the apparent unwillingness of the African population to register births and deaths with colonial authorities led to a dearth in the vital statistics needed to justify future expenditures on maternal and child care programs (TNA 34300:7).[21]

In a letter he sent out to all provincial medical officers in 1947, Sneath questions the economic feasibility of providing hospital-based maternity care for every pregnant native woman, citing the financial costs of resuming its prewar responsibilities of inspecting and ensuring the quality of health care provided in hospitals and clinics throughout the Territory. He accuses the "so-called Maternity and Child Welfare effort" of not being so much concerned with preventive measures such as prenatal, postpartum, and child care as it was with increasing government funding for hospital-based births and creating a dependence on Western medicine:

> [Lying-in facilities] have become so popular, that the purposes of ante-natal, post-natal and child welfare have either been lost or have never been incorporated into the program. Infant and child welfare work, where such is to be found in conjunction with maternity work, appears in the majority of instances to consist in the treatment of sick infants and children. The argument that I have met in defence of this, has been that mothers *require* that medicine be provided or they will think they are not getting anything for their effort. . . . [T]o follow this course as part of an infant and child welfare function, is to perpetuate in a malleable community, all of the iniquity and fraud of our own kind, whose views of treatment may be erected upon the shrine of the bottle and syringe. I believe the time has come when the African mother should be "weaned" from this worship of false gods, and that Infant and Child Welfare should be made an integral part of the whole Maternity Scheme. To popularize ante-natal efforts and competent institutional or domiciliary deliveries of African women . . . and to fail in making it clear to the mothers . . . that their part in the programme is to raise a healthy child and ours to provide facilities for guidance and direction to that end, is to waste effort and miss the target. (TNA 34300:11a–b; emphasis in the original)[22]

TABLE 2.1.   **Distribution of Infant and Maternity Health Services Available to the African Population by Type of Health Facility in Tanganyika, 1946**

Type of Institution	Government	Missions	Native Authorities
Hospitals (medical practitioner in charge)	62	16	—
Dispensaries[a]	25	70	—
Special maternity clinics	5	32	6

Source: TNA 34300:4a.

[a]Sneath noted that only one or two of these dispensaries provided maternal and child health services.

The issue of the provision of government-funded maternity service for nonnative women was also raised in the late 1940s. In a letter to the chief secretary on September 2, 1947, Sneath seems irritated by what he characterizes as a "vocal community of officials' wives [who] appear to be assembled, and to have used the controversy about the sick bay as a means to air various other matters" (TNA 34300:35). He continues:

> The fundamental demand of the women-folk concerned is that the same kind of service as is available in the United Kingdom should be available here, upon the assumption that this Government is oblig-ated to provide and is capable of providing the benefits of complete social security envisaged in the United Kingdom in the near future. Under prevailing circumstances the absurdity of this postulate is patent. It appears to be recognized that Government for some time to come will be unable to provide Lying-in Services within convenient range of every non-native woman who is liable to become pregnant, and to proceed to term in the Territory . . . I am of the opinion that the "complaint" of greatest significance to the minds of proponents of this thesis rests with the lack of hostel, hotel, boarding-house or guest house facilities at lying-in centres for the interval between expected and actual confinement, and the distress and expense of leaving domestic coverage for husbands and families left at home. I regret that while I can appreciate the logic of holding the state responsible for the costs of delivery of its future citizen, I have been reared in another tradition and find myself out of sympathy with the reasoning. (TNA 34300:35)

The overcrowding of maternity services led the Colonial Medical Department to reassess their policy toward the management of births. The emphasis began to shift from that of a concern with "harmful native birth customs" to stressing that normal births should take place at home, so as to free up maternity beds for women experiencing birth complications (TNA 34300:74). In 1953, the member of local government of the Secre-tariat in Dar es Salaam sent a letter to all provincial commissioners in Tan-ganyika asking for their comments on the government's proposed policy on government-funded maternity services. The new policy, while acknowl-edging an appreciation for the benefits of maternity services, was designed to stem the growing use of those services for uncomplicated cases. Five changes with respect to maternity care were proposed: (1) an emphasis on prenatal and postnatal care with hospitalization for complicated maternity cases only, (2) a curb on the uncontrolled expansion of institutional midwifery services, (3) encouragement of domiciliary births for normal cases, (4) development of domiciliary services in rural areas, and (5) the training of native midwives for domiciliary work (TNA 34300).

But this attempt to shift the emphasis away from hospitalization for normal births did not go unchallenged, as we see in this letter dated September 23, 1953, from the acting provincial commissioner from Arusha in the Northern Province:

> In effect the essence of the Medical Department's advice is that we should now try to "soft pedal" a demand we have been striving to create for the past 15 years or more. We must now, it seems, change our tune and urge the expectant mother to use the clinic for ante and post natal advice only. In urban areas such as Townships or other thickly populated areas such as Kilimanjaro where there has been little or no Administrative popularizing propaganda, I agree that the emphasis should be on domiciliary services and ante and post natal care. In rural areas, however, it is quite a different picture and I am averse to the suggestion that the "tendency" to use the wording of the Circular "towards uncontrolled expansion of institutional midwifery services should be resisted." The fact that the number of trained midwives, be they certified or not is so small itself "resists" any possibility of uncontrolled expansion. (TNA 34300:96)

Responses from the Provincial Offices in Dar es Salaam, Lindi, and Tanga raise similar misgivings, while responses from the Mwanza, Nzega, and Dodoma Provinces, although more supportive, nevertheless anticipate resistance from native mothers toward a policy stressing domiciliary births, especially in areas where overcrowding on hospital maternity wards was not yet a problem.

According to the archival records for Tanganyika, it appears that the definition of risk in the context of maternal health underwent a change over the span of less than thirty years. The concentrated effort to address the dangers of native customs and traditions in the 1920s and 1930s was transformed, due to economic and personnel constraints by the late 1940s and early 1950s, into a concern with the new danger of relying on the "false gods" of Western medicine.

Risk and Colonial Culture

In what ways is Mary Douglas's claim that communities have their own constructions of risk and danger relevant to the colonial situation in Tanganyika? And whose constructions of danger are relevant? If it is true, as Douglas suggests, that "someone" already unpopular is going to be blamed, who were those somebodies in the colonial context?

In Blacklock's document we saw how social problems were portrayed in part as a result of backwardness, and thus the education of young women and mothers was seen as the solution. Those members of society seen as incapable of being educated, that is, older women, were simply bypassed in the development process. "Native motherhood" was also seen as posing risks to the successful development of the colonized societies. We saw how motherhood as a category of risk was addressed through programs, modeled after European notions of motherhood, that sought to transform native mothers into "useful" mothers by teaching them how to maintain "healthy and happy homes." Archival documents provide only glimpses of how some of the colonial development programs were perceived by members of the local population, but the glimpses we are provided—for example, that women were reluctant to attend some of the health education courses offered—suggest that some local people may have seen the colonial project as a threat to the structure of daily life as they knew it.

In the case of the Shinyanga District specifically, we saw how attempts were made to undermine local structures of authority, a system that values age over youth, when older women were defined as being "contaminated by native customs" and thus bypassed in the colonial efforts to train health-care workers. "Uncontaminated" young girls were also ineligible for training programs outside of their home areas because they were seen as susceptible to the temptations of big-city life. Although the district officer acknowledged that girls who obtained training might abandon their new profession upon marrying, he nevertheless appears consoled by the fact that "some useful and intelligent mothers have been given to the community."

It is also important to point out that the meaning attributed to women's aversion to giving birth far from home is different depending on whether women were African or European. African women's aversion to giving birth in hospitals was interpreted in both Blacklock's article and

Tanzanian archival documents as natives' suspicions of "strange foreign customs" as well as the strange customs of their own. In contrast, European women's aversion to traveling long distances to give birth was interpreted by the director of medical services as "the distress and expense of leaving domestic coverage for husbands and families left at home." The former reaction is seen as a lack of education, while the latter is seen as understandable, albeit irritating.[23]

Are the points of disjuncture between government health development agendas and local populations examined in this chapter still relevant today? To begin to answer this question, let us turn now to a discussion of the components of a specific health development agenda in the contemporary context: the Safe Motherhood Initiative. It is through the various recommendations of this initiative that some of the educational, medical, and social problems of third world mothers are officially addressed today.

CHAPTER 3

The International Community:
Making Motherhood Safe from Afar

It is the purpose of this Conference to heighten awareness and concern
among governments, agencies and non-governmental organizations
about the neglect of women's health, particularly in the developing
world, and to elaborate strategies to remedy this desperate situation.
We do not pretend to have all the answers, but we do believe that we
have the scientific knowledge and the means to cut maternal mortality
in half in the next ten years at a cost affordable to most developing
countries. In order to strengthen the hand of those responsible for
health care we will examine together how best to apply this knowledge
in order to make pregnancy and childbirth safe for all the world's
women.
> —Joint statement issued by the World Bank, WHO, and
> UNFPA on the occasion of the first Safe Motherhood
> Conference, February 10–13, 1987, Nairobi, Kenya

The agendas of major development donor institutions are made to
seem like the only possible way to deal with problems of poverty and
social inequality. Faced with the moral discourse of "saving lives," we
have to be careful to distinguish between evaluation of the medical
initiatives being promoted and evaluation of the actual social and
institutional means through which these medical techniques are
introduced . . . Relations of power, as well as states of health, are at
stake in health development encounters.
> —Stacy Pigg, "Acronyms and Effacement"

Since the mid-1980s, international attention has increasingly focused on
the high levels of maternal mortality in the Third World. This new attention to maternal health was itself an outcome of the United Nations'
"Decade for Women 1976–1985," a decade in which women's issues were
made visible through the volume of research generated about women during that period (Escobar 1995; Kabeer 1994; Ong 1988; Royston and Armstrong 1989).[1] One result of this new gaze directed toward women was the
increased attention paid to maternal mortality.[2]

In chapter 2, we examined the risks of motherhood as they were defined by colonial administrators and missionaries working in the Tanganyikan health-care setting. In this chapter we turn our attention to how maternal health risks were defined in the Safe Motherhood Initiative.

WHO and the Safe Motherhood Initiative

> In the industrialized countries maternal deaths are now rare: the average lifetime risk for a woman of dying of pregnancy-related causes is between 1 in 4000 and 1 in 10,000. For a woman in the developing countries the average risk is between 1 in 15 and 1 in 50. These countries commonly have maternal mortality rates 200 times higher that those of Europe and North America—the widest disparity in all statistics of public health. Why have these inequities in maternal death rates only recently become apparent and a cause of grave concern to governments and to WHO? The main reason is that until lately the size of the problem was largely unknown.
>
> —Dr. Halfdan Mahler, Director-General
> of WHO, *The Safe Motherhood Initiative*

Much of the literature produced during the first decade of the Safe Motherhood Initiative included the disturbing statistic that 500,000 women died every year from complications associated with pregnancy and childbirth, and that approximately 99 percent of those deaths occurred in developing country settings.[3] One WHO publication puts those 500,000 maternal deaths in "real" terms:

> Every four hours, day in, day out, a jumbo jet crashes and all aboard are killed. The 250 passengers are all women, most in the prime of life, some still in their teens. They are all either pregnant or recently delivered of a baby. Most of them have growing children at home, and families that depend on them. (WHO 1986:175)

Similar to the story of Mrs. X, this vivid image of a plane, filled with 250 women, crashing every four hours, catches the reader's attention, making the hard-to-conceptualize number of a half-million deaths of women easier to grasp. It also helps underscore the point that women in the developing world face incredible risks every time they become pregnant.

As noted by the Director General of WHO above, a primary concern of the Initiative was the disparity in maternal deaths between rich and poor countries. Maternal death rates attempt to measure a woman's risk of dying from a given pregnancy in a particular country or regional setting. Although considered an estimate due to the lack of accurate data, this health indicator is nevertheless used by health development agencies as an estimate of the health status of women in a given country.

One article that appeared early in the first decade of the Initiative notes that maternal mortality is a function of a country or region's patterns of mortality and fertility: "If levels of mortality and fertility are high, and life expectancy low, mortality among women of reproductive age can be expected to be high" (Boerma 1987:552). Generally speaking, if few women die from pregnancy-related causes, the overall health of women in that country is assumed to be relatively good.

But what is a maternal death? And what is the relationship between that concept and maternal mortality rates and ratios? In the tenth revision of the International Classification of Disease (ICD-10 1992), a maternal death is defined as

> the death of a woman while pregnant or within 42 days of termination of pregnancy, irrespective of the duration and the site of the pregnancy, from any cause related to or aggravated by the pregnancy or its management but not from accidental or incidental causes.[4]

Ideally, the maternal mortality rate should reflect the number of maternal deaths in terms of the number of pregnancies within a specified period of time (usually a year). Due to factors such as self-induced abortions, unattended births in many rural areas, or incomplete hospital records, however, many pregnancies are not recorded (Royston and Armstrong 1989). Given this dearth of reliable data on pregnancies, the next best measurement of mortality is the maternal mortality ratio, often incorrectly referred to as a rate.[5] The maternal mortality ratio is calculated by dividing the number of maternal deaths by the number of live births within a given country. Usually expressed per 100,000 live births, this measurement makes it possible to compare maternal mortality ratios across national borders. It is this latter measurement that I am referring to when presenting maternal mortality statistics in this chapter.

Maternal Mortality and the Language of Statistics

The myriad statistics generated with regard to maternal mortality are overwhelming and oftentimes confusing, especially for the uninitiated nonspecialist. Duden (1992) has noted the same overwhelming nature of the statistics used to describe the "population problem." Statistics, she notes, seem to function as outsiders in the context of language, as

> immigrants into ordinary speech outside of their original context. They are used to generate the semblance of a referent which may only be a pseudo-reality, but which at the same time gives the impression of something very important and obvious, and which the layman cannot understand without an explanation by experts. (149)

The problem with relying exclusively on the information produced by statistics, Duden notes, is that it may lead some planners and policymakers to assume that people can be managed, manipulated, and controlled just like the dependent and independent variables in a study (1992:148).

Others have called attention to the homogenizing effects of statistical representations. Although such representations can quantify the material of everyday practices, they do not capture their form:

> Statistical inquiry, in breaking down those "efficacious meanderings" into units that it defines itself, in reorganizing the results of its analyses according to its own codes, "finds" only the homogenous. The power of its calculations lies in its ability to divide, but it is precisely through this ana-lytic [sic] fragmentation that it loses sight of what it claims to seek and represent. (de Certeau 1984:xviii)

Others have sounded a cautionary note regarding the reliability of maternal mortality statistics specifically. Mauldin (1994), for example, notes that there are striking differences in how maternal mortality statistics are presented in three publications produced by international organizations: the *1993 World Development Report* (World Bank 1993), the *1993 Human Development Report* (UNDP 1993), and WHO's *Global Factbook on Maternal Mortality* (WHO 1991a). Given the problems associated with calculating reliable estimates of maternal death—for example, underregistration of births, underreporting of maternal deaths—as well as the large margin of statistical error associated with calculating death rates of a relatively rare event, "maternal mortality data," Mauldin suggests, "should be presumed guilty until found innocent" (1994:421).

Despite the above misgivings regarding the clarity and reliability of statistics, the dominant message emerging from the large number of maternal statistics generated during the first decade of the Safe Mother-hood Initiative is a clear one: there is a striking disparity between maternal mortality indicators for first and third world countries. But, as Ravindran and Berer (1988:5) have noted elsewhere, the way in which information related to maternal mortality is interpreted affects how it will be used to prevent deaths. What does this mean exactly? To answer this, let us see what kinds of questions emerge when information about maternal mortal-ity is presented differently. I use the statistics presented in two different sources on maternal mortality during the early years of the Safe Mother-hood Initiative as examples.

In table 3.1, we see how maternal mortality and fertility rates are pre-sented in a table adapted from a 1993 World Bank publication. The authors of this document (Tinker and Koblinsky 1993) note that this information is drawn from several sources. The world is divided up in sev-eral ways: into two broad categories of industrialized versus developing countries, and again into the regions/subregions of Africa, Asia, South America, North America, Europe, Oceania, and the Commonwealth of Independent States. But dividing the world up in this way raises some important questions. Into what region do Caribbean countries and Cuba belong? Other types of information are also obscured. Why, for instance, is the maternal mortality ratio reported for Oceania high—an estimated 600 maternal deaths per 100,000 live births—when the region as a whole has a reported fertility rate of only 2.6 children per woman? And why are the maternal mortality ratios consistently similar in "East, Middle, and West Africa"? Is this indeed the case? Does our perspective on the mater-nal mortality problem change when the measures of maternal mortality are presented differently, for example, in smaller units, according to specific countries as opposed to larger geographic regions?

To answer these questions, let us turn to a different publication, the "Special Issue in commemoration of the International Day of Action for Women's Health, May 28, 1988," produced by the Women's Global Net-work on Reproductive Rights and the Latin American and Caribbean Women's Health Network. In that issue, Ravindran (1988:40–41) com-piled a much more detailed account of maternal mortality ratios world-wide, drawing upon a variety of sources.[6] In tables 3.2 through 3.4 I pre-sent adapted versions of Ravindran's compilation of maternal mortality ratios by country. As we can see, the maternal mortality statistics that appear in this latter publication provide more detail than the World Bank–based table 3.1. Not only do we get country-specific information, but we also learn where the ratios occur within each country. With the more detailed information provided in these tables, we can ask different kinds of questions. For example, when Oceania (which is grouped with Developed Countries in table 3.1) is broken down into separate countries, we learn that the maternal mortality ratio for Papua New Guinea is 100 times the ratio reported for Australia. And although the ratios for Latin America and the Caribbean presented in table 3.3 are similar to the ratios presented in the region identified simply as "South America" in the World Bank table, in Ravindran's presentation of data we see that the maternal mortality ratio for Cuba—31 maternal deaths per 100,000 live births—is

TABLE 3.1. Selected Measures of Maternal Mortality by Region and Subregion

Region/ Subregion	Maternal Mortality Ratio, 1988 (per 100,000 live births)	Total Fertility Rate, 1991[a]	Lifetime Risk of Maternal Death
World	370	3.4	1 in 67
Industrial countries	26	1.9	1 in 1,687
Developing countries	420	3.9	1 in 51
Africa	630	6.1	1 in 22
North	360	5.0	1 in 47
East	680	6.8	1 in 18
Middle	710	6.0	1 in 20
West	760	6.4	1 in 18
South	270	4.6	1 in 68
Asia	380	3.9	1 in 57
East	120	2.2	1 in 316
Southeast	340	3.4	1 in 72
South	570	4.4	1 in 34
West	280	4.9	1 in 61
South America	220	3.3	1 in 115
North America	12	2.6	1 in 2,671
Europe	23	1.7	1 in 2,132
Oceania	600	2.6	1 in 54
Commonwealth of Independent States	45	2.3	1 in 805

Source: Adapted from Tinker and Koblinsky 1993.

[a]Included along with the table is the following definition: "The total fertility rate is the number of children a woman would bear if she lived to the end of her childbearing years and bore children at each age in accordance with prevailing age-specific fertility rates. Sources: For lifetime risk, Herz and Measham 1987; for maternal mortality ratio, WHO 1991b; for total fertility rate, Haub et al. 1991" (Tinker and Koblinsky 1993:1).

not so different from the 26 maternal deaths per 100,000 live births presented in the World Bank table for industrialized countries. Yet Cuba has significantly fewer economic resources than industrialized countries. To take a third example, the data presented in table 3.2 enable us to see that the maternal mortality ratios for selected sub-Saharan African countries vary a great deal. Although the reported maternal mortality ratio for Cameroon is high—130 maternal deaths for every 100,000 live births— this ratio is, nevertheless, dramatically lower than that reported for the North Bank in The Gambia: 2,362 maternal deaths for every 100,000 live births. What is going on in Cuba? In Papua New Guinea? In Cameroon? In The Gambia?

According to WHO, differences in maternal mortality ratios are related to women's exposure to the risk factors associated with maternal death. Below, I present summary descriptions of these risk factors as they were articulated during the early years of the Safe Motherhood Initiative. Since part of my attention in this book is focused on the discourses and practices surrounding maternal health that predominated during the early

TABLE 3.2. Maternal Mortality Ratios for Selected African Countries

Region/Country	Area	Year	Ratios	Data Type
Africa	Region	1983	640	WHO
Ethiopia	Addis Ababa	1982–83	566	Community
	Addis Ababa	1981–83	1,268	Hospital
Kenya	Nairobi	1977	510	Hospital
Mauritius	National	1982	90	Official
Tanzania	National	1986	342	Hospitals
Zambia	National	1980–83	142	Official
Egypt	National	1981	500	WHO
	Upper Egypt	1981–83	1,950	Hospitals
Sudan	Khartoum Province	1972	320	Community
	West Country	1974–78	2,270	Hospital
Gambia	North Bank	1981–83	2,362	Community
Nigeria	National	1981–83	1,500	Official
Senegal	National	1981–85	600	Official
Cameroon	Yaounde	1980–85	130	Hospital
Zaire	Karawa	1981–83	630	Hospital
Libya	Benghazi	1981–84	21	Hospital
South Africa	National (all)	1980–82	84	Hospitals
	Pietermaritzburg (black)	1973–75	454	Hospital

Source: Adapted from Ravindran 1988.

years of the Initiative, and because the literature produced during this period is quite extensive, my discussion of the risk factors for maternal mortality will be drawn primarily from two early WHO publications, "Maternal Mortality: Helping Women Off the Road to Death" (WHO 1986) and *Prevention of Maternal Deaths* (Royston and Armstrong 1989). The conclusions reached and recommendations made in these two publications are representative of much of the early Safe Motherhood literature.

TABLE 3.3. **Maternal Mortality Ratios for Selected Latin American, Caribbean, and Asian Countries**

Region/Country	Area	Year	Ratios	Data Type
Latin America/				
Caribbean	Region	1983	270	WHO
Guatemala	National	1984	79	Official
Mexico	National	1982	91	Official
Cuba	National	1984	31	Official
Haiti	National	1984	230	WHO
Bolivia	National	1973–77	480	WHO
Brazil	National	1980	154	Estimate
Ecuador	National	1980	162	WHO
Chile	National	1984	37	WHO
Argentina	Abortion only	1981	25	Official
Paraguay	Abortion only	1984	34	Official
Trinidad and Tobago	Abortion only	1981	41	Official
Asia	Region	1983	420	WHO
Burma	National	1985	135	Community
Indonesia	Bali	1980–82	718	Community
Philippines	National	1985–86	242	Hospitals
Vietnam	National	1983–85	576	Hospitals
China	National	1984	44	Community
Japan	National	1983	15	Official
Bangladesh	Tangail District	1982–83	566	Community
India	Anantapur (urban)	1984–85	545	Community
	(rural)		830	
Iran	National	1985	233	Estimate
Nepal	Jumia District	1981	1,657	Community
Pakistan	National	1982	957	Hospitals
	Larkana	1982	5,006	Hospital
Sri Lanka	National	1980	90	Official

Source: Adapted from Ravindran 1988.

"Official" Definitions of Maternal Health Risk

Although the direct causes of maternal mortality—hemorrhage, infection, obstructed labor, and eclampsia, as well as unsafe abortions (to be discussed below)—are the same worldwide, WHO noted that women living in developing countries face an average lifetime risk of dying from a pregnancy-related cause between 1 in 15 and 1 in 50. This is striking when compared to the average lifetime risk of between 1 in 4,000 and 1 in 10,000 for women living in developed countries (Royston and Armstrong 1989:9).[7] If the causes of maternal death are the same, one might ask, why is pregnancy more life-threatening for women living in the Third World? According to the WHO literature, the answer becomes obvious upon examination of the risk factors associated with maternal death. At the same time, this literature also acknowledges that the degree of risk faced by women—even among those living within the same social setting—can vary (Royston and Armstrong 1989; WHO 1986). Below is a summary of how risk factors for maternal mortality were defined in the early years of the Safe Motherhood

TABLE 3.4.   **Maternal Mortality Ratios for Selected North American, European, and Oceanian Countries**

Region/Country	Area	Year	Ratios	Data Type
Developed Countries	Region	1983	30	WHO
North America				
United States	National (white)	1983	6	Official
	(black)		18	
Canada	National	1980–84	5	WHO
Oceania				
Australia	National	1980–84	9	WHO
Aotearoa (NZ)	National	1980–84	12	WHO
Papua New Guinea	National	1980	900	Official
Europe				
Romania	National	1980–84	152	WHO
Austria	National	1980–84	11	WHO
Bulgaria	National	1980–84	20	WHO
France	National	1980–84	14	WHO
Portugal	National	1980–84	19	WHO
Netherlands	National	1980–84	7	WHO
Sweden	National	1980–84	4	WHO

Source: Adapted from Ravindran 1988.

Initiative. I first present WHO's notion of reproductive and socioeconomic risk factors. I then examine how these risks are linked to the direct and indirect causes of maternal death.

Reproductive Risk Factors

Age
Worldwide, women younger than 20 years of age or older than 35 years of age generally have a higher risk of experiencing pregnancy complications than do women in the 24–34 age range. In one of its publications, WHO cites data from eight studies conducted in developing countries that show that "women aged 35–39 years old were 85%–461% more likely to die from a given pregnancy than women aged 20–24" (1986:179). A woman's age is seen as a particularly significant risk factor for maternal mortality in countries in which women are married at a very young age and begin bearing children before their bodies have physically matured.

Previous Pregnancies
According to the WHO publication edited by Royston and Armstrong, the "safest pregnancies" are generally the second and third ones (1989:39). A woman's chance of experiencing complications rises after the third birth. Mortality has been found to be higher in women who have had more than three pregnancies. One study in Jamaica showed that women who had five to nine births were 43 percent more likely to die during pregnancy than were women who had given birth to two children (39). According to WHO, women who have had more than six births are at three times the risk of dying from a given pregnancy than women who have had only two previous births (WHO 1986:179). From WHO's perspective the dangerous consequences of high fertility are particularly relevant in the African context where the average number of births per woman is six or seven.

Unwanted Pregnancy
Unwanted pregnancy, according to WHO (1986), is a major cause of maternal mortality. This is thought to be a significant problem in societies where it is often noted that women have little or no control over their own reproductive decisions. WHO notes that unwanted pregnancy can be detrimental to a woman's health in two ways: (1) it can lead to unsafe, illegal abortions; and (2) women with unwanted pregnancies may be less likely to seek prenatal care in the biomedical setting.

Unattended Births

Another contributing factor to the high maternal mortality ratios seen in developing countries, according to WHO, is that many of those births are not attended by a trained health professional. In 1986, WHO estimated that only 34 percent of all births are attended by health professionals in Africa versus 98 percent in developed countries (WHO 1986; see also Boerma 1987). WHO notes that several factors determine whether or not a birth will be attended, such as the distance a woman lives from a health facility and whether or not transportation to a health facility is available. Findings from studies conducted in the early 1990s raised the possibility that factors other than geographical distance affect women's access to care. Some of that literature suggests that women might be less willing to travel the distance to a health facility if they anticipated being treated poorly by clinic or hospital staff or if they knew they would have to wait long hours before receiving treatment (MotherCare 1998; Okafor and Rizzuto 1994; Sundari 1992; see also Thaddeus and Maine 1990).

Socioeconomic Risk Factors

This broad category of risk addresses the educational and economic issues that have a bearing on women's status in any given country. Female illiteracy, for example, is identified as a risk factor for pregnant women, as it is closely related to both high infant and high maternal mortality. According to WHO (WHO 1986), illiteracy can negatively affect the health of women in at least three ways: (1) women who can not read have less access to health information and, therefore, may be unaware of the need for prenatal care; (2) their job opportunities are usually limited to low-skill labor at low wages, which means less money for health care; and (3) lower wages lead to greater economic dependence on a spouse or mate, which may result in less autonomy for individual women. This lack of autonomy, according to WHO, often means that women have less input into decisions that affect the number of children they will have (1986).

Medical Risk Factors: Direct Causes of Maternal Death

WHO estimates that a large percentage of maternal deaths can be avoided if proper intervention takes place at some crucial point during a woman's pregnancy or labor. These avoidable deaths, according to WHO, are further classified into categories of direct and indirect deaths. In 1986, an estimated 50 to 98 percent of the maternal deaths were thought to be the result of direct causes, that is, obstetric complications having to do with pregnancy, labor, and the postpartum period. These include hemorrhage, sepsis (infection), obstructed labor, eclampsia (high blood pressure), and illegal abortion (1986). According to the book edited by Royston and Armstrong (1989:75), direct deaths together with complications associated with anemia account for 80 percent of maternal deaths in developing countries. To understand why these deaths are seen as preventable, it is helpful to look at their underlying causes as defined by WHO.

Obstructed Labor

Although the term *obstructed labor* has, in some instances, been described as a relative term,[8] in sub-Saharan Africa it is estimated that 3 to 17 percent of all maternal deaths are due to obstructed labor. This occurs when there is a disproportion between the space in the mother's pelvis and the size of the infant's head (Royston and Armstrong 1989:79–82). When the infant's head is much larger than the mother's pelvis, a vaginal delivery is difficult and sometimes impossible, and cesarean section is required. Small pelvis size is a result of two different factors. One is tied to inadequate diet during childhood, which results in poor growth of the female child (and thus future mother). Obstructed labor also occurs when the mother is young and has not finished growing. Prolonged labor, an outcome of obstructed labor, can occur during the first or second stages of birth and has implications for the survival of both the birthing woman and the fetus. For the mother, prolonged labor can result in a rupture of her uterus, which, without emergency treatment, can result in her death by hemorrhage. Prolonged labor can also result in the compression of the umbilical cord, which in turn may cut off the supply of oxygenated blood to the fetus, resulting in its death.

Hemorrhage

According to WHO, death from hemorrhage is one of the most frequently cited causes of maternal mortality (Royston and Armstrong 1989). It can occur either during or after labor, and sometimes even during pregnancy. The underlying causes of hemorrhage depend in part on when it occurs: hemorrhage that occurs during labor, for example, is often a result of obstructed labor, while hemorrhage after labor usually follows prolonged labor. In prolonged labor, the uterine muscles become weak from their extended contraction and thus can not effectively expel the placenta. It is the retention of the placenta that is a major cause of hemorrhage. Retention of the placenta is also common among women whose uterine muscles are otherwise weakened from malnutrition or repeated pregnancies. Hemorrhaging that occurs in late pregnancy is a result of placenta previa, a condition that occurs when the placenta prematurely detaches from the uterine walls. According to WHO, placenta previa is found mainly among women who have had severe scarring of the uterus secondary to infections, among woman who have heavy work loads during pregnancy, and among women whose cervix or pelvic muscles are too weak to support the weight of a growing fetus (WHO 1986).

Eclampsia

Death from eclampsia, or pregnancy-related hypertension, is linked both to poor weight gain and abnormally excessive weight gain during pregnancy. Symptoms of eclampsia-prone patients are easily detected, and death from this condition could be avoided through adequate prenatal care. According to WHO, identifying these high-risk women rests on an early recognition of eclampsia's symptoms, which include swelling of the face, hands, and feet; abnormally high blood pressure; and the presence of protein in the urine. Untreated eclampsia can result in convulsions and coma, ultimately leading to the woman's death (WHO 1986; Royston and Armstrong 1989).

Sepsis

Maternal sepsis, the potentially lethal presence of infectious organisms in the bloodstream, is often a consequence of an infection of the genital tract following labor or abortion and is highly associated with unsterile conditions. High levels of sepsis occur in situations such as obstructed labor, difficult delivery, and invasive procedures such as episiotomies, cesareans, and abortions. Unsterile hands and instruments are often identified as the main culprits. In addition, the potential for contracting sepsis is exacerbated in the malnourished woman whose resistance to infection is greatly lowered. According to WHO (1986; see also Boerma 1987) the reliance on untrained traditional birth attendants with their unhygienic practices has often been associated with a high incidence of maternal death resulting from sepsis or tetanus.

Abortion

Deaths due to illegal abortions are a serious problem in Africa, where abortion is legal (for reasons other than saving the life of the pregnant women) in only seven countries (Tietze and Henshaw 1986, as cited in Coeytaux

1988:186).[9] Deaths from illegal or unsafe abortion are usually a result of sepsis, hemorrhage, or a perforation of the uterus. Some of the early Safe Motherhood literature estimated that abortion accounted for 50 percent of all maternal deaths (Royston and Armstrong 1989:107–36). A more conservative estimate put the number at 25 to 30 percent of all maternal deaths in the Third World. According to Coeytaux (1988:186), in the 1980s, relatively little was known about the actual number of women who survive self-induced abortions, because under the Reagan administration the U.S. government denied funding to any international health project that was even remotely associated with abortion services. This funding freeze led to a dearth of accurate data collected on the subject. The information available at the time, however, was disheartening. Studies conducted in Zairean and Kenyan hospitals indicated that since the early 1970s, hospitalizations for women who attempted to abort had more than tripled, from 2,000 to 3,000 a year to a reported 10,000 (Coeytaux 1988:187). One study in East Africa showed that 60 percent of the beds allocated to gynecology in one Kenyan hospital were being occupied by women who had self-induced abortion (Aggarwal and Mati 1982, as cited in Boerma 1987:555–56).[10]

Medical Risk Factors: Indirect Causes of Maternal Death

As suggested above, many of the direct causes of maternal death have their basis in various indirect factors that undermine the overall health of pregnant women. Indirect causes of maternal death—for example, anemia, malnutrition, and malaria—are seen as taking their toll on women long before they become pregnant. According to WHO, indirect causes of maternal death are often traced to poor nutrition in early childhood.

Nutrition
Hemorrhage, sepsis, and hypertension are linked to poor nutritional status of the mother (Royston and Armstrong 1989). An earlier related study suggested that maternal malnutrition among women in developing countries was the rule rather than the exception (Omolulu 1974). The problem of poor nutrition is said to begin in childhood when, in some countries, boys get preferential treatment with regard to food and medical care. This preferential treatment, however, is usually presented as an Asian, rather than African cultural phenomenon (cf. Caplan 1989).[11] Poor nutrition in the African context, in contrast, is often portrayed as an outcome of cultural norms whereby children are often the last to eat at mealtime, thus receiving a smaller portion of food.

Poor nutritional status is exacerbated in adulthood for women as a result of their heavy work loads and high fertility rates; energy requirements during pregnancy are also thought to be rarely met for these women. On the average, pregnant women are expected to consume an additional 300 kcal per day and at least 30 grams of protein to achieve an overall desired weight gain of ten to twelve kilos during pregnancy (Hamilton et al. 1984). However, the literature at the time estimated that malnourished pregnant women, on the average, were gaining only five to seven kilos during pregnancy. According to WHO (1986; Royston and Armstrong 1989), the combined effects of heavy work loads during pregnancy and traditional practices that limit the types of food pregnant women are allowed to eat result in an overall poor nutritional status for pregnant women. The resulting malnutrition leaves these women more susceptible to disease and, subsequently, vulnerable to complications during pregnancy.

Anemia
Anemia, defined as a deficiency in the quantity or quality of red blood cells that carry oxygen in the blood, has been linked to serious complications in the pregnant woman (Royston and Armstrong 1989:85–88). Anemia is a result of metabolic as well as nutritional deficiencies; cultural practices such as food taboos that limit women's intake of nutritious foods were often identified as the culprits (Royston and Armstrong 1989:85–88; Starrs 1987). In addition to insufficient dietary intake of iron and folic acid, anemia can also result from, or be exacerbated by, high levels of parasites (Hamilton et al. 1984). The resultant anemia in the pregnant woman leaves her more susceptible to postpartum hemorrhage, not to mention leaving her exhausted and less able to care for her other children as a result of a lowered work capacity. As a result, some women may require blood transfusions to treat their anemia and/or consequent hemorrhage. Blood transfusions have been associated with an increased risk of acquiring HIV infection, hepatitis, and malaria in some rural areas in Africa where blood is not always screened at health facilities due to the scarcity of the required laboratory materials.

Malaria
Some early studies suggested that pregnancy decreases a woman's immunity to malaria (Kortmann 1972; see also Foster 1996), while others suggested that pregnant women are more susceptible to cerebral malaria (Royston and Armstrong 1989:161). In addition to exacerbating anemia,

malaria in the pregnant woman is also associated with a high degree of miscarriage and low birth-weight infants (161).

Tetanus

According to WHO (1986), tetanus is a major problem in countries that are heavily dependent on the services of untrained midwives. Unhygienic practices, such as the use of unsterile instruments or improper care of the umbilical cord, can lead to high rates of neonatal and maternal mortality due to tetanus (Boerma 1987:556).

Reproductive Tract Infections and Sexually
Transmitted Diseases

Left untreated, reproductive tract infections (RTIs) and sexually transmitted diseases (STDs) can lead to serious complications for both the mother and the newborn infant (Royston and Armstrong 1989; Wasserheit 1989). According to Wasserheit (1989:146), untreated lower reproductive tract infections such as chlamydia and gonococcal cervicitis or bacterial vaginosis can ascend into the upper reproductive tract, causing severe lower abdominal pain (also known as pelvic inflammatory disease [PID]). Untreated reproductive tract infections can also lead to infertility (see also Dixon-Mueller and Wasserheit 1991). It has been noted that infertility is sometimes as high as 30 to 50 percent of all couples in some sub-Saharan African communities (Wasserheit 1989:160; Belsey 1976).[12] This is in sharp contrast to what at the time was the "generally accepted 'core infertility' rate of 7% attributable to genetic, anatomic, or endocrine factors" (Wasserheit 1989:160). Untreated venereal diseases can result in the scarring of the fallopian tubes, resulting in life-threatening ectopic pregnancies, pregnancies that implant in the fallopian tubes rather than in the womb (147). Ectopic pregnancies require surgical treatment and can be fatal if access to adequate medical facilities is limited. Gonorrhea in the birthing woman is linked to eye infection in the newborn infant, which, if left untreated, often causes permanent loss of vision.

International Recommendations

In February 1987, WHO, UNFPA, and the World Bank, with support from UNICEF and the Population Council, jointly sponsored the Safe Motherhood Conference in Nairobi, Kenya. Representatives from thirty-seven countries participated, including the ministers of health from five countries, the director-general of WHO, the president of the World Bank, the administrator of the United Nations Development Program (UNDP), the assistant executive of the United Nations Fund for Population Activities (UNFPA), and staff from fourteen nongovernmental organizations and seven bilateral aid agencies (Mahler 1987:668; Starrs 1987). Four essential cornerstones of a maternal health program were identified as the strategy to combat maternal mortality in the developing world:

> First, adequate primary health care at all levels and an adequate share of the available food for girls from infancy to adolescence, and family planning universally available to avoid unwanted or high risk pregnancies; second, after pregnancy begins, good prenatal care, including nutrition, with efficient and early detection and referral of high-risk patients; third, the assistance of a trained person for all women in childbirth, at home or in a hospital; and fourth, women at higher risk and, above all women in those dire emergencies of pregnancy and childbirth, must all have effective access to the essential elements of obstetric care. (Mahler 1987:669)

In other words, the solutions to the problem of maternal mortality initially proposed in the early years of the Safe Motherhood Initiative included recommendations for the implementation of programs that would increase women's access to family planning, promote the value of prenatal care, increase a pregnant woman's access to emergency treatment should complications during pregnancy or childbirth arise, develop programs to train traditional birth attendants, and increase access to health facilities in general. It was through the implementation of programs based on these cornerstones that the overall goal of reducing the number of maternal deaths in developing countries by half by the year 2000 was seen as attainable.

What happens when these general categories of problems and solutions are taken to the national level? Are all of these categories viewed as equally relevant by the host country health officials or do new categories of problems and solutions emerge? In the next chapter we explore how key aspects of this internationally conceived initiative are discussed at the national level in Tanzania. We examine the government's official position on maternal health-care issues as it is articulated in the literature produced by and for the Tanzanian Ministry of Health. We will then see how the issue of maternal mortality is taken up as a cause by a Tanzanian nongovernmental women's media organization that sees itself as speaking in the interest of all Tanzanian women. In what ways are the issues raised in these two distinct national contexts similar? In what ways are they different? And to what extent do these Tanzanian agendas appear to mirror those put forth by policymakers and health experts at the international level?

CHAPTER 4

The National Community: Making Motherhood Safe in Tanzania

In reviewing Tanzania's commitment and progress in SMI [the Safe
Motherhood Initiative] it is appropriate to look into each of the items
contained in the Call for Action adopted at the Nairobi Safe
Motherhood Conference in February 1987. However, it may be stated
from the outset that in the Tanzanian context SMI is essentially a call
for review of the long established national integrated MCH/FP
[Maternal and Child Health/Family Planning] program with the
objective of strengthening the maternal health component and
development of a comprehensive multisectoral approach. Most of the
actions that constitute SMI are embodied in the national health plan.
—M. Kaisi, *The Safe Motherhood Initiative in Tanzania*

In February 1989, Dr. M. Kaisi, a Tanzanian obstetrician and gynecolo-
gist, was asked by Tanzanian Ministry of Health officials to prepare pro-
posals for the development of a Tanzania-specific Safe Motherhood Initiative. That initial request resulted in *The Safe Motherhood Initiative in
Tanzania: Role of the Health Sector,* which, according to its descriptive
subtitle, was an assessment of "unmet need, recommendations and proposed activities [for reducing maternal mortality in Tanzania]" (Kaisi
1989). As noted in the epigraph that opens this chapter, the Safe Motherhood Initiative was seen as a means of strengthening the government's
already existing MCH/FP program rather than developing a new, separate
program altogether. Kaisi makes the point, however, that the MCH/FP
program—which was launched in Tanzania in 1974—received most of its
funding through foreign aid, and therefore its success or failure depended
on the availability of those funds (1989:25). Moreover, as less and less of
the government's total budget was being allocated to health programs,
"the success of SMI will initially very much depend on program funding
from external sources" (25).

Kaisi begins the document by tracing the history of the Safe Motherhood Initiative at the international level: its inception, its definition of the problem, and its general recommendations for reducing maternal mortality in the developing world. He includes the story of Mrs. X ("a real life account," he notes) along with a drawing of the road to maternal death that summarizes both the causes of and recommended solutions for maternal mortality.

Having covered the major points of the Safe Motherhood Initiative, Kaisi then moves to a review of the literature on maternal mortality in Tanzania specifically. Most of those studies were hospital-based. Although he noted that they provided useful information on the causes of maternal deaths in Tanzania, he also points out that they did not shed much light on how home-based births may also contribute to maternal mortality (1989:7). Nevertheless, he identifies five important findings of those hospital-based studies: (1) hemorrhage, sepsis, anemia, eclampsia, and prolonged/ obstructed labor are the leading causes of maternal death in Tanzania; (2) factors such as lack of blood for emergency transfusion, late arrival at the hospital, poor management after arrival at the hospital, and lack of "self-discipline and commitment among health personnel" all contribute to these deaths; (3) maternal mortality experiences yearly fluctuation within every region; (4) significant variations in maternal mortality rates occur between regions; and (5) the level of maternal mortality rates for Tanzania overall had remained the same in the past fifteen years (7–8). Kaisi notes that this latter piece of information is ironic given that this period of fifteen years also corresponds to the existence of the government's MCH/FP program.

Tanzania's unmet needs, according to Kaisi, include those that relate to policy, program planning, training, research, and financial support. He also notes, in a manner similar to the early Safe Motherhood literature, that the measures needed to reduce Tanzania's maternal mortality rates include both long-term and short-term strategies (1989:11). The long-term strategies are nonmedical, such as the implementation of educational and legal policies with the goal of improving the overall status of women. The short-term measures, on the other hand, focus on more immediate medical concerns such as improving the quality of care in government health facilities, implementing the Tanzanian National Blood Transfusion Services program (first proposed in 1985), and improving people's access to health care by training laypersons as village health workers (VHW) and traditional birth attendants (TBA).

To reach these goals and to increase the public's awareness of maternal mortality in Tanzania, Kaisi proposed a multisectoral approach that included the participation of key governmental and nongovernmental organizations working on various related issues such as health, family planning, women's status, nutrition, information and education, and research. He also proposed the formation of a Safe Motherhood Committee comprised of members from these various sectors who would work together to develop a coherent Safe Motherhood strategy for Tanzania. This committee, which became known as the Safe Motherhood Task Force, developed the Draft Strategy for Safe Motherhood, a document that was discussed at the Tanzanian National Safe Motherhood Conference in August 1990. Recommendations coming out of that conference led to the creation of a final document, *Safe Motherhood Strategy for Tanzania,* which was published by the Tanzanian Ministry of Health in March 1992.

Overall, Kaisi's categories for both causes and solutions to the problem of maternal mortality in Tanzania are similar to those presented in the early Safe Motherhood literature. But how did the initial categories of problems and recommendations for solutions in Kaisi's 1989 document hold up under closer scrutiny? When the issue of maternal mortality was debated in public forums organized at the national level in Tanzania, did completely new categories of causes and solutions emerge?

In the following two sections, I present a discussion of two such forums. The first is a workshop on maternal mortality organized in 1988 by an association of Tanzanian female journalists and media professionals. The second forum was The National Conference on Safe Motherhood in August 1990 mentioned above. To what extent do the definitions and recommended solutions that emerged from these two different forums anticipate the pregnancy-related concerns articulated by women at the local level?

The Tanzania Media Women's Association

The number of maternal deaths at the Muhimbili Medical Centre (MMC)[1] maternity block in Dar es Salaam may be more than triple this year if a sudden upsurge recorded in the first quarter is not arrested, it has been learnt. According to an official report by the MMC's Obstetrics and Gynecology Department obtained by the *Daily News* . . . 71 mothers died in the first three and a quarter months of this year compared to a constant 65 to 70 deaths recorded annually in the past. . . . According to the report, 42 of the 71 deaths this year were of mothers aged between 15 and 25 years. Thirty-two deaths or 45 per cent of the total occurred within 24 hours of admission at MMC.

The MMC Director of Hospital Services . . . acknowledged the existence of the crisis at the maternity block when contacted by the Daily News this week but said he was not prepared to make a public comment on the matter.

—Excerpt from the Tanzanian newspaper
Daily News, May 6, 1988

In August 1990, I was given a photocopy of the above newspaper item, along with a bundle of other photocopied articles on the issue of maternal mortality in Tanzania, by the chairperson of the Tanzania Media Women's Association (TAMWA).[2] When, during the course of our conversation, she learned that my future dissertation research would address some aspect of maternal mortality in Tanzania, she told me that it was TAMWA, in fact, that had been responsible for organizing Tanzania's first "Day of Action for Women's Health" seminar in May 1988. Hearing this, I mentioned that I had just returned from Tanzania's National Conference on Safe Motherhood and that I had copies of all the papers presented at the conference. Her interest was piqued, and she offered to strike a deal. She told me that she had not been able to attend the National Safe Motherhood conference due to her prior commitments. She offered to exchange copies of TAMWA's documents addressing the issue of maternal mortality for copies of the papers I had collected at the National Safe Motherhood Conference. I agreed, and we exchanged our copies a few days later.

Many of the documents she gave me were from the TAMWA-sponsored workshop "1988 Day of Action for Women's Health." In addition to her written report of that event, I also received texts of the papers presented at the workshop. These included two papers on the general issue of maternal mortality written by physicians from the Muhimbili Medical Center (Justesen 1988; Kaisi 1988), another paper on unwanted pregnancy presented by a German physician working with a German development project located on the grounds of Muhimbili Hospital (Nachtigal 1988), and a paper written by a woman involved with the training of traditional birth attendants in the Tanga Region (Zimbwe 1988).

TAMWA's summary report provides some background information on how TAMWA members first became aware of the issue of maternal mortality in Tanzania and why they decided to organize a "Day of Action" around that theme:

We in TAMWA were discussing what to do [on the International Day of Action for Women's Health]. In *Sauti*[3] on page 28 [one of TAMWA's members] did an article based on material received from Global Network on fact and figures and importance of the issue. . . . The article was well received and it seemed women wanted to discuss the issue of maternal mortality first and foremost. In other words, put it on the agenda. (Alloo 1988:1)

The Global Network publication mentioned above is the May 28, 1988, special issue "A Call to Women for Action" jointly produced by the Women's Global Network on Reproductive Rights (WGNRR) and the Latin American and Caribbean Women's Health Network/ISIS International.[4] The "Day of Action for Women's Health" called for by these two organizations had its genesis in a conference held in Costa Rica in 1987. As noted in the opening pages of the WGNRR and ISIS special issue on maternal mortality:

> Maternal mortality should be an issue of concern to everyone in the world. Because it is central to the struggle for reproductive rights, the Women's Global Network on Reproductive Rights and the Latin America and Caribbean Women's Health Network of Isis International decided to organize an international campaign on the prevention of maternal mortality. . . . The decision to organize this campaign was taken at the Fifth International Women and Health Meeting, held in Costa Rica in May 1987, by feminist groups active in the international women's health and reproductive rights movement. Throughout that meeting, the deaths of women in relation to all aspects of reproduction and health were a central issue. Women who are working to make pregnancy and childbirth safe in their countries, and women who are working for safe contraception and abortion came together, sometimes from very different groups, and reaffirmed that our focus and aims are in common, reflecting all the varying needs which women have. (WGNRR and ISIS 1988:2)

That the initial impetus for TAMWA's decision to focus on the issue of maternal mortality in Tanzania came from outside of the country is interesting in itself and important to note. My concern for the moment, however, is with how the problem of maternal mortality was defined during the TAMWA-sponsored workshop of 1988.

The report notes that men and women from thirty-five organizations based in the capital were invited to the workshop, although fifteen people declined due to prior commitments at other "women's issues" conferences taking place in Tanzania during the same period.[5] Regarding the format of the seminar, the report includes the following observation:

> Two weeks before, the issue of maternal mortality had broken in the press and there was a lot of controversy on the issue [see excerpt from *Daily News* above]. We went to see the doctors involved and invite them to speak and to our surprise they agreed. We discussed the topic and they chose how they wanted to put it. (Alloo 1988:1)

The chairperson's report provides a summary of the major points raised at the seminar including whether maternal mortality is a medical or social issue, the relevance of family planning and the spacing of births to reducing mortality, the problems of inadequate health centers and facilities, the lack of transport to health facilities, illegal abortion and its consequences for women, women's mistrust of some health practitioners who "want money only and will do anything," the institution of marriage and women's choice within it, and finally a discussion as to whether or not maternal deaths occur primarily among poorer women. With regard to this latter question the report notes: "The answer was that the doctors in hospitals failed to trace it [the effect of economic factors on maternal death] because in Tanzania, no one can live on salaries."[6]

The workshop participants concluded that the problem of maternal mortality was many-sided: individual, institutional, and national. The summary concludes with the following set of recommendations:

> This question of maternal mortality should be put to the nation. We *need education* at [the] conceptual level. Traditional practices also which [are] detrimental to women's health need to be exposed. We *need changes* at [the] institutional level. We *need involvement* at [the] national level where resources are allocated—priority [needs] to be given to this question. We need education that women need *a choice.* Strong religious sentiments have been an obstacle to legalize abortion yet they are taking place and women are dying from what can be a safe operation, if legalized. We need *reintroduction of traditional sex education* and in primary schools for both boys and girls. Naivety is a cause of a lot of schoolgirl pregnancies. It is a national issue. We need to look into *laws* which are detrimental to women's right to choose.

We *need research* into the rate of maternal mortality in the country as a whole so that we know where to start to deal with it. *Birth control availability* at demand is necessary. Women should not be asked for husbands' permission when they do go to get birth control. Also *traditional birth control* needs to be enhanced. *Training of birth attendants* who have and are performing a very important task and they must be given weight at a national level. It seems that this question needs a *mass campaign*. Does society know about the maternal mortality rate in our country? Why not? This year is the year of Safe Motherhood. What does that mean? (Alloo 1988:3; emphasis in the original)

Another shorter summary of the seminar accompanied the report. Its tone was quite different. Written by a TAMWA member who had been involved in research on teenage pregnancy, this second summary seemed less a simple list of topics discussed at the seminar than it was this woman's personal reflection on the wider issue of female oppression. Her summary portrays Tanzanian women as passive victims of male patriarchy. Women, she suggests, have been duped into believing that their primary role is to bear children. Furthermore, they are not even aware that they are oppressed:

Although the day was to discuss maternal mortality it became clear to me that there was another, more important discussion arising out of this meeting and this is the discussion related to the construction of gender. Peoples' attitudes towards sexuality, sex, childbearing and rearing are socially constructed and are not part of a "natural" desire for procreation. Because this is so women do not even own their bodies and are not aware, because of a constant barrage of male-centered propaganda, that the power to choose whether or not they want children lies in their hands and nowhere else. . . .What the issues did was to make me think of ways of effectively challenging the patriarchy and exposing it as an illegitimate system. (Alloo 1988: Appendix X)

Her summary concludes with her analysis of some problems with the forum. She felt that it was too short and that it did not achieve its initial purpose of eliciting ideas to reduce maternal mortality. The seminar also failed to develop any concrete plans of action to address maternal deaths. She ends her summary by calling on TAMWA to establish women's action groups and support networks for keeping women's issues alive.[7]

To what extent are the issues raised at the TAMWA-sponsored workshop on maternal mortality similar to how the problem of maternal mortality was discussed by health-care professionals engaged in determining Safe Motherhood policies for Tanzania as a whole? To answer this, let us examine some of the issues that unfolded at the National Conference on Safe Motherhood, held in Morogoro, Tanzania, in August 1990. As already mentioned above, the conference was organized in order to finalize the recommendations raised in the Draft Strategy for Safe Motherhood in Tanzania. The document discussed at the conference was very similar to Kaisi's 1989 document; he was, in fact, the head of the Safe Motherhood Task Force that developed the draft. The recommendations coming out of the Morogoro conference would, in turn, be forwarded first to the prime minister's office and, at a later date, to the Tanzanian Parliament for approval.

The National Safe Motherhood Conference

> In Tanzania, like in most other developing countries, reproduction is an extremely risky endeavor. Maternal morbidity and mortality are among the leading public health concerns. Maternal mortality, for example, represents an area in public health with the widest disparity when comparisons are made with rich countries. Women's health in general, and reproductive health in particular, bears unique significance in Tanzania. This is so because women's contribution to the national economy as well as family income is greater than that of men. In addition women in Tanzania play a major role in family health promotion and well-being. Child survival is largely dependent of the health of mothers.
> —Excerpt from the *Draft Strategy for Safe Motherhood in Tanzania,* presented and discussed at the National Safe Motherhood Conference, August 1990

The National Conference on Safe Motherhood, which was held at a hotel in Morogoro, Tanzania (a three-hour drive from the capital city), was well-attended. Approximately fifty to sixty Tanzanians from all around the country participated, and there seemed to be an equal number of men and women present. The participants included physicians, regional coordinators of the maternal health programs at government hospitals, and representatives from religious organizations, from the government's family planning organization, and from the national women's organization, as well as Tanzanian representatives from UNICEF and other UN programs. The non-Tanzanians present included myself and one other American college student (as observers) and two American women from the American-based nongovernmental organization that was providing logistical support for the conference.[8] The only other non-Tanzanian present was the Swedish director of UNICEF, who took an active role throughout the conference.

The structure of the three-day conference was as follows: papers addressing the various issues involved with maternal mortality were presented in the morning, and preassigned key topics relevant to maternal mortality were discussed in small groups in the afternoons. On the morning of the third day the draft plan for a national policy for Safe Motherhood was presented, then the small groups reassembled to discuss the plan and suggest changes, additions, or recommendations for action. In the afternoon the whole group reconvened in order to arrive at a consensus as to the appropriate format for a national Safe Motherhood policy.

The issues raised throughout the conference were similar in many ways to those raised in the seminar sponsored by TAMWA. At issue throughout were the topics of gender, abortion, teenage pregnancy, education, and family planning. In the small groups these themes were discussed in more detail.

The theme of the first group discussion I sat in on centered around the issues of the legal, economic, and social factors that affect women's well-being and thus ,their health status. The institution of marriage was discussed at length. Polygyny, age at marriage, the custom of brideprice, and women's lack of relative power vis-à-vis their husbands in marriage were key topics.[9] Many women in the group felt that the custom of brideprice was responsible for women's heavy work loads, as the husband usually expected to be compensated through his wife's work. Some women also felt that the custom of brideprice was also responsible for high rates of wife beating, in that oftentimes the husband is angry for having had to pay a high price. It was also noted that wives must obtain permission from their husbands before receiving birth control from government hospitals.

Another issue discussed as problematic for women was the age of marriage. It was noted that in Tanzania, the legal age of marriage was fifteen years for females and eighteen years for males. A female participant from Zanzibar, the predominantly Muslim-populated island off the coast of mainland Tanzania, mentioned that oftentimes girls as young as thirteen years are married to older men (see Katapa 1994).[10] The problem of obstructed labor, common in pregnancies of young girls due to the small size of their pelvis, was associated with this type of marriage arrangement (cf. WHO 1986).[11] There was a consensus in the group that the legal age of marriage for females should be raised to eighteen years, although many acknowledged there would be strong opposition from Muslim leaders. The need for legalized abortion was also raised but dropped because those present felt there would be too much opposition, again from Muslim leaders (see Rwebangira 1994).[12]

The government policy of expelling pregnant girls from school permanently was also sharply criticized and identified as one of the factors responsible for the high rates of deaths from botched abortions among schoolgirls. Many of the female participants at the conference wanted to see some sanctions imposed against the men or schoolboys who had "caused" those pregnancies (see Puja and Kassimoto 1994). The issue of legally mandated child support was also raised, and it was noted that "currently" (in 1990) men were only required to pay the one-time fee of 100 Tanzanian shillings (equivalent at the time to about 50 U.S. cents) for pregnancies resulting from their sexual relations with unmarried females.

The decline in traditional forms of sex education, referred to in many parts of Tanzania as *unyago* (Shaba and Kituru 1991), was also seen as responsible for high rates of pregnancy. The group recommended that such practices be revived (see Tumbo-Masabo and Liljeström 1994; cf. Allen 2000).[13] How this was to be accomplished, however, was not discussed.

There was also concern about the practices of traditional birth attendants. It was noted that an estimated 50 to 60 percent of births in Tanzania take place outside of the hospital environment, with the number possibly reaching as high as 90 percent in some rural areas. Several doctors mentioned that herbs used by traditional birth attendants often caused uterine rupture.[14] Shortages at hospital blood banks were mentioned as a significant factor contributing to maternal mortality in that many women are severely anemic and need blood transfusions either during pregnancy or after giving birth. Lack of prenatal care, distance to health facilities, and shortages of medicine were also identified as factors that negatively affected the survival of pregnant and birthing women in Tanzania.

National Recommendations

Overall, the issues raised at the National Safe Motherhood conference and in the TAMWA report were quite similar to those identified in the Safe Motherhood Initiative discussed in chapter 3 and in Kaisi's 1989 Safe

Motherhood document. At the national level in Tanzania, childbirth is seen as a risky event in the lives of many women who suffer from poor health and, as a consequence, experience life-threatening complications during pregnancy and birth. A lack of access to biomedical resources, the need for family planning, and harmful traditional practices such as bride-price were highlighted.

There were two notable differences, however. In the TAMWA report, there was no direct mention of the harmful practices of traditional birth attendants per se, just that the training of birth attendants, who were noted as "performing a very important task," needed to receive national attention. The TAMWA report also explicitly mentioned unethical practices of health-care personnel who "want money only and will do anything." Although Kaisi's document mentions a lack of "self-discipline and commitment among health personnel," there was no mention of this at the National Safe Motherhood Conference in Morogoro, nor was it raised as an issue in the early WHO literature. Economic hardships experienced by medical doctors and other health-care personnel were not mentioned either.

Despite these differences, participants at both the TAMWA "Day of Action" and the National Safe Motherhood Conference appear to have echoed the major concern articulated in the Safe Motherhood Initiative: the survival of pregnant and birthing women. Although the stated reasons for that concern may be different—the government sees women as an economic asset to be invested in, while TAMWA presents the issue as one of women's survival and basic human rights—there nevertheless appeared to be general agreement that maternal mortality in Tanzania must be reduced. It is worth mentioning again, however, that many of the categories of problems and proposed solutions to address maternal mortality in Tanzania are similar to those proposed by outside international organizations such as WHO and, in the case of TAMWA, the Women's Global Network for Reproductive Rights.

It remains to be seen whether some of these same categories of problems are also acknowledged by people living at the local level and, if they are acknowledged, whether they are prioritized in the same manner. As a way of beginning, in the next two chapters I provide a description of the local level, the community of Bulangwa, from a historical and contemporary perspective.

CHAPTER 5

Situating the Fieldwork Setting: The Shinyanga Region in Historical Perspective

It seems that most of my interaction so far has been with the non-Sukuma members of the community. This town center is actually a mixture of people from different parts of the country. For example, one of the Tanzanian women with whom I have become friends is a Jaluo woman from the northern part of the country. Although her husband is Sukuma, he comes from a different district. . . . [N]eedless to say, my first week here I was feeling a bit anxious as I wasn't meeting any Sukuma women. But that in itself is interesting, I suppose, and I also realize that I have only been here one week.
—Letter from Bulangwa, November 24, 1992

When I originally selected the Shinyanga Region as the site for my fieldwork, my decision was based on two main factors. First, maternal mortality in the Shinyanga Region during the 1980s was quite high: for every 100,000 live births, approximately 300 women died from complications associated with pregnancy, childbirth, or the postpartum period (Kaisi 1989; Mandara and Msamanga 1988). Second, although the Sukuma people are the predominant ethnic group living in the region, the majority of the most recent studies from which information on Sukuma women's health-care practices could be gleaned were at least twenty years old and had taken place primarily in the Mwanza Region to the north (Lang and Lang 1973; Reid 1969; Varkevisser 1973). By selecting a rural community in the Shinyanga Region as the site for my study, my goal was to address the apparent gap in the literature: pregnancy and childbirth among the southern Sukuma.

The anxiety that is hinted at in the above excerpt from one of my first letters from the field reflects my initial concerns that I had somehow ended up in the wrong place: a predominantly *non*-Sukuma community. What I gradually came to realize over the course of my fieldwork is that despite the multiethnic makeup of Bulangwa, or perhaps because of it, certain aspects of Sukuma culture seemed to serve as a cultural backdrop against which everyday interactions in the community took place. This seemed especially true with regard to healing strategies in general and local practices surrounding pregnancy and childbirth in particular. Since returning from my fieldwork and immersing myself once again in the historical and anthropological literature for that part of the country, I have come to understand the cultural heterogeneity I observed in Bulangwa in a different light: not as a possible aberration but, rather, as a present-day reflection of past historical processes in west central Tanzania.[1]

In this chapter I begin to situate contemporary social relations in Bulangwa within their historical context. In doing so, my aim is to show how past social and cultural formations in west central Tanzania continue to be reflected in today's cultural landscape of Bulangwa in general and, in later chapters, especially in women's pregnancy-related experiences. Appadurai's (1996:181) observation that there is a historical and dialectical relationship between how local subjects and neighborhoods are "produced, named, and empowered to act socially" seems particularly relevant to what I am trying to accomplish in this chapter. My discussion of some of the major themes in the history of west central Tanzania—early migrations, changes in the role of the chief, trading networks, interethnic relations, the impact of British colonial rule—is not meant to be a mere recounting of historical facts but, rather, an exploration of how locality was actively produced and maintained in west central Tanzania during the past. This chapter sets the stage for an examination of social relations in Bulangwa in the contemporary setting and, in later chapters, for a discussion of how the particularities of locality have shaped the management of motherhood and maternal health risk in the ethnographic present.

For example, given the place that some female figures occupied in the social life of contemporary Bulangwa, whether as healers or as ancestors seen as capable of affecting the fertility of their living kin, what does the historical record suggest about women's participation in the ritual and political life of their communities (Berger 1976; Boddy 1989)? Although we don't read much about women in the history books that mention this part of Tanzania, we know that women certainly must have been present. What were they doing? Why, for that matter, does sorcery figure so significantly today in rural women's perceptions of risks to their fertility? Is the disproportionate amount of sorcery accusations currently directed at women in this part of Tanzania a reflection of gender relations in the past, or does their frequency point instead to a transformation in the character of gender relations over time (Gabba 1989, 1990; Mesaki 1993, 1995; Tanner 1970)? These are just a few of the questions that emerged during my fieldwork and that are important to keep in mind as we examine the historical record.

In the following section I describe the Shinyanga Region in terms of its geographic location and overall cultural identity. I then review some of the historical literature for west central Tanzania, starting with the early migrations into the area and ending with the early years of British colonial rule.[2]

The Shinyanga Region: Past and Present Boundaries

The Shinyanga Region—which is made up of the six administrative districts of Shinyanga Urban, Shinyanga Rural, Maswa, Bariadi, Meatu, and Kahama—is interesting for a variety of geographical, cultural, and historical reasons. Geographically, Shinyanga lies approximately 100 miles to the south of Mwanza town, the capital of the Mwanza Region, and 125 miles to the north of the town of Tabora, the capital of the Tabora Region. Taken together, these three regions—Mwanza, Shinyanga, and Tabora—are considered the home of the culturally and linguistically related Sukuma and Nyamwezi, an agropastoral people who, according to one author, accounted for over four million people in 1990, the largest ethnic grouping in Tanzania (Brandström 1990).

During the earlier years of British colonial rule in Tanganyika, Shinyanga had the administrative status of a district; at various points in time it fell within the administrative boundaries of two different larger regions, or provinces as they were referred to then. From 1916 through 1926 Shinyanga was a subdistrict of the Tabora District. From 1926 through 1932, Shinyanga was one of the four districts of the Tabora Province with Tabora, Kahama, and Nzega as the other three. In 1932, Tabora Province was renamed the Western Province, but from 1932 through 1962 the Shinyanga District became part of Lake Province to the north, which included Mwanza town. Lake Province was subsequently renamed the Lake Region in 1962. Shinyanga eventually became a region in its own right in the mid-1960s.

The area that makes up the present-day Shinyanga Region has also been associated with two different cultural identities. During the periods of German and British colonial rule, for example, parts of west central

Tanganyika were referred to either as Sukumaland or Nyamweziland. Sukumaland (Usukuma), according to several authors, consisted of the Mwanza and Kwimba Districts of the present-day Mwanza Region and the Maswa and Shinyanga districts of the present-day Shinyanga Region (Austen 1968; Cory 1952; Holmes and Austen 1972; Holmes 1969; Itandala 1979; Malcolm 1953; Maguire 1969; Shoka 1972), while Nyamweziland (Unyamwezi) included the Kahama District of the present-day Shinyanga Region and the Nzega and Tabora districts of the present-day Tabora Region (Abrahams 1967; Blohm 1933; Bösch 1930; Brandström 1990; Roberts 1968b).

The issue of cultural identity in terms of geographic location speaks to one of the recurring themes in the anthropological and historical literature for west central Tanzania: do the Sukuma and Nyamwezi ethnic groups represent two distinct peoples? Several authors have noted the similarities between the Sukuma (the predominant ethnic group living in the Shinyanga and Mwanza Regions) and the Nyamwezi (the predominant ethnic group in the Tabora Region) with respect to language, cosmology, and cultural institutions (e.g., healing and other secret societies) as well as aspects of social and political organization during the precolonial period (Abrahams 1967; Brandström 1986; Cory 1960; Holmes and Austen 1972).

Per Brandström, a Swedish anthropologist whose work in the Tabora Region spans a period of nearly thirty years, suggests that the concept of ethnic identity among what he refers to as the "Sukuma-Nyamwezi peoples" is fluid and changing rather than fixed.[3] The term *Nyamwezi,* he notes, is a reflection of "outsider/insider" classification:

> The terminological confusion of the early visitors to this region can be explained by the fact that they encountered two different sets of systems of classification, one for insider/outsider-relations and the other for insider/insider-relations. A person became, so to speak, a Nyamwezi in the inclusive sense only in confrontation with the outer world. (Brandström 1986:4)

In other words, *Nyamwezi* is a term linked to the nineteenth-century caravan trade routes that linked the interior of Tanzania to its eastern coast, a system that will be discussed in more detail below. Upon arriving at the coast African traders and porters are said to have referred to themselves as having come "from the west" or "from where the moon comes" (*ya mwezi* in Kiswahili, *ng'wa ng'weli* in Kisukuma), and thus they became known as the Nyamwezi (see also Burton 1860; Cory 1952).[4]

Brandström describes another way that ethnic identity has been referred to among the Sukuma and Nyamwezi peoples, a method he refers to as "insider/insider classification":

> Directional terms are applied as the most inclusive way of classifying closely related people. People are recognized as Basukuma, Badakama, Banang'weli and Banakia, which simply means northerners, southerners, westerners, and easterners. Their criteria for identification are here, above all, linguistic characteristics. All the dialects spoken in Usukuma and northern Unyamwezi are mutually comprehensible. However, there are differences in intonation and vocabulary disclosing area of origin. Furthermore, there are variations in habits and customs, marking out differences between the various groupings, and there are stereotypes in the form of stories people tell about each other. The easterners, for example, in a jokingly manner, are said to be outspoken, quarrelsome and cunning people, while, at the same time stories are told about how timid and gullible the southerners are. (Brandström 1986:7)[5]

Although some people in Bulangwa also referred to themselves in a manner similar to that described by Brandström above, such references to ethnic identity were not very common. Regardless of their own ethnicity, people in the community tended to refer to people from Tabora as Nyamwezi rather than Dakama (from the south), although in the formal interviews I conducted with women about their experiences during pregnancy and childbirth (see chap. 6), a few of the older women referred to themselves as either Dakama or Kiya (from the east). When I asked people about the differences between the Sukuma and Nyamwezi peoples, I was often told that the dialect spoken by the Sukuma, the word for "north" in the Kisukuma language, was harder (*ngumu*) or more clipped than the softer dialect of the Nyamwezi.[6]

The Sukuma in West Central Tanzania:
Early Migrations

> The Sukuma of today are the products of an extensive long term agglomeration of disparate, Bantu-speaking people intermixed on a small scale with intrusive Highland Nilotes, especially Tatoga, and to a

somewhat greater extent with immigrants from the interlacustrine region . . . They are Sukuma by virtue of their language, laws and customs as well as their supra-ntemiship [chiefship] kinship ties and long term residence in Usukuma more than anything else. To a great extent pre-colonial Sukuma history is the story of how these people of various backgrounds made contact and experienced an assimilation process which brought forth the modern Sukuma.
> —Holmes and Austen, "The Pre-colonial Sukuma"

The historians Holmes and Austen have suggested that the "agglomeration of disparate, Bantu-speaking peoples," which is said to have taken place in western Tanzania over the course of the first millennium A.D., was, for the most part, peaceful (1972:379–81). They identify two main patterns of migration into the area during this period. The first consisted primarily of Bantu peoples from the south who came and settled in scattered communities, most likely clan groups, without any centralized system of political authority.[7] The second pattern of migration included Bantu and Highland Nilotic peoples. It was during this second wave of migration that cattle are believed to have been introduced into the area, apparently by ancestors of the present-day Taturu people (Holmes and Austen 1972:380; see also Sutton 1968; Were 1968).

According to Were (1968), invasions of Lwoo-speaking peoples into Buganda (in present-day Uganda) in the sixteenth century set off a third wave of migrations westward that eventually arrived in Usukuma (see also Roberts 1968b:120). Cory (1952) suggested that these new immigrants had been part of the ruling elite in Buganda and because of their "intellectual superiority" eventually occupied similar positions of power in their adopted homeland. Holmes and Austen, however, see these positions of power as a result of mutual accommodation rather than conquest:

Beginning as early as the first decades of the seventeenth century particular groups of immigrants who were able to offer fresh, effective solutions to both old and new problems began to appear on the scene. Somewhat inadequate analyses of the traditions concerning the arrival of these people have in the past identified them as immediate immigrants from the interlacustrine region where more centralized political systems were in existence. . . . Somewhat closer to the truth is the suggestion that these immigrants had previously experienced and preferred the institutions of more centralized control similar to the interlacustrine region. The assumption that they were "pure" Hima

or Hinda as the legends attempt to establish, is not conclusively sup-
portable, nor is the rather arrogant value judgement that their inherently superior physical and mental powers were decisive factors. It is
much more likely that those who brought new concepts of political
control to the Sukuma were also by-products of the ubiquitous Bantu
assimilation process, one which in this case had been applied to
Nilotes and Cushites who had intruded into the regions west of Lake
Victoria generations ago. (Holmes and Austen 1972:381)

The Tanzanian historian Itandala, in contrast, suggests early migrations into this area were anything but peaceful:

Contrary to prevailing theory, that pastoralists peacefully infiltrated
an area and gradually incorporated the agriculturalists into an almost
voluntary clientage system, the process of subjection was accomplished by the bloodiest of military clashes when the agriculturalists
had been decimated by starvation. The only alternative to clientage
was migration. (1979:152–53)

Despite the differences in scholarly opinion as to the nature of the
migration of new peoples into this area, historians for the most part seem
to agree that these series of movements of people resulted in a change,
gradual or otherwise, in the way that society was organized. As we will see
later in this chapter, the structure of early society in west central Tanzania
was eventually transformed from one characterized by widely scattered,
autonomous clan-based settlements into one that reflected a more centralized form of political and social organization.

The Role of Chief

There are three themes in the institution of chiefship among the Sukuma
and Nyamwezi peoples.[8] One theme describes the initial role of chief as
being magico-religious in nature. According to Roberts (1968b:119),
chiefly power was primarily concerned with the ritual health of society,
while the real political power rested in the hands of the chief's council of
elders (*banang'oma*) and headmen (*banang'wa*). Holmes and Austen hold
a similar view of the power of the early chiefs, noting that the first chiefs
were "sacerdotal rulers, high priests in an ancestral cult, who exercised few

administrative powers and duties" (1972:383). The second theme notes that prior to the development of extensive internal and external trading networks, chiefdoms were clan-based, widely dispersed over a sparsely populated area and in terms of political organization, characterized by a system of autonomous rule in relation to neighboring chiefdoms. The subsequent changes in social and political organization were accompanied by a transformation in the nature of the authority of the chief, eventually resulting in the secularization of his powers (383).

A third theme related to the role of the chief centers around the nature of succession to the chiefship itself. Prior to 1905, succession to chiefship in some of these autonomous chiefdoms was matrilineal: new chiefs were chosen among the sons of a sister of the ruling chief, or in some cases, brothers of the ruling chief (Austen 1968:52; Brandström 1990:184, n. 11; Holmes and Austen 1972:385; TNA 3387). Holmes and Austen (1972:384) suggest that matrilineal succession to chiefship served "as a means to prevent succession intrigues" as well as "an institutional balance in the exercise of authority" (cf. Douglas 1969). This latter suggestion merits further discussion as it raises questions regarding characteristics of gender relations and modes of social power in the past and their relevance to present-day Bulangwa.

The Gender of Chiefs

Very little of the scholarly work available on the institution of chiefship among the Sukuma and Nyamwezi people mentions gender as a factor. Brandström provides one of the few exceptions in a footnote to his 1990 article on the relationship between fertility and ancestor veneration among the Sukuma-Nyamwezi peoples:

> In the past, women were not in principle even excluded from chiefly position, and they could rise to great fame as potent diviners and healers. . . . [T]his theme was presented to me, during a field study in 1975, in my encounter with a renowned female *mfumu* [healer] in central Sukumaland who, like the female chiefs in the past (cf. Bösch 1930:497) had provided *nsabo*, "wealth," "groomwealth" we may say in this case, for her husband. (Brandström 1990:185, n. 13)

Where other references to female chiefs are made in the literature, however, the reason for their succession is downplayed. In his comments on the role that gender played in the selection of chiefs among the Nyamwezi, the historian Roberts states the following:

> In many chiefdoms, succession was matrilineal, but there are several chiefdoms where the succession has been transferred to the male line. Personal ability and popularity as well as kinship were important qualifications for chieftainship; and a woman was sometimes chosen *if there was no suitable male available.* (1968b:119; emphasis added)

Some of the ethnographic and archival data that I collected during the period of my fieldwork challenges the impression left by Roberts's work that women were merely passive players in the process of succession to chiefship among the Sukuma. I happened upon this information two months after I moved to Bulangwa, when I was invited by the government cultural officer (*bwana utumaduni*) to sit in on an interview he was conducting with two elder men in the community.[9]

One of the men being interviewed was a renowned healer in the area. He told us that he was a small boy around the time the Germans left Tanzania (ca. 1916). He then made the offhand comment that when the Germans arrived among the Sukuma, they found female chiefs. When I expressed my surprise that women had been chiefs in the past, he responded by saying it had actually been a common practice in some areas. He mentioned one female chief in particular, a woman who lived in Busanda and whose daughters were chiefs of Kizumbi, Busanda, Tinde, Busule, Mwantini, and Usiha (communities in the present-day Shinyanga Region). According to his version of the events, sisters of chiefs were often quite active in trying to ensure that a chief's successor would be female. Apparently, they did this by killing their sons so that their daughters would succeed to the chiefship instead. He explained that this practice was a result of the tradition that a chief's own children could not succeed him as chief; candidates for the position of chief were chosen instead from among the children of a chief's sister. If a chief had no nephews, his sister's daughters would be eligible to succeed him as chief. It was by this rule of succession, he noted, that women initially became chiefs.

Even female chiefs were known to kill their own sons, he told me, citing the case of one female chief who gave birth to a son who eventually fled the community before she could kill him. The son went to Kizumbi, where people expressed their desire that he become their chief, which he did. The healer noted that it was as a result of this particular incident that the rules regarding the selection of new chiefs began to change from matrilineal to patrilineal succession. In other words, according to this healer's version of the events (and in contrast to Holmes and Austen's characterization of matrilineal succession), the rules regarding succession to the chiefship changed *as a result of* the possibility for political intrigue under the matrilineal system. When I told him that I had read somewhere that the Germans had been the ones who had initiated the change in the rules of succession, he disagreed, stating emphatically that the Germans had left the institution of chiefship alone. Subsequent changes in the succession to chiefship, he assured me, had occurred *after* the arrival of the British. Although other historical sources refute this healer's version of the events, dating the change to patrilineal succession to 1905 when the Germans were still in power (Austen 1968:52; TNA 3387), it has also been noted that the Germans didn't venture often into southern Sukumaland, as their headquarters were in Mwanza to the north (Austen 1968; Maguire 1969).[10]

I was intrigued by this elder man's rendition of history for several reasons, but mainly for the suggestion that in former times some Sukuma women held public positions of ritual and political power. I also thought it possible that his version of the events might be a reflection of contemporary male attitudes regarding women's leadership abilities and women's status in the community in general. It is equally possible that his version of the events regarding the untrustworthiness of female chiefs merely reflects his own personal bias regarding women in public roles of authority.[11]

The Tanzanian historian Itandala, whose work traces the origin of the Babinza clan of eastern Usukuma, also makes reference to the positions of authority and practices of political intrigue by the foremothers of modern Sukuma women (Itandala 1979). Despite their marginal position implied by the title of his article "Ilembo, Nkanda and the Girls: Establishing a Chronology of the Babinza," Itandala's work provides evidence that some Sukuma women did, in fact, occupy significant positions of political power in the past. Although he doesn't suggest that women had been chiefs, he does, nevertheless, provide evidence from oral history that "the girls," along with their brother, had been founders of new chiefdoms:

One group of the traditions maintains that Ilembo [the son of a chief near Lake Victoria in the late sixteenth century] and his sisters were the first immigrants from Lukalanga to enter Usukuma. These were then followed by Nkanda, the great conqueror and founder of the Babinza *luganda* [clan]. Another group of traditions claims that

Nkanda and his sisters were the first immigrants from Lukalanga to settle in Usukuma. (1979:153)

Another version of this story, which he presents in the same article, posits that Ilembo set off on his own, to be followed later by four of his sisters:

> After Ilembo's arrival in Seke, a group of immigrants consisting of his four sisters followed him. One of them settled in what became Sukuma on the lakeshore, the other three went to eastern Usukuma where one settled in what became Ntuzu, and the other two settled in what became Ng'wagala [in the eastern part of Shinyanga Region]. (1979:154; cf. Beidelman 1993; Varkevisser 1971)[12]

And contrary to Holmes and Austen's assertion that matrilineal succession would protect the process of succession from intrigue, the oral history of the Babinza clan suggests otherwise:

> The tradition states that before the two sisters established the *butemi* [chiefdom in Kisukuma], they first went to Ng'wagalankulu in Seke and stole Ilembo's *ndeji* [symbol of chiefly powers].[13] It was Mbuke [Ilembo's sister] who appropriated it but while on their way home, her younger sister, Holo, stole it from her and went to install her son Mangula as *ntemi* [chief] with it. Naturally, her action caused discord between her and Mbuke which was only resolved by offering the latter's children the position of *batemi bahoja* [community elders] in their area of Sang'ombe. (Itandala 1979:158)

Iris Berger's work on religious movements in precolonial East Africa provides further evidence that some Sukuma women occupied significant positions of ritual power in their communities in the past (1976). Although she notes that female subordination was a common characteristic of social life during the nineteenth century, at the same time her work shows that religious activity, such as participation in possession cults, was one area in which some women commanded considerable social power as spirit mediums (Boddy 1989; Giles 1987; cf. Lewis 1971).[14] Citing written accounts by nineteenth-century travelers to the area, she suggests that many of these female spirit mediums were respected and feared. Berger's examination of the literature for the area also reveals that many of these spirit mediums were Sukuma and Nyamwezi women, and that women's participation in such cults, whether as medium or client seeking treatment, was often related to problems they were experiencing with their fertility (1976:167). Her discussion of the various techniques used by these spirit mediums to mark their authority, such as the clothing worn and the behavior adopted while possessed, brings to mind Appadurai's observation that the production of locality requires "hard and regular work . . . to produce and maintain its materiality" (1996:180–81). In later chapters, we will return to a discussion of modes of female power and authority when we examine the role played by some women within the contemporary context of healing.

The Impact of Trade

By the eighteenth century, African peoples living in the interior had begun to establish trade networks that extended northward to Lake Victoria (Hartwig 1970) and southwest to the kingdoms of Kazembe and Lunda (Boahen 1987), resulting in a continual influx of new peoples and new ideas into central Tanzania (Holmes and Austen 1972).[15] Holmes and Austen have noted that the subsequent development of a complex trading economy also led to transformations in the nature of chiefly authority, from that of ritual specialist seen in early times to a new position as "trader-chief" and then, along with the development of the notion of territoriality, to that of "warlord" (1972:389–94; Koponen 1988:141). According to the historian Alpers (1968), prior to 1800 very little contact took place between the coastal peoples to the east and the people living in the interior regions of Tanzania. Trade networks within the interior that involved primarily the Sukuma and Nyamwezi peoples and their neighbors to the north, west, and south, however, were extensive, characterized by trade in items such as iron, salt, beads, fish, local agricultural goods, and ivory (1968:238–40; Gray and Birmingham 1970; Hartwig 1970; Holmes and Austen 1972:386–88; Kjekshus 1977; Roberts 1968b, 1970).

As already noted above, by the early nineteenth century, Nyamwezi traders began to make their way to the coast, a development that was to have later repercussions for the stability of the interior. Although many people living in the Tanzanian interior eventually became involved in these trading networks, Nyamwezi men were particularly well known as porters (*wapagazi*) in the caravan trade. Holmes and Austen (1972:388) posit that although there is not much evidence that the northern Sukuma were involved as porters in the caravan trade, it is quite possible that the southern Sukuma—those living in the present-day Shinyanga Region—also became involved as porters. They also note that much prestige was attached to the role of porter, prestige that was due not only to the increase in economic opportunities available to the porters, but also because porters began to be looked upon as "the most cosmopolitan people," as their participation in these long-distance caravans led to contact with new peoples, products, and ideas (1972:390).

The wealth of goods brought from the interior to the coast via the caravan trade stimulated the interest of Arab and Swahili peoples living in the coastal regions, many of whom moved to the interior around the middle of the nineteenth century and established trading outposts of their own (Bennett 1968). Arabs arrived in the Unanyembe chiefdom (in the present-day Tabora Region) in 1858 and established what was to become a major trading outpost in the nineteenth century, an outpost in which various lines of the caravan route converged (Roberts 1968b:131).

Utani: Joking Relationships

One important effect of the establishment of trade links between the interior and the east coast was the creation of joking relationships (*utani*) between diverse ethnic groups, a social institution that is still relevant today. As noted by Roberts:

> It was the caravan trade which brought about the joking relationships which now exist between the Nyamwezi [and also Sukuma] and the peoples living along their route to the coast, especially the Zaramo. Such *utani* regulated behavior between the Nyamwezi and the people among whom they constantly passed to and fro, and ensured that the travellers could expect hospitality (cf. Beidelman 1993). (1968b:130)[16]

Abrahams gives a more detailed example of the character and social implications of these joking relationships:

> The relationships typically involve privileged verbal abuse, and in the past at least considerable horseplay, between those participating in them, and it is important that such joking partners should not take offense at what is said or done to them. In the past there was also typ-

ically an exchange of services, accompanied by such abuse, on ritual occasions such as funerals. According to most accounts the partnerships arose originally out of an earlier state of hostility between members of the participating groups, and it seems possible that they were modelled upon similar forms of relationship between chiefdoms, dynasties and clans within the groups concerned. Their function . . . appears to have been the establishment of peaceful and fruitful interaction between groups of people whose relationships to each other could otherwise easily be marked by unpredictability, tension, and violence. (1981:124)

These joking relationships were also relevant within the context of my fieldwork in Bulangwa and existed between groups other than the Sukuma and Nyamwezi. It was not unusual, for example, to hear Jaluo and Haya members of the community refer to each other as *mtani* (joking partner).[17] It is interesting that although the Arabs were also heavily involved with the caravan trade in the nineteenth century, no *utani* relationship has been noted between the African and Arab peoples in Tanzania. Given the tension that exists between these latter groups in the contemporary setting of Bulangwa, the absence of a joking relationship between Arab and African peoples is notable.

Conflict in the Interior

With the involvement of the Arabs, the character of trade shifted from one concerned primarily with the movement of agricultural goods to the coast and luxury items such as cloth to the interior, to one in which slaves and ivory became important export commodities to Zanzibar and guns became important commodities that were imported into the interior (Bennett 1968; Holmes and Austen 1972; Roberts 1970).[18] Not all of the Arabs living in the interior, however, became directly involved in the caravan trade. Maguire (1969:4) notes that by the late nineteenth century, Lalago in eastern Usukuma was a large trading outpost for Arab businessmen whose trade was limited to small items such as cloth, oil, utensils, spices, and local native produce, a description that still holds true for the Arab shops found in small and large towns throughout the Shinyanga region today.

The movement of Arab and Swahili peoples into the interior of Tanzania also corresponds to an increase in interethnic warfare that intensified by the end of the century, although the reason for this phenomenon is not always agreed upon by scholars (Koponen 1988:139–50). Several historians note that the increase in struggles over control of trade routes was significant, as chiefs controlling the routes that fell within the boundaries of their chiefdoms were able to extract high fees (*hongo*) that guaranteed not only safe passage but also access to water and the food needed to feed the large numbers of porters.[19] Some historians associate the increase in interethnic warfare with the influx of guns supplied by Arab traders concerned with keeping the caravan routes open.[20] The increase in arms, in turn, is linked to an increase in conflict, as chiefs in the interior regions engaged in struggles to control the trade routes (Holmes 1971; Roberts 1968b; cf. Kjekshus 1977).[21]

By the second half of the nineteenth century, interethnic warfare became quite significant for the southern Sukuma. From 1850 to 1870 a series of conflicts known as *vita mhamila* took place among the various southern chiefships (Holmes 1971:487). According to Holmes and Austen (1972:392), these wars had a major impact on the social and economic structure of the southern Sukuma in that this area, once characterized by widely scattered settlements, underwent a transformation in which a clustering of villages became the norm. Although first initiated for defense purposes, the authors note that this eventually led to changes in social organization when, as a result of the clustering of villages, the pooling of agricultural labor also became common (Gluckman 1963; Noble 1970).[22]

Cattle raiding between the Sukuma, Taturu, and Maasai peoples (a practice that still continues today, although to a limited extent) is also said to have increased during the latter part of the nineteenth century. The colonial records for 1919 also mention the history of warfare between these three groups in southern Sukumaland:

There are quite a large number of Wa-Nyramba who have moved from their own country during various famine years also some Wa-Taturo with large herds of cattle. The lat[t]er tribe are nomadic people with customs akin to the Maasai. They originally invaded the District via the Manonga River Valley but were driven out within the last 30 years by Wanyamwezi and Maasai combined. Those remaining are the remnant of the invading force. They occupy the eastern end of Usiha where there is some fine cattle country very suitable for their needs. They do not intermarry with either the Wa-Nyramba or Wa-Sukuma. (TNA 2551:14–15)

Scholars disagree on the character attributed to the cattle raiders. Citing the work of several authors, Kjekshus (1977:18) points out that the common portrayal of the Maasai as "perpetrators of wanton destruction" has been contested, stating that these characterizations have no basis in reality, but are merely examples of "tribal lore" (see also Jacobs 1967). Galaty (1993), however, provides a countercritique (especially of Jacobs's work), noting that the Maasai's reputation as fierce warriors was warranted (cf. Koponen 1988:141–43). Other scholars (Holmes and Austen 1972:387, but also Kjekshus 1977) suggest that the increase in cattle raiding may have been a result of an increasing scarcity of land with adequate grazing and water resources.

Whether the portrayal of the Maasai as "perpetrators of wanton destruction" is warranted or not, peoples' perceptions of the Maasai as warriors and cattle raiders continued into the twentieth century. One result of local peoples' fear of the raiding capabilities of the Maasai can be seen in an incident that occurred on February 8, 1936, in the Magu chiefdom in the Mwanza region. According to the author of an article that appeared in a 1936 issue of *Tanganyika Notes and Records,* a rumor of an impending "ferocious Maasai raid" set off a panic that resulted in masses of Sukuma people fleeing the area with thousands of their cattle (Hone 1936:98; TNA 23384). The source of the rumor, it was eventually learned, was a frightened young boy who, while tending cattle, had been surrounded by what appeared to him to be a band of the "dreaded" Maasai warriors. What the young boy actually witnessed, the author tells us, was part of a healing rite that consisted of a mock cattle raid. According to the author, the mock raid had been organized by an old Sukuma woman who was related by marriage to the Maasai. The "raid" was part of a healing rite for the old woman, who had been sick for a long time, and in order to ensure that the ritual would be successful, she and the "raiding party" (which, we are told, consisted mainly of women and girls) proceeded to

> array themselves in Maasai war costume . . . and arm themselves with such weapons as they could lay their hands on. . . . Carefully they stalked their fictitious prey, then suddenly sprang from the cover of the bushes, brandishing their weapons and uttering the fearsome cries enjoined upon them by their instructress. (Hone 1936:99–100)

Archival documents supply the additional information that although this particular event was a rumor, an actual Maasai raid occurred seven months later on September 9, 1936, in Meatu, located in eastern Usukuma (TNA 23384). As we will see later in chapter 8, past tensions between the Sukuma, Maasai, and Taturu peoples continue to play out in people's experiences of illness and possession in the contemporary setting.

The Early Years of British Colonial Rule: Shinyanga in the 1920s

Austen (1968:4) has characterized the periods of German and British colonial rule in Tanganyika (1890–1916 and 1916–61 respectively) as "ruling indirectly," although he notes that the term had slightly different meanings in each case.[23] According to Austen, "ruling indirectly" under the German colonial administration was characterized by "a general paternalistic notion of native policy" without ever actually being called "indirect rule" per se (4).[24] The British form of "ruling indirectly," however, was an actual policy known as "indirect rule" that was modeled after British colonial policy in Nigeria, whereby local chiefs were incorporated into the colonial administration.

In his analysis of the consequences of British colonial policy in Sukumaland, Maguire (1969:7) notes that despite an apparent colonial effort to preserve the traditional forms of political power by incorporating chiefs into a system of Native Authorities, the policy of indirect rule ultimately resulted in the transformation of what constituted the "traditional." Indigenous chiefs, whose authority had originally come from the consensus of their people,

> found themselves increasingly estranged from this traditional context as they became simultaneously tied to and empowered by an alien colonial superstructure. . . . At the same time the chief lost the position of preeminence which his new employer, the British Government, now enjoyed. In the eyes of both chief and people, the local incarnation of alien rule, the District Commissioner, assumed an aura of authority and the prerogatives of power. (1969:8; see also Gluckman et al. 1949)

Although the appointing of chiefs not originally from the area was a common practice of colonial administrators in the Lake Province to the north (Mwanza Region of the present day), this was not the case among the Sukuma living to the south (in present-day Shinyanga Region). The fact that this had not been the practice in Shinyanga is a major theme in the colonial records for 1919 through 1926, where we see frequent references to the reason why the local people were "behaving" themselves:

> The natives of this sub-district are both docile and law-abiding. A great deal of the latter is no doubt due to the fact that there are no alien Chiefs in this sub-district and from time immemorial the natives have looked to their Chiefs as rulers by "Divine Right." (TNA 1733/20:89)

Other transformations linked to the imposition of colonial rule were also occurring. According to Bates, these included transformations in people's notions of identity:

> If the average African did not yet think of himself as a Tanganyikan, he did think of himself as an African in contrast to the Europeans, Asians, and Arabs who also inhabited the country. (1965:636)

Despite the references to the "docile and law-abiding" Sukuma natives in the Annual Reports covering the period of 1919 through 1926, there were occasional references to the presence of non-Sukuma peoples living in the area as well, references that indicate that movements of peoples into the area did not stop with the imposition of colonial rule. A 1919 Tabora District Report, for example, notes that Sumbwa, Taturu, Kamba, Nyiramba, and Tusi were also significant groups in the area. Trade, an important vehicle for the coming together of peoples in the past, continued to be significant in the early twentieth century (TNA 2551). The annual report for 1923 mentioned that the new colonial government had established a system of trade centers (TNA 1733/14), and that by the year 1925, thirty-nine trade centers with a total of 289 shops were in business (TNA 1733/20).

The railroad reached Shinyanga town in 1926, an event that would further open up the interior, an opening-up that wasn't without its consequences. An entry in the Tabora Province Annual Report of 1926, for example, blamed the recent increase in the crime rate for the Shinyanga District to the "large influx of natives [working] on the railway construction and in connection with the [gold] prospecting which has been going on near Shinyanga for the last year" (TNA 1733/9).[25] Of the sixty-five "natives" accused of crimes in 1926, the report continues, only eighteen were inhabitants of the Shinyanga District.

But movements out of the area, as in former times, also continued to be significant. In 1923, 3,500 male laborers were recruited to work on clove plantations in Zanzibar, while an additional 2,000 went to the coast on their own. This movement to the coast, which had been a means of garnering prestige in the past, became, by 1923, a source of resentment for the chiefs who complained that those returning "tend to regard themselves as having thereby acquired a degree of civilization superior to that of their chief and are prone to ridicule and defy him" (TNA 1733/14:3). Missionary activities were also blamed for giving rise to the natives' disdain for chiefly authority, for "detach[ing] natives from their tribal allegiance" (2). As a result, "every responsible chief in the district dreads any extension of missionary activity and regards every labor recruiter with the deepest mistrust" (3).

This colonial record of chiefs' suspicions of the missionaries' intentions is somewhat different from what others have written with regard to the relationship between these two groups, and what we learned with respect to the Kolondoto mission in chapter 2. Although some scholarly accounts suggests that Sukuma people were resistant to the missionizing attempts of European Christians (Alpers 1968; Austen 1968; Holmes and Austen 1972; Mesaki 1993; Tanner 1969), others have pointed out that chiefs were more likely than others to convert (Bakinikana 1974).[26] We will revisit the issue of religious affiliation in the next chapter when we examine the fieldwork setting in the contemporary context.

In 1923 the colonial government launched a massive tsetse fly control campaign and by 1926, 15,000 Africans were involved in the campaign, which included the burning down of trees and bush in the surrounding countryside (TNA 1733/9), a practice that undoubtedly contributed to the soil erosion that plagued the area in subsequent years (Austen 1967:598; Bates 1965:627). Drought in 1924 and 1925 caused significant damage to local crops, resulting in a poor harvest, but the 1926 Annual Report for the Tabora Province notes that rains were heavy in 1926, and despite flooding in some areas, the harvest that year was good (TNA 1733/9:69).

To what extent do the processes that shaped the past social and cultural life in west central Tanzania continue to be reflected in contemporary times? To begin to answer this, let us turn now to a description of the community of Bulangwa in its contemporary setting.

CHAPTER 6

The Community of Bulangwa

[Southern Sukumaland] is the commencement of a most beautiful
pastoral country, which terminates only in the Victoria Nyanza [Lake
Victoria]. From the summit of one of the weird grey rock piles which
characterize it, one may enjoy that unspeakable fascination of an
apparently boundless horizon. On all sides there stretches toward it the
face of a vast circle replete with peculiar features, of detached hills,
great crag-masses of riven and sharply angled rock, and outcropping
mounds, between which heaves and rolls in low, broad waves a green
grassy plain whereon feed thousands of cattle scattered about in small
herds.

—Henry M. Stanley, *Through the Dark Continent*

Despite a puzzling lack of reference to the presence of any people, the
above description of the physical landscape of southern Sukumaland is
still somewhat recognizable over a century later, although the cattle and
the grassiness of the rolling plains are no longer as abundant as this entry
in Stanley's journal for February 17, 1875, suggests.[1] Descriptions of this
same landscape by forestry officials and development agencies working in
the Shinyanga Region during the 1990s are filled with references to the
serious problem of soil erosion in the area, a problem they link to the over-
grazing of cattle and local people's never-ending search for available
sources of firewood (cf. Austen 1968; Bates 1965).[2] Periods of drought
during the early 1980s, in 1993, and again in the early part of 1994 wreaked
additional havoc on the environment. The resulting poor harvests and
death of large numbers of cattle brought much hardship to rural households in the region. Bulangwa, the rural community that served as my
home base from November 1992 to July 1994, is situated within this part
of the country.

This chapter introduces the reader to the fieldwork site in its contemporary setting. I begin by providing some preliminary observations about
social relations in the community and the available biomedical and non-

83

biomedical sources of maternal health care. I then introduce the reader to the sample of 154 women who spoke with me about their pregnancy and birth-related experiences. This chapter sets the stage for the examination of the unofficial definitions of maternal health risk that are presented in chapters 7 through 11.

The Research Setting

Bulangwa is best described as a small rural settlement—larger than a village, but not quite a town—where cold bottles of Coca-Cola and Pepsi products were always available in the only two local shops equipped with kerosene-run refrigerators.[3] Throughout the course of my fieldwork, people would often wax nostalgic about how Bulangwa used to be quite a bustling center and a great place for business ("There even used to be several Indian shopkeepers and a guest house here!"), while noting in the same breath that it has experienced a gradual economic decline since the late 1970s.[4]

The community, with its approximate population of 4,000, was served by fourteen shops, two butcheries, five churches, two mosques, one government clinic, two private clinics, two primary schools, one secondary school, three motor-run mills for grinding local grains, and a weekly outdoor market. These amenities, excluding the primary schools, also serviced those living in nearby villages.[5]

The center of town was dominated by the presence of seventeen Arab households. Of the fourteen shops in the community, eight were owned by Arab families; two others closed in 1993 due to poor business. Two of the three mills were also owned by Arab families; the third was run by an African man who rented part of the needed machinery from an Arab man in the community. Eight of the twelve cars in town were owned by Arab shopkeepers, one belonged to me, one to a Sukuma man, one to the secondary school, and one to a local UNICEF project. The primary mode of transportation for other members of the community included transportation by bicycle, bus, ox-drawn cart, or foot. Privately owned cars could be rented out for a fee when emergencies arose and immediate transportation was needed.

Electricity came to Bulangwa in 1993, although only those living in the center of town, or very nearby, had access to it. This latter fact was a function of both financial and physical restrictions. In addition to the large down payment required (8,000 TSH), electricity could only be installed in houses whose roofs were made of corrugated iron. The majority of these types of houses were owned by Arab shopkeepers and located in the center of town, mine included. Most of the houses located outside of this central location had thatched roofs.

Subcommunities

One of the defining features of everyday life in Bulangwa was its cultural heterogeneity, evidence of which could be found in its social differentiation, in the various subcommunities embedded within the larger community. Although not always geographically nor physically distinct, these subcommunities functioned as cultural spaces in which multiple and simultaneously occurring identities often came into play. The result was a fluidity in everyday social interactions, a fluidity that often transcended ethnic, cultural, or religious boundaries.

Ethnicity
Although the Sukuma people constituted the largest ethnic group in the community, a variety of other ethnic groups gave Bulangwa a distinctly multicultural feel. In general, however, issues related to ethnicity were not overtly stressed in the public context. When people did discuss matters related to ethnicity, the way in which they did so was often contextual (Arens 1978; Brandström 1986).

People might, for example, broadly refer to themselves as being African or Arab when speaking about themselves in relation to others in the community. The question of who was or was not Arab or African was itself also contextual. Although some members of the Arab community were born of African mothers or had African grandmothers, they referred to themselves as Arab and were regarded as such by Arab and non-Arab members of the community alike. They participated in all aspects of Arab culture including dress, food preparation, marriage practices, and overall worldview.

There were others in the community, however, who, although they had Arab fathers and African mothers, were not regarded as Arab at all: they didn't act like them, they didn't dress like them, they didn't even think like them. They referred to themselves and were referred to by others as African. The key to whether a person assumed an Arab identity was whether their Arab father had publicly acknowledged his paternity *and* brought the child into his home as a member of his household. If this latter act did not take place—if the child lived with its mother in an African household—the child was considered African, even if his or her father lived in the same community.[6] The two general categories of African and Arab were differentiated further when a person wanted to distinguish him- or herself by a specific African or Arab ethnicity.

Muslim and Non-Muslim Distinctions

Two other subcommunities, Muslim and non-Muslim, maintained a presence in the community. The subcommunity of Muslims was further differentiated along ethnic lines: although all Arabs in Bulangwa were Muslim, not all Muslims in Bulangwa were Arab; African Muslims in the community were generally referred to as *Waswahili,* or Swahili people (Eastman 1971). The subcommunity of non-Muslim people of African descent included Christian and non-Christian alike.

One of the striking differences between these two subcommunities was how festivities associated with their respective holidays temporarily transformed the social life in the center of town. During the Muslim holy month of Ramadan the usually quiet evenings in Bulangwa were temporarily transformed. Once the sun had set and the day-long period of fasting ended, members of the Muslim community, both Arab and African, congregated on the verandas outside Arab shops in the center of town, eating, talking, and playing cards well into the night. As midnight approached, Muslim youth visited Muslim households in the center of town, to beat their drums and announce that the time for the final meal was drawing near. Festivities marking the Muslim holidays of Idi el Fitr and Idi el Hadj, on the other hand, were a bit more subdued. On those days, all the Arab-owned shops remained closed for business. Special holiday meals—usually *pilau* (a spicy rice and meat dish) or *boku-boku* (a dish of pounded rice and goat meat mixed together and accompanied by a fruit jam relish)—were prepared and eaten together with family members and African Muslim friends in Arab homes, while throughout the day Muslim children, African and Arab alike, knocked on neighbor's doors in the center of town, asking for the treats handed out to the young on those special occasions.

Social life in the center of town on Christmas, New Year's, and Easter holidays, in contrast, was dominated by non-Muslims who lived in Bulangwa or who traveled from surrounding villages. Arab-owned shops, which remained open throughout the day, played music and sold countless cold soft drinks to the crowds of people who converged on the town's center to dance, drink, and have their picture taken by the only photographer in town.

Religion

Some might regard the presence of five churches and two mosques in Bulangwa surprising given that much of the historical and ethnographic literature on the Sukuma people characterizes them as a people generally resistant to religious conversion. According to Mesaki (1993), a Tanzanian anthropologist, this characterization of an almost inherent Sukuma aversion to organized religion remains true even in contemporary times. As evidence, he provides statistics cited by the regional commissioner of the Shinyanga region who was interviewed for a Tanzanian newspaper in 1992:

> For a long time the Sukuma shunned conversion to either Islam or Christianity and in a recent interview, the Regional Commissioner (Sunday News: March 8, 1992) of Shinyanga Region confided that "roughly out of a population of two million only 6% have a formal religion and 94% of Shinyanga people are animists." An inquiring priest (Kirwen 1979:128) found that 58% of those he interviewed were traditionalists; Catholics formed 24% and the Protestant "Africa Inland Church" accounted for 10%; Seventh Day Adventist 6% and other 2%. (Mesaki 1993:197)

The regional commissioner's estimation that only 6 percent of the population belonged to a formal religion is quite different from the religious affiliations claimed by the sample of women I interviewed in 1994, a sample whose characteristics will be described in greater detail below. Among the 154 women I interviewed, 52.6 percent (*n* = 81) claimed affiliation with a formal religion, while 47.4 percent (*n* = 73) did not. In terms of the former, 35 women (22.7 percent) stated they were Catholic, 26 (16.9 percent) said they were Muslim (of these 26 women, 14 identified their ethnicity as Arab), 17 (11.1 percent) worshiped at the African Inland Church, two women (1.3 percent) were Seventh-Day Adventist, while one woman said she was Lutheran. Whether claiming adherence to a formal religion means anything in terms of a woman's experience of pregnancy and childbirth, however, is another issue entirely and will be taken up again later at various points throughout the book.

Livelihood
The manner in which people in the community earned their living constituted another category of social differentiation, or subcommunity, in Bulangwa. Agriculture and animal husbandry served as the primary source of livelihood for the majority of Bulangwa's inhabitants. Maize, millet, sorghum, peanuts, sweet potatoes, and, to a lesser extent, cassava were the main food crops planted, both for subsistence as well as for extra cash when the harvest was good. Cotton also provided a source of cash for local farmers, as did the selling of milk by those who owned cattle. As noted already at the beginning of this chapter, periods of drought and famine, which were frequent in this part of the country, brought much hardship to those whose sole source of income came from the land. Others in the community depended on more regular sources of income for their livelihood, working as nurses, medical assistants, primary and secondary school teachers, and in the civil services, or earning their living through privately owned medical clinics or family-owned shops.

Most of the Arab families in Bulangwa earned their living through this latter type of occupation. Although many of the Arab families in the community were considered to be well-off financially in comparison to African members of the community, not all those belonging to the class of the more financially secure were Arab, nor were all Arabs well-off. Some Arab families in Bulangwa received additional financial assistance from relatives living abroad in Oman, a fact that contributed to income differentials within this latter group.

Gender
Different perspectives on the proper role of women in the community provided another form of social differentiation. Major distinctions within this category mirrored some of the differences between the Muslim and non-Muslim subcommunities described above. Although both African and Arab Muslims spoke about women in terms of their level of modesty and respectability, there nevertheless appeared to be much more social control placed on Arab women. Generally speaking, a self-respecting Muslim woman (*anajiheshima*) is one who stayed close to home. This was especially true of the Arab women in the community, who were rarely seen walking around in the community on their own unless on their way to visit female relatives or neighbors who lived nearby. Muslim women as a whole were also expected to dress in a modest manner, which included covering their heads in public and wearing dresses with long sleeves and high neck-

lines. To behave otherwise was to invite the scorn of Muslim friends, neighbors, and relatives alike.[7]

Other distinctions among the women living in Bulangwa were evident in terms of their level of education and relation to the land. Of those women who had received some level of formal education, most had not continued their education beyond primary school. Further distinctions could be found between Arab and non-Arab women, both Muslim and non-Muslim, in this regard. In a manner that seems to mirror concerns of the "Mohammedans" described by a colonial administrator in the Shinyanga District in the 1920s, Arab women tended to speak about placing limits on young girls' education as how Arab parents could ensure their daughters' modesty. Once an Arab girl completed primary school, she stayed at home (helping out in the family-run shop if one existed) until she married.[8] Limits that African parents placed on their daughters' schooling were spoken about differently: not as a means of ensuring a young girl's modesty per se but, rather, as a reflection of her family's economic hardship. Either they were not able to afford school fees or they needed the additional household labor.

The level of women's engagement with agricultural work was another means of social differentiation among women in the community. As noted above, most of the people in the community depended on farming for their livelihood; women were primarily responsible for the planting and harvesting of crops. Two groups of women in the community provided exceptions to this general rule: women who earned monthly salaries and Arab women. Women who earned regular wages might also farm a small plot of land for their household's consumption. Most of the Arab women in the community did no farming per se, although a few tended small plots of corn directly behind their homes for their families' use. Most of the Arab families in the community hired African men (and sometimes women) to cultivate their land for them.[9]

It is important to note here that most of my conversations that touched on issues related to sexuality, fertility, and women's pregnancy-related concerns were with women; the contexts in which I felt comfortable discussing these topics with men were limited. Given the restricted amount of informal contact between men and women within the Arab members of the community, for example, I never felt comfortable engaging in conversations on sexuality with Arab men. I did, however, feel comfortable sitting with older men in the Arab community and would do so for hours, although these conversations usually took place outside in the open and never touched upon issues of sexuality or reproduction. In the non-Muslim community, where informal contact between men and women wasn't as strictly regulated as it was in the Muslim community in general and the Arab community specifically, I did, from time to time, engage in conversations about issues of sexuality and reproduction with men, but those conversations were themselves contextual and often took place in mixed company. Conversations with male healers constituted a different category altogether. With them I felt completely comfortable talking about anything, ranging from specific aspects of male and female sexuality, to the ingredients of the various love medicines used by both men and women, to the topic of male-female relations in general.

Beliefs Regarding Sorcery and Witchcraft

Despite the numerous churches and mosques in Bulangwa as well as the high percentage of self-identification with a formal religion, many people, regardless of their religious affiliation, sought protection against the effects of *uchawi,* the Kiswahili word for both sorcery and witchcraft (Arens 1987). In Bulangwa, both sorcerers (who could be male or female, kin or nonkin) and witches (who could be male or female, kin or nonkin) were talked about in terms of their ability to affect the health or fertility of a person through the use of harmful medicines (Mesaki 1993). Given that both sorcerers and witches were spoken about as being able to affect a person's fertility, I use the more general term *sorcery* throughout this book. Having stated this, however, it is also important to note that people made distinctions with regard to the power of each. One major distinction between witches and sorcerers was that witches, in addition to being able to affect the health or fertility of people, were also talked about as having the power to steal people's souls, turn them into zombies, and make them work as farm laborers without pay (see also Mesaki 1993:33). People also spoke about witches' ability to make themselves invisible. It was also generally "known" that witches traveled at night by hyena to a secret location, where they met with fellow witches and danced naked under the moonlight.

People's descriptions of the source of "witchness" in Bulangwa were in sharp contrast to what Evans-Pritchard noted regarding the etiology of witchness among the Azande peoples. In the latter case, witches were described as being born as such and containing the substance of witchness within their bodies, sometimes unknowingly (Evans-Pritchard 1937). In Bulangwa, people weren't talked about in terms of being born witches, but in terms of having actively sought out "witchhood" by agreeing to kill a family member, usually a blood relative.[10]

Although the essence of being a witch wasn't spoken about as an inherent quality per se, many people often noted that witches were predominantly women because of the inherent quality of being female. Apparently, women are more likely than men to be witches because women, as a general rule, are inherently stingy, jealous, and mean-spirited beings (*Wanawake wana roho ndogo*). Although I often tried to argue this latter point with various friends and neighbors—male and female, Sukuma and non-Sukuma, African and Arab alike—I was always given counterexamples to disprove my claim that women weren't really such bad people at all. One such example was the connection between women's stinginess and salt. "Even salt!" many of the women I spoke with would tell me. "A woman will refuse to lend you even salt!" (*Hata chumvi! Atakunyima hata chumvi!*).

Mesaki (1993) has linked the increase of witchcraft accusations in Sukumaland in recent years to a decline in the significance of ancestor worship in people's daily lives as well as to government economic policies that have resulted in a decrease in people's standard of living. Both of these factors, according to Mesaki, have led to a subsequent "expansion and commercialization of divination" (221). He notes further that in contrast to what is seen in other parts of the country, the majority of those accused and subsequently killed as witches in Sukumaland are female (Gabba 1989, 1990; Tanner 1970). Of the 2,246 witch killings that occurred in Mwanza and Shinyanga between 1970 and 1988, 83.2 percent (*n* = 1,869) were women (Mesaki 1993).[11]

Biomedical Sources of Maternal Health Care

Government and Nongovernment Health Facilities

Administratively, mainland Tanzania is divided into twenty regions.[12] Each region, in turn, is divided into districts, districts divided into divisions, divisions into wards, and, in rural areas, wards comprised of several villages. The distribution of health facilities throughout the country closely follows this administrative pattern. In terms of the Shinyanga Region specifically, the largest government health facility, the hospital, could be found in the capital cities of five of Shinyanga's six administrative districts, including the larger regional hospital which is located in Shinyanga town.[13] The rural health center, the next level in the health-care system, is located at the division level. Maternal and child health (MCH) clinics, a smaller category of health facility, are located at the division levels within government clinics. Dispensaries, the smallest government health facility, can be found throughout the region, usually at the village level, but also in some neighborhoods in larger towns.

Nongovernment health facilities, both hospitals and privately run clinics or dispensaries, also provided an important source of health care. In terms of the Shinyanga Region specifically, two mission hospitals were located in two of the region's districts. Privately run dispensaries were found at the level of division or ward, and in larger towns at the level of the neighborhood. Summary data for the formal health sector in the Shinyanga Region as a whole are presented in tables 6.1 and 6.2.

Maternity Care

Pregnant women who lived in the same division in which the community of Bulangwa was located had several options for maternity care within the biomedical system. In theory, they could either give birth at one of the MCH clinics located throughout the division, at the eight-bed maternity ward at the division health center, at the regional hospital in Shinyanga town, or at the Kolondoto mission hospital.

For women living in Bulangwa specifically, birth at the health center in the division was not very feasible as it was located off the beaten path, about a six- to seven-hour walk away. Instead, many women gave birth at the two-bed maternity clinic within the government clinic in Bulangwa. Women who experienced obstetric complications at the clinic were referred out to a higher-level facility: either to Kolondoto hospital or to the regional hospital located in Shinyanga town. The former was located approximately an hour's drive away, while the latter was located an additional thirty- to forty-five-minute drive beyond that. My observations of births within the biomedical setting were primarily limited to these two latter settings.[14] These facilities were similar in that both had operating rooms on their premises in which life-saving emergency obstetric procedures could be performed. There were some differences between these two health facilities: although the maternity ward at Kolondoto hospital usually appeared fairly clean, the maternity ward at the regional hospital was less so (see chap. 10).

Fees for Service
Although up until 1993, services at government health facilities were technically "free,"[15] women were nevertheless required to bring medical supplies along with them when they came to give birth. Women wanting to give birth at a government facility were required to bring the following items: two pairs of latex examining gloves (1,000 TSH per pair), two vials of ergometrine to prevent postpartum hemorrhage (250 TSH per vial), and one syringe for its injection (60 TSH). This meant a minimum cost to each woman of 2,560 TSH. Women needing suturing, either because they had torn during birth or had had an episiotomy, had to supply those materials as well. Women who needed cesarean sections at the regional hospital in Shinyanga town were required to supply at least two liters of IV solution (1,500 TSH per liter). In other words, a "free" birth at a government facility could cost a woman between 2,500 and 6,000 TSH.

Women who gave birth in private facilities were not required to bring their own supplies; they paid fees for services rendered. At the Kolondoto

TABLE 6.1.   Shinyanga Region Health Profile (1993 data)

Area	50,764 sq km
Population	2,060,630
Hospital	7 (Government)
	2 (Nongovernment)
Population per hospital	354,000
Hospital beds	1,157
Population per bed	1,780
Doctors	34
Medical officers	17
Assistant medical officers	17
Population per dispensary	12,000

Source: Shinyanga Regional Hospital.

TABLE 6.2.   Health Facilities in the Shinyanga Region (1993 data)

Type of Facility	Government	Nongovernment
Hospital	7	2
Rural health center	19	—
MCH clinic	194	—
Dispensary	146	42

Source: Shinyanga Regional Hospital.

hospital, a vaginal delivery cost 700 TSH, while a cesarean section cost 10,000 TSH. There was also an additional 500 TSH charge per day of hospitalization. Women who preferred staying in a semiprivate room paid 1,100 TSH per day. Meals were not included in the cost of the room. Those who stayed overnight at the hospital (or for several days) either had meals brought to them by family members or purchased food sold by local vendors on the hospital compound.

Transportation

Transportation was another cost associated with birth in the hospital or clinic setting. These costs varied from 400 to 800 TSH for a bus ride to Kolondoto or Shinyanga town to 8,000 to 30,000 TSH for women needing emergency transport via private car, tractor, or oxcart. Health personnel I spoke with told me that it wasn't unusual for transportation costs to exceed even those amounts if the emergency was considered life-threatening.

Births before Arrival

During my fieldwork, I visited all of the government MCH clinics that were located in the same division as Bulangwa. I wanted to get a sense of how many women gave birth at these facilities during a year compared to the number of women who brought their newborns to the clinic for registration after they had already given birth. These latter cases were referred to as births before arrival, or BBA (see table 6.3). Although a total of 142 (approximately 11 percent) of the 1,311 registered births at the MCH clinics in the division took place outside of the clinic setting during 1992, table 6.3 also shows a wide variability between the number of such births. For example, almost 20 percent of the births at three of the clinics (clinics B, F, and J) took place outside of the clinic setting, whereas that number was less than 10 percent at four other clinics (clinics A, G, H, and I). My point in presenting these numbers is to underscore the fact that a variability in women's birth experiences exists even between rural settings. A variety of factors might have contributed to this level of variability, including the distance from a woman's home to the clinic, the timing of the birth, or even the quality of interactions between health-care personnel at specific clinics and their clientele. We will take a closer look at some of these explanations when we examine the case studies presented later in this book.

Although the practice of registering BBAs also takes place at the regional and mission hospitals, their numbers are much lower (see table 6.4). While the percentages of out-of-hospital births registered at the regional and mission hospitals are much lower than those recorded for the government MCH clinics, we can also see that a slightly higher number of births before arrival were registered at the Kolondoto hospital. Again, this might be a reflection of various factors. For example, the mission hospital is located in a relatively rural area, surrounded by several villages, outside of the boundaries of a large town. The regional hospital, in contrast, is located in the regional capital itself. The lower numbers in table 6.4 might also mean that women are simply more likely to register out-of-hospital births at a clinic near their homes.

Cesarean Sections

As noted in chapter 3, cesarean sections are often life-saving procedures, especially in settings where obstructed or prolonged labor is common. As we will see later in chapter 10, the low percentage of cesarean sections presented for the two hospitals in table 6.5 does not necessarily reflect a small number of cases of obstructed births but, rather, may actually be a

TABLE 6.3.   Comparison of Clinic Births and Registered Births before Arrival (BBA) at Ten Government MCH Clinics in One District of the Shinyanga Region, 1992

MCH Clinics	Births Attended	BBA	Total Births	BBA (%)
Clinic A	169	14	183	7.7
Clinic B	109	27	136	19.9
Clinic C	91	16	107	15.0
Clinic D	86	10	96	10.4
Clinic E	105	—	105	—
Clinic F	61	14	75	18.7
Clinic G	76	7	83	8.4
Clinic H	95	9	104	8.7
Clinic I	314	30	344	8.7
Clinic J	63	15	78	19.2
Total	1,169	142	1,311	10.8

TABLE 6.4.   Comparison of Hospital Births and Registered Births before Arrival (BBA) at the Shinyanga Regional and Kolondoto Mission Hospitals in 1992

Health Facility	Births Attended	BBA	Total Births	BBA (%)
Shinyanga regional hospital	3,927	51	3,978	1.3
Kolondoto mission hospital	1,025	27	1,052	2.6

reflection of an absence of funds or medical supplies to conduct such operations.

Nonbiomedical Sources of Maternal Health Care

Local Cultural Options for Prenatal and Obstetric Care

As suggested in tables 6.3 and 6.4, not every woman living in the division gave birth in the hospital or MCH clinic. Sometimes women made the conscious choice to stay away from such settings or had family members who made the decision for them, while at other times women did not reach such facilities because of the economic costs of doing so. Women who chose to give birth outside of the clinic or hospital setting might do so either at home or at the home of healer known for her midwifery skills. But, as we saw in chapter 2 and as we will see again in the next, traditions related to the practice of midwifery have never been that well-established in this part of the country. Although some women were known to possess such skills, they were, apparently, few and far between.

As we will see in chapters 8 and 9, some women sought biomedical and nonbiomedical forms of prenatal care simultaneously. Nonbiomedical options for prenatal care included those offered by herbalists, diviners, spirit mediums, or specialists in maternity care. Mwana Nyanzanga, the pseudonym for the healer whose work I observed from December 1992 to July 1994, is an example of this latter category of healer. She was well-known throughout the surrounding area, both within and outside of the division, and many people traveled long distances to seek care with her. Although she was not Sukuma, many of the women who consulted with her about their pregnancy-related concerns or who gave birth at her home were. Some initial remarks about the setting of her midwifery and healing practice are appropriate here.

TABLE 6.5.   Cesarean Sections Performed at the Shinyanga Regional and Kolondoto Mission Hospitals in 1992

Health Facility	Total Births	Number of Cesarean Sections	Cesarean Section (%)
Shinyanga regional hospital	3,927	137	3.5
Kolondoto mission hospital	1,025	39	3.8

Mwana Nyanzanga's Hospitali

Mwana Nyanzanga's home, which was similar in appearance to the other houses in her village, was a series of separate buildings constructed of mud brick, some covered with thatch or corrugated iron roofs. One of these buildings, which she referred to as her *hospitali* (hospital), was situated farther away from the other structures, a bit off on its own. Like most of the other buildings on her compound, her *hospitali* was made of mud bricks with a thatched roof. It was a three-room structure consisting of an examining room/postpartum room, a room for dispensing medicines, and a birthing room. Although both men and women numbered among her clientele, the *hospitali* was almost exclusively the domain of women, reserved for prenatal consultations, births, postpartum care, or other reproductive health concerns.

In the remainder of this chapter I describe the sample of 154 women who took part in my formal survey. I preface those remarks with a brief description of a different research project among Sukuma women that addressed some of the same research questions as my own. This latter study, which was conducted by the Dutch anthropologist Corlein Varkevisser in the mid-1960s, took place in the Mwanza Region to the north. Varkevisser was primarily concerned with Sukuma customs and beliefs, and thus her informants were Sukuma. My study, in contrast, was focused on women's pregnancy-related experiences irrespective of their ethnicity.

Categories of Women, Categories of Risk: A Note on Methodology

Traditional versus Modern Mothers

Varkevisser's research among the Sukuma took place in the Mwanza Region from February 1965 through April 1967 (Varkevisser 1973). Her study was similar to other research projects among the Sukuma during the 1960s in that it was trying to assess how a traditional Sukuma way of life was adapting to modernity.[16] Scattered throughout Varkevisser's work are references to change; the Sukuma were either beginning to abandon practices associated with a strict adherence to the tenets of traditional religion and cultural taboos, or they had already done so.

Varkevisser characterizes her study as heavily influenced by the "new" field of psychological anthropology. Although she was primarily concerned with "the cultural context in which the socialization of the Sukuma child takes place" (1973:6), she devotes one chapter of her book to the beliefs and practices surrounding pregnancy and childbirth.

She identified what she saw as two distinct categories of Sukuma mothers between the ages of twenty and forty: the "traditional, illiterate" and the "literate, Christian." In her analysis, the traditional Sukuma mother is represented by the data collected from her interviews with six-teen women who had never attended school and who did not belong to any Western-based religion. The modern Sukuma mother is represented by her interviews with a group of sixteen Christian women with at least a fourth-grade education.

In retrospect, however, this juxtaposing of traditional and modern behaviors (or "mentalities," as Varkevisser referred to them) is prob-lematic in that one is left with the impression that a person's behavior and beliefs can be predicted by knowing into which of these two distinct analytical categories he or she fits. That categories, however they may be defined, are fluid is a point that emerged quite clearly in my own fieldwork. I learned, for example, that Christians in the community who were respected as church elders might (unbeknownst to church leaders) run a secret healing practice based on herbal and spiritual medicines out of their homes, or that a school-educated nurse working in the govern-ment clinic might, for a fee, show traditional birth attendants the ingre-dients of an herbal remedy used to treat cases of prolonged labor "caused" by a pregnant woman's promiscuity. I also learned that devout African and Arab Muslim women were not averse to using local medicines as protection against sorcery, or that a primary school teacher might use a local love medicine in the hope of causing her hus-band to fall out of love with his current mistress. Despite the difficulty in defining what exactly constitutes traditional versus modern behavior, these distinctions continue to be made by policymakers, health-care workers, and community members alike. As we will see later in chapters 7 through 11, such labels often function as barriers to women's access to maternal health care.

Unlike Varkevisser's research design, which set out to examine the beliefs and practices of two predetermined categories of Sukuma mothers, I interviewed a sample of women and then analyzed the results according to the categories that emerged from the data themselves. Summary char-acteristics of the sample I interviewed are presented below.

The Bulangwa Study: Methods and Descriptions

One hundred and fifty-four women agreed to participate in my formal survey. Ninety-four of these women were randomly selected from a list of households in Bulangwa, while 46 women were randomly selected from a list of the households in the village where I observed Mwana Nyanzanga's work. The one exception to the randomness of my sample is a subset of 14 Arab women, all of whom lived in houses located in the center of Bulangwa and who therefore might not have been represented in a purely random selection of households.

A tendency to want to group similar responses into larger encompassing categories is something that I struggled with in deciding how to present the data from my interviews. To try to counteract the homogenizing effect of such groupings, I have used women's own words to create some of the analytical categories themselves. As a result, some of the numbers I present in this and subsequent chapters would not be considered powerful or statistically significant because many of the categories I present often contain only one woman's experience. In addition, some of the results I present throughout this book reflect missing data. Although my formal survey included interviews with 154 women, I didn't always ask every woman every question. There were several reasons for this. If, for example, a woman seemed uncomfortable with a particular question, I didn't press for an answer, but moved on to the next question instead. In other cases, new questions emerged as a result of issues women raised within the context of my interviews.

Age
Ideally, exact age should be a factor in my analysis. This was a problem, however, because some of the women did not know the date of their birth. As a result, some of the women's ages I recorded were estimated or guessed ages, based on the timing of specific life events, such as puberty, marriage, or first birth, in terms of local historical events. When I began to analyze the results of my formal interviews, it became apparent that two main categories of women had been interviewed: a subset of 104 younger women who were still in their reproductive years and a subset of 50 older women who were not. This was good, I initially thought, as it would enable me to get a sense of whether practices during the prenatal period had changed or remained constant over time, and whether differences in

knowledge, practices, and perceptions of risks during pregnancy were talked about differently by younger and older women. For the purposes of my analysis, I defined women as younger if they still experienced their monthly menses and older if they had already reached menopause (i.e., they appeared older, were no longer experiencing their menses, and were not pregnant).

Within the subset of younger women, three main categories of formal education emerged: women who had never attended primary school, women who had attended but didn't finish primary school, and women who had attended and completed primary school. Given these distinct differences within the younger subset of women, I have chosen to present some of my analyses in terms of four groups of women: (1) older women; (2) younger women with no formal education; (3) younger women who had not finished primary school; and (4) younger women who had completed their primary education. The characteristics of these four groups are summarized in table 6.6. As the table shows, 94 percent of the ages listed for older women were guessed ages, producing an estimated average age of 62.5 years and an age range of 45 to 90 years. None of the women in this group had ever attended school.[17] The education level among the younger group of women falls into three categories: (1) never attended primary school ($n = 43$); (2) attended some years of primary school ($n = 20$); and (3) completed primary school ($n = 41$), three of whom had attended secondary school for a short period of time. Seventy percent of the ages of younger women with no formal education were guessed ages, with an average age of 35 years and a range of 23 to 50. Women with some years of primary education had an average age of 33 years, with a range of 17 to 47 years. Thirty percent of their ages were estimated. The average age for younger women who had completed primary school was 28 years, with a range of 19 to 45. Only 5 percent of the ages in this latter group were estimated.

Having identified my main categories of analysis, I then wanted to see in what ways these women were similar or different. Did they differ, for example, in their ethnicity, marital status, religious affiliation, and place of residence? Answers to some of these questions in terms of the categories of older and younger women are presented in table 6.7.

Ethnic Categories
The majority of the women stated their ethnicity was Sukuma. The percentages of older and younger women who claimed to be of either Sukuma

or Nyamwezi ethnicity were about the same: 78.4 and 79.8 percent respectively. The striking difference within this particular category is the difference in how ethnicity was specified. Some of the older Sukuma women made directional references with regard to their ethnicity, for example, *Dakama* to indicate they came from an area to the south or *Kiya* to indicate they came from an area to the east, which, as we saw in chapter 5, is a Sukuma-Nyamwezi way of referring to identity that Brandström describes as "insider/insider classification" (1986). Younger women did not use these terms. Instead, they used the term *Nyamwezi,* a way of referring to people who come from the Tabora Region to the south.

Marital Status
Most of the younger women (82.7 percent) were in some type of relationship with a man, as opposed to 45 percent of the older women. Among the younger women currently in a relationship, 80 percent (*n* = 69) stated it was their first such union, 17 percent (*n* = 15) said it was their second, one woman said it was her third, and one woman said it was her fourth. These numbers differed from the older subset of women wherein 39 percent (*n* = 9) said it was their first such relationship, 39 percent (*n* = 9) said it was their second, and 22 percent (*n* = 5) said it was their third. Of the eighteen younger women currently not in a relationship, 72 percent (*n* = 13) said they had only been in one such relationship before, while five women, or 29 percent said they had been in two previous relationships with a man. Of the older women not currently in a relationship, 39 percent (*n* = 11) said they had been in one previous relationship, 39 percent said they had been in two, 18 percent (*n* = 5) had been in three, and one woman had been in four previous relationships with a man. This suggests that marriage is not necessarily a stable institution in the community, with younger as opposed to older women more likely to be in a current relationship with a man. Older women have been in more relationships than the younger women, a

TABLE 6.6.   **Distribution of Age and Education of Survey Respondents (*N* = 154)**

Group	Number of Women	Age Range	Average Age	Percent Guessed	Formal Education
Older women	50	45–90	62.5	94	None
Younger women	43	23–50	35.0	70	None
	20	17–47	33.0	30	Quit primary school
	41	19–45	28.0	5	Completed primary school

TABLE 6.7. Selected Descriptive Characteristics for the Subsets of Older and Younger Women (N = 154)

	Older Women (n = 50)		Younger Women (n = 104)	
	n	%	n	%
Ethnicity				
Sukuma/Nyamwezi-related				
Sukuma	30	58.8	80	76.9
Kiya	1	2.0	—	—
Dakama	9	17.6	—	—
Nyamwezi	—	—	3	2.9
Other African				
Nyiramba	6	11.8	1	1.0
Kerewere	1	2.0	1	1.0
Jita	—	—	1	1.0
Kimbu	—	—	1	1.0
Kuria	—	—	1	1.0
Nyasa	—	—	1	1.0
Taturu	—	—	1	1.0
Ngoni	—	—	1	1.0
Tusi	1	2.0	—	—
Zanaki	1	2.0	—	—
Non-African				
Arab	1	2.0	13	12.5
Marital Status				
Currently married or				
living with a man	23	44.0	86	82.7
Divorced or widowed	28	56.0	17	16.3
Never married	—	—	1	1.0
Religious Affiliation				
No affiliation	37	74.0	36	34.6
Catholic	5	10.0	30	28.8
African Inland Church	2	4.0	15	14.4
Muslim	6	12.0	20	19.2
Seventh-Day Adventist	—	—	2	1.9
Lutheran	—	—	1	1.0
Place of Residence				
Bulangwa	32	64.0	76	73.1
Village	18	36.0	28	26.9

finding that is not surprising given that older women have lived longer and thus had more life experience.

Four categories of living relationships between men and the younger and older subsets of women emerged: (1) "traditional," with no church or civil service, but bridewealth was paid; (2) religious ceremony, a category that included Arab and African Muslim women for the most part; (3) lived together, no formal arrangement made; and (4) ran away together (*kupulwa* in Kisukuma). This latter category was similar to elopement. Sometimes bridewealth was paid at a later date (Brandström 1990).[18] The majority of the older and younger women currently in a relationship described it as being the first type, 69.6 and 57.0 percent respectively.

Marriage Payments

In chapter 4, we learned that these types of payments were referred to as *brideprice* at the national level. But following Evans-Pritchard's discussion regarding the misuses of that term, I substitute the term *bridewealth* instead below (see chap. 4, n. 9; Evans-Pritchard 1931:36).

Whether bridewealth was paid and, if so, how much proved to be a sensitive topic, similar to what has been noted about survey questions related to income. If a woman seemed uncomfortable answering my question about bridewealth payments, I did not pursue it further. Some told me they didn't know how much bridewealth was paid, because it was handled by the elders (*wakubwa*). Given those limits on the interpretation of this data, it is nevertheless interesting to note that the older women were less likely than the younger women to have had their bridewealth paid in money. This is consistent with earlier observations that by 1945 in Tanganyika, bridewealth transactions were increasingly conducted in cash as opposed to cattle (Bates 1965:630).

Religious Affiliation

The information regarding religious affiliation is a bit more problematic. When I asked the question "*Una dini?*"—which literally means "Do you have religion?" and contextually means "Do you belong to an organized religion?"—one-third of the younger women and almost three-fourths of the older women said they did not. Generally speaking, Christians and Muslims in the community spoke about people who do not affiliate with an organized religion in terms of what their "not belonging" meant: they are referred to either as pagans (*wapagani*) or as people who have not seen the light, literally "people in darkness" (*watu wa giza*). Some people linked their own Christianity with modernity by referring to themselves as belonging to the category of people who had "woken up" (*nimeamka*). In terms of the religions mentioned, thirteen out of the twenty younger Muslim women were Arab, while one out of the five older Muslim women was Arab. Of the remaining religions cited, Catholicism and the African Inland Church seem to be more popular than either the Seventh-Day Adventists or the Lutherans for both groups of women. The seeming indifference to these two latter religions may have more to do with their geographic location in the community than to anything else. Both the Catholic and African Inland churches were located on the side of Bulangwa where I conducted my formal survey. Had the sample of women I interviewed been selected instead from the other side of town, we might have seen a difference in these numbers.

Religion as a category of analysis is problematic for another reason: what can be assumed about those women who said of themselves, "I don't have a religion" (*Sina dini*) or "I don't pray" (*Sisali*)? Do we immediately classify them as adherents to traditional religion or animists, as Kirwen did in the Mwanza study referred to by Mesaki above (1993), or as having "traditional mentalities," as Varkevisser did in her study conducted in the mid-1960s (1973)? In chapter 8 we will examine the role that ancestors play in people's lives in this particular region of the country. We will see that a belief in the ability of ancestors to affect their descendants' health is not always strictly a function of a person's ethnicity nor of his or her religious affiliation. Also important to note is that a belief in a world of nonliving kin is not talked about by the people in the community as a religion per se; it is just simply the way things are (Needham 1981). Because of the ambiguity in the meaning that can be attributed either to a person's religious affiliation or to their lack of affiliation, I excluded religion as a category of analysis.

Level of Education

Compared to religion, the category of formal education was less ambiguous. As already noted, the levels of formal education between these two groups of women were quite different: none of the older women I interviewed had ever attended primary school. Still, almost half of the younger women had never attended school either. Older and younger women with no formal education responded differently to my inquiries as to their level of formal education. When I asked whether they had ever attended primary school, literally "Have you ever studied?" (*Umewahi kusoma?*), some of the older women told me they had not because "a long time ago" (*zamani*) only boys went to school. One elderly woman whose relative had been a chief told me that in the past, only the sons of chiefs attended school; she herself had only attended a Koranic school.

Some of the younger women who had not been to school seemed embarrassed by the question, while a few others were mildly amused. When I asked if they had ever studied, some responded by saying that they had "watched over cattle" or had been "herders of cattle" instead (*Nimechunga ng'ombe; Mimi nilikuwa mchungaji wa ng'ombe*). Their answers are similar to what the regional head of the national women's group Umoja wa Wanawake wa Tanzania (UWT) in Shinyanga told me

TABLE 6.8.   Selected Descriptive Characteristics of Women according to Age Category and Years of Formal Education (*N* = 154)

	Older Women		Younger Women					
	(*n* = 50) (0 years)		(*n* = 43) (0 yrs)		(*n* = 20) (< 7 yrs)		(*n* = 41) (7 yrs)	
	n	%	*n*	%	*n*	%	*n*	%
Ethnicity								
Sukuma	30	58.5	39	90.7	14	70.0	27	65.9
Dakama	9	17.6	—	—	—	—	—	—
Kiya	1	2.0	—	—	—	—	—	—
Nyamwezi	—	—	—	—	1	5.0	2	4.9
African/Non-Sukuma	9	17.8	1	2.3	3	15.0	4	9.8
Arab	1	2.0	3	7.0	2	10.0	8	19.5
Marital Status								
Currently married/ living with a man	23	44.0	36	83.7	17	85.0	33	80.5
Divorced or widowed	28	56.0	7	16.3	2	10.0	19	19.5
Never married	—	—	—	—	1	5.0	—	—
Religious Affiliation								
No affiliation	37	74.0	28	65.1	4	20.0	4	9.8
Catholic	5	10.0	6	14.0	9	45.0	15	36.6
African Inland Church	2	4.0	5	11.6	4	20.0	6	14.6
Muslim	6	12.0	4	9.3	3	15.0	13	31.7
Seventh-Day Adventist	—	—	—	—	—	—	2	4.9
Lutheran	—	—	—	—	—	—	1	2.4
Place of Residence								
Bulangwa	32	64.0	27	62.8	15	75.0	34	82.9
Village	18	36.0	16	37.2	5	25.0	7	17.1

during my first visit to the Shinyanga Region in the summer of 1990. She noted that the level of literacy was particularly low among Sukuma women because many young girls were kept out of school to tend cattle.

In table 6.8, I revisit some of the descriptive categories presented above in terms of women's age and level of formal education. Again, we see that the percentage of women who defined their ethnicity as Sukuma is larger than the percentage of either non-Sukuma African women or Arab women, although a larger share (34 percent) of the women who had finished primary school listed their ethnicity as other than Sukuma. It is also in this particular group that we see a higher percentage of Arab women than in the other three groups of women. In addition, a higher percentage of the women who have had some formal education acknowledge affiliation with an organized religion than do either the older or younger women who never attended school before. In terms of place of residence, in all four groups a larger percentage of the interviews were conducted in Bulangwa as opposed to the village setting. However, we also see that even in the latter setting, younger women without formal education are more similar to the older women in this regard than to the other two groups of younger women with some formal education.

Having introduced both the community of study and the women who took part in the formal survey, let us now turn to an examination of how risks to maternal health are spoken about at the local level. In the next chapter, we revisit a factor that figured significantly in colonial, international, and national definitions of maternal health risk: the risk of tradition.

CHAPTER 7

Risk and Tradition

Members of the international development elite can talk at length, with
tremendous conviction, about the "real" medicinal value of traditional
healing—without ever having observed or interacted with any actual
healers. They *already* know what these healers do because development
lore and literature synthesizes and summarizes data from particular
places, molding it into a powerful mythology of traditional healing and
its hidden worth.

—Stacy Pigg, "Acronyms and Effacement"

Tradition is an ambiguous concept. It has been invoked both to stigmatize
as well as to celebrate African cultural practices. In chapter 2, we saw how
native practices were often portrayed as "backward" and "harmful." Such
perceptions led government officials to implement policies that sought to
transform traditional native cultural practices into those seen in the more
developed parts of the world. Chapters 3 and 4 showed how negative
aspects of tradition have also been highlighted in the contemporary health
development literature. In regard to the Safe Motherhood Initiative
specifically, tradition has been implicated in the low status accorded
women in the developing world, in poor outcomes when births are managed outside of the biomedical context, and in cultural practices that
adversely affect pregnant women's overall health.

But tradition has also been invoked at the international and national
levels to convey beneficial aspects of African culture. Some population
experts, for example, have noted that, in the past, cultural prohibitions on
sexual relations during the postpartum period enabled women to safely
space their births (Lesthaeghe et al. 1981). Others have pointed out that
past rituals of initiation at puberty in Tanzania served a positive function
in that they facilitated adolescents' transition from childhood to social
adulthood and taught them about proper sexual behavior (Ntukula 1994;
Rwebangira and Liljeström 1998; Tumbo-Masabo and Liljeström 1994;
cf. Allen 2000).[1] The problem arises when development experts' assump-

tions about the widespread applicability of certain cultural practices serve as the rationale for particular kinds of projects that are implemented everywhere, irrespective of the context (Ferguson 1990; Grillo and Stirrat 1997; Pigg 1995).

In this chapter we take a closer at some of the assumptions that informed Safe Motherhood interventions in Tanzania. Our focus will be on two specific Safe Motherhood policy recommendations that targeted tradition: (1) the need to train traditional birth attendants, and (2) the need to eliminate harmful cultural practices that negatively affect pregnant women's nutritional status. The first recommendation, which approaches tradition as a solution to draw upon, is based on the assumption that the cultural category of indigenous midwife is relevant throughout the developing world. The second recommendation, which approaches tradition as a problem to be eliminated, is based on the assumption that the poor nutritional status of pregnant women is a direct result of cultural practices that limit women's intake of nutritious foods. As we will see in the following pages, some of the Initiative's assumptions about these traditions were not relevant to everyday life in Bulangwa, while others were relevant in unexpected ways.

Tradition As Solution: The Traditional Birth Attendant

Traditional birth attendants are often the first (if not only) health care workers with whom pregnant women in poor countries have contact. Therefore, it is essential that they be made as effective as possible through training, supervision and support.
—WHO 1986. "Helping Women off the Road to Death"

A traditional birth attendant (TBA) is a person who assists the mother during childbirth and initially acquired her skill by delivering babies herself or through apprenticeship to other traditional birth attendants. A family TBA is a TBA who has been designated by an extended family to attend births in the family. A trained TBA is a TBA or a family TBA who has received a short course of training through the modern health care sector to upgrade her skills.
—WHO 1992. *Traditional Birth Attendants*

One example of an intervention that portrays traditional practices as a solution to tap into can be seen in the Safe Motherhood Initiative's recommendation to train the traditional birth attendant (TBA). Based, in part, on the primary health-care movement launched at the Alma Ata Conference in 1978 as well as on a growing body of literature in the late 1970s and early 1980s that examined cultural practices related to child-bearing, health development organizations began to look for alternative sources of health-care delivery in areas characterized by a shortage of health-care professionals and medical facilities (Pigg 1995:50–52; WHO 1978a, 1981).[2] In targeting what was assumed to be a category of traditional healer found throughout the developing world, policymakers and program planners sought to improve maternal health outcomes by transforming existing harmful midwifery practices into good ones through "retraining" (Maglacas and Simons 1986; Verderese and Turnbull 1975; WHO 1979).

Similar hopes regarding the potential of the TBA were expressed at the national level in Tanzania during the late 1980s and early 1990s. One of the Tanzanian obstetricians I spoke with at the 1990 National Safe Motherhood Conference, for example, explained to me that the urgency to train TBAs lay primarily in the need to train harmful practices out of them. He was particularly concerned with what he believed to be TBAs' use of herbs to induce or speed up labor. He told me that when a woman with a ruptured uterus arrives on the maternity ward of the hospital in central Tanzania where he worked and her stomach is pumped, the remains of herbs are usually found. When I asked if any chemical analyses had been conducted to establish a direct link between the contents found in those women's stomachs and their uterine ruptures, he said he didn't think so (Price 1984).[3]

Another Tanzanian obstetrician I spoke with who worked at a large referral hospital in Dar es Salaam was more cautious about linking cases of uterine rupture to the use of herbal remedies specifically. He told me that he didn't know whether herbal remedies actually caused uterine rupture, pointing out that the chloroquine tablets given to pregnant women as a means of preventing malaria also had oxytocic properties.[4] He was also a bit skeptical about the widespread use of the terms *traditional birth attendant* and *traditional midwife,* noting that in many cases the women who assisted with births were not midwives at all, but simply the oldest woman living in the pregnant woman's household or in the community.

As we will see later in chapter 10, herbal remedies were indeed sometimes given to women in the hope of facilitating labor. Such remedies, which come in a variety of different forms, were given to pregnant women by healers or self-administered by the pregnant woman herself. That such remedies exist indicates difficult labor is recognized as a maternal health risk by members of the community. One cannot assume, however, as the doctor I spoke with at the National Safe Motherhood Conference in 1990 did, that herbal remedies *cause* uterine rupture. Some of the life-threatening conditions associated with birth may be the result of delays in treatment, delays that, as we will see in later chapters, often have nothing to do with traditional practices at all.

In order to explore how decontextualized generalizations about traditional practices are problematic, how they can lead to the implementation of development interventions that have very little relevance in particular local contexts, I turn to a case study of sorts. I say "of sorts" because my aim here is not to present the case of one specific woman. I present, instead, the group experience of a particular set of women in one part of the Shinyanga Region—women who were identified as traditional birth attendants and who participated in a UN-funded project to train TBAs. Who are these women? Whose tradition is being invoked here? And what is the relevance of traditional midwifery to the Shinyanga Region specifically?

Tradition and Midwifery among the Sukuma

The Sukuma custom of giving birth apart by oneself has impeded the accumulation of systematic knowledge about birth and attendant disorders. Modern prenatal clinics have hardly any functional equivalent in traditional society.

—Corlien Varkevisser, *Socialization in a Changing Society*

It will be interesting to hear the results of the Mwanza training course for domiciliary midwives. It was originally a stopgap measure to help Native Authorities by giving a three-week course to illiterate traditional midwives in the simplest side of hygiene (clean hands and the use of a basin and scissors) and could hardly be said to turn out certificated tribal midwives. The difficulty seemed to be to find enough women who knew enough about midwifery to be worth giving a three week course in simple hygiene. Perhaps it has become more ambitious since then.

—Excerpt of a letter from the Provincial Office of the Eastern Province to the Member for Local Government, Dar es Salaam, August 5, 1953 (TNA 34300:82)

One of the recurring themes in the ethnographic literature on Sukuma healing practices is that there has never been a distinct tradition of midwifery. Some healers knew how to treat infertility or certain conditions that arose during pregnancy, both of which will be discussed in later chapters, but no indigenous category of midwife existed per se.[5] Many women simply gave birth alone, cutting the umbilical cord themselves (see Sargent 1982).[6] Others gave birth in the presence of a female relative who cut the cord. In some cases, this relative was the woman's mother or mother-in-law (Lang and Lang 1973; Reid 1969; Varkevisser 1973). If problems arose, such as a retained placenta, an *nfumu* (healer in Kisukuma) might be called for assistance. My own interviews with women about their birthing experiences, which will be addressed in more detail in chapters 10 and 11, corroborate this earlier ethnographic literature.

How to Become a Traditional Birth Attendant
in Ten Easy Lessons
Postcolonial efforts to train traditional birth attendants (*wakunga wa jadi*) in Tanzania began in 1985 (Kaisi 1989:21). By 1988, the Ministry of Health had finalized the specifics of the training program, and workshops began to be held around the country. The first TBA training workshop in the Shinyanga Region took place in 1986.[7] From 1986 through 1989, the workshops were funded by UNICEF. From 1990 until I left the field in 1994, UNFPA provided the funds for TBA training.

I observed two TBA training workshops at the beginning of my fieldwork in September and October 1992. The first was a three-day refresher course for women who had undergone the introductory training six months earlier. The second was the introductory ten-day training workshop. By the end of 1992, fifty-eight women residing in one administrative division of the Shinyanga Region had attended at least the initial ten-day training. In 1993 I interviewed forty-four of these women in their homes. I was specifically interested in whether they had ever assisted with a birth prior to participating in the TBA training and, if so, how they had initially acquired their midwifery skills.

One woman, with much retrospective amusement, told me that when she and her neighbor were selected by the village government official to attend the first TBA training workshop in 1986, her neighbor, a healer who had never attended a birth before, showed up later at her home "trembling with fear" (*ametetemeka*). She was quite frightened and worried about their collective fate once they arrived "at that place." It appears that the government official in their village had not explained the exact purpose of the training workshop to them; perhaps he didn't understand it clearly himself. He merely told them that they had been selected to represent their village at the training and therefore they must go.

When I asked the forty-four women I interviewed whether they had ever assisted with another woman's birth prior to attending the TBA training course, approximately 30 percent ($n = 13$) said they had not. One woman, who attended her first TBA training in April 1992, told me that she had only been selected to attend because other women in her village refused to go. Another told me that although she had never assisted with anyone else's birth, she was selected because she herself had given birth ten times and thus was considered to have a lot of experience. Still another woman told me she was selected for training because she had helped a neighbor with a retained placenta by pushing on the woman's "stomach." She wasn't very happy that she had been chosen because, as she pointed out to me, she had never attended an actual birth. She went anyway because local government officials told her it was for the good of the village. Although none of these thirteen women had prior experience delivering babies, a few of them were selected because they were known in the community either for their knowledge of fertility medicines or as healers in general.

But some of the women who were selected to participate in the training workshops did have prior experience assisting with births. The extent of their experience varied, however, from one Sukuma woman who assisted with a woman's birth in the 1960s but never again (she had learned to assist births from watching her husband, who worked as a medical assistant at the local government clinic), to the experience of Mwana Nyanzanga who had delivered over 100 babies in 1992. Mwana Nyanzanga, the midwife and healer whose work I observed over the course of my fieldwork, came from a family of female healers and had acquired her midwifery skills by assisting with the births her mother attended in their village.[8] Unlike the majority of the other women I interviewed, however, Mwana Nyanzanga was not Sukuma. She had been born in a different region to the north and claimed to be of a different ethnicity. In table 7.1 I present a summary of how these women acquired their initial experience attending births.

Several surprising results emerged from my interviews. Although much of the development literature on TBAs suggests that lay midwifery skills are passed on to women through a period of apprenticeship with an experienced traditional midwife, only eight of the forty-four women I interviewed learned from a relative, neighbor, or friend. But even this bit of information is misleading; most of those women had not acquired their midwifery experience over a long apprenticeship, but, rather, from hands-on experience with the births of relatives or neighbors instead.

One woman's first experience assisting with a birth occurred before she had even reached puberty. Her mother, who had gone into labor at home, had sent her husband to ask the health worker at the government dispensary to come and assist with her birth. But she birthed before the health worker arrived, so she called out to her young daughter (who was waiting just outside the door) to come and help her cut the cord. Another woman learned to deliver babies from her mother who had been taught by nurses at a mission hospital many years previously.

This latter case highlights another surprising result from my interviews: almost half ($n = 21$) of the women who had been identified by the government as traditional birth attendants had acquired their initial experience assisting with births either directly or indirectly from health-care personnel in hospitals or clinics. In other words, these so-called traditional birth attendants acquired their "traditional" midwifery skills via the biomedical system. When placed within the context of past colonial maternal health policies in Tanganyika, this finding is not surprising. We already saw that much government effort during that time was directed at training native women to attend births. Seven of the women I interviewed specifically mentioned learning either directly or indirectly from African nurses at the Kolondoto mission hospital, while others mentioned learning at hospitals and clinics in general.

TABLE 7.1.   **Level of Prior Experience Attending Births among Women Participating in Training Seminars for Traditional Birth Attendants ($N = 44$)**

Level of Experience	Number of Responses	Percent of All Responses
No prior experience	13	29.5
Taught by nurses at the hospital/clinic	11	25.0
Taught by/learned from watching relative, neighbor, or friend	8	18.2
Taught by relative who is health-care-provider	5	11.4
Taught by relative who learned from nurses	3	6.8
Worked as nurse or nurse's assistant	2	4.5
Is a village health worker[a]	2	4.5
Total	44	100.0

[a]These two village workers were quite young: one was nineteen years of age, while the other was in her early twenties.

Most of the women who learned to deliver babies in hospital and clinic settings expressed a lot of fondness for their instructors. One woman told me that she learned how to assist with births from nurses who befriended her when she was hospitalized at the government hospital in Shinyanga town for a broken arm. During her month-long stay, they took her to the labor ward where she learned to deliver babies by first observing, then practicing what she had learned on the birthing women. Another woman learned to deliver babies as a result of her own birth experience at Kolondoto. She had been the only woman to give birth to a boy that day, and, as a result, the nurses began to refer to her affectionately as their mother-in-law. She ended up staying at the hospital for a week, during which time her newly acquired "daughters-in-law" showed her how to deliver babies. Many years later, when her own daughter went into labor, she brought her to the government clinic in their community. The nurses on duty, however, refused to assist with her daughter's birth because she had not brought along a current record of her prenatal care. The woman and her daughter returned home. Remembering what the nurses at the mission hospital had taught her many years previously, she delivered her grandchild herself.[9]

When I asked people in Bulangwa about the concept of the traditional birth attendant, several described it as a recent phenomenon, with some specifically linking the first appearance of the Kiswahili term *wakunga wa jadi* in the area to the first training for traditional birth attendants in 1986. As one Sukuma woman who was in her mid-forties and who had attended a TBA training herself put it: "A long time ago there weren't any traditional birth attendants. That is only a recent thing!" (literally of "these days") (*"Zamani, hawakuwa na wakunga wa jadi. Ni kitu cha siku hizi tu!"*). She herself had learned both from her mother and also while working at a government clinic dispensing medicine. Her mother, she told me, had given birth by herself "like all women did in the past." She was also of the opinion that women who gave birth in the past experienced far fewer complications than women giving birth "these days" did.[10]

Pregnant women were not fooled by the term *traditional birth attendant* either. While observing births at Mwana Nyanzanga's home, I noticed that some of her clients traveled from villages in which women who had been trained as TBAs also lived. When I asked them why they didn't just stay at home and birth with the trained TBA in their village, they scoffed at such an idea, stating that this or that particular TBA had never assisted with a birth before and therefore did not know what she was doing.

The issue of TBA training programs has become a hotly contested topic among maternal health advocates in recent years (Kasonde and Kamal 1998; Starrs 1998). Those in favor of continuing such programs often argue that TBAs remain the only source of delivery care for many women in the developing world (Fortney 1997, as cited in Starrs 1998:30). Those who are less supportive of TBA training claim there is no hard evidence that such programs have actually reduced maternal mortality (Fortney 1997). This latter position, which has received some support from WHO, UNICEF, and UNFPA, holds that the benefits of TBA training programs are modest at best, and because of this, scarce resources should instead be redirected to improving the skills of health-care personnel and the health-care system's ability to respond to emergencies (WHO 1999).

This all-or-nothing approach to TBA training—either advocating that all such programs be continued or declaring that all TBA training is ineffective—is precisely where the problem lies. To claim, for example, that "training traditional birth attendants didn't work" overlooks the fact that in some cases the women who participated in TBA training courses were not traditional birth attendants at all. Many had no prior experience attending births, nor did they have any intention of attending births in the future. As the case study of TBA training in the Shinyanga Region reveals, in some cases the term *traditional birth attendant* simply served as a synonym for "rural African woman," rather than as a reflection of a distinct tradition of midwifery per se. When women who have had no prior experience delivering babies are somehow turned into traditional birth attendants within the span of a ten-day training course, it is hardly surprising that TBA training programs have not produced the results policymakers and program planners originally intended. Nor is it surprising that pregnant women residing in rural areas perceive some of these TBAs as risks rather than as sources of labor support when birth is imminent.

The results of my interviews with women trained as TBAs in Shinyanga also indicate that the success or a failure of such training programs may be mixed. Some of the women who attended TBA training workshops in the Shinyanga Region were indeed providing an important source of maternal health care to pregnant women. Mwana Nyanzanga, for example, delivered more births at her home in one year than the nurses who worked at the government clinic located less than five miles away. In her case, resources expended to retrain her in more hygienic birthing practices were well spent.

Have other assumptions regarding the widespread applicability of traditional practices missed their mark in the context of women's pregnancy-related experiences in Bulangwa? To answer this, let us turn our attention to health-care interventions that approach tradition as a problem to be eliminated.

Tradition as Problem: Cultural Prohibitions during Pregnancy

There was a considerable variability in how the 154 women I interviewed talked about cultural prohibitions, or taboos, during pregnancy (*mwiko* in Kiswahili, *ng'wiko* in Kisukuma), a variability that others who have conducted research on Sukuma women's pregnancy-related experiences have noted as well (Varkevisser 1973). Some women told me that taboos varied according to clan, while others described the differences in pregnancy-related taboos in terms of religious distinctions. Several women stated that although they were aware of pregnancy-related cultural restrictions, they did not follow them personally, while others told me they adhered to a particular taboo at the insistence of older female relatives. I also heard that pregnancy-related taboos were not taken seriously anymore and therefore were no longer followed. The diversity of opinion expressed by the women I interviewed indicates that even within one small rural community, the definition of what is and is not taboo and who adheres to it depends on a variety of factors, such as ethnicity, religious affiliation, or the influence of particular family members.[11]

Although many of the women I spoke with were able to list a number of pregnancy-related taboos, in some cases they were merely telling me what they had heard was culturally prohibited, not what they necessarily believed or adhered to themselves. In addition, most did not know the specific meaning underlying a particular taboo, other than as a general protection against miscarriage. Among the thirty-nine older women I asked about cultural prohibitions during pregnancy, 59 percent ($n = 23$) stated there were no pregnancy taboos at all, while 60 percent of seventy-five younger women whose answers were recorded ($n = 45$) told me there were no pregnancy taboos. In table 7.2 I present the categories of pregnancy-related taboos that emerged in my interviews. All the taboos mentioned by older women were mentioned by the younger women, although the reverse is not the case. This reflects the fact that almost twice as many younger than older women answered this question, and it should not be interpreted as an indication that new categories of cultural prohibitions during pregnancy have emerged in recent years. For example, although no older women in my formal survey mentioned the category "Can't carry stone on head," several of the older TBAs I had interviewed the previous year had mentioned this particular pregnancy-related taboo, with one recounting her personal experience with this contraindication. Many years ago, when she was a young mother and still breast-feeding a child, she realized, unhappily, that she was pregnant again. In desperation, she walked around for weeks with a stone on her head, hoping that such behavior would cause her to abort. Her attempts to purposely miscarry were unsuccessful, however, and she ended up carrying that pregnancy to term.

The pregnancy-related taboos listed in table 7.2 are also striking for what they do not mention. In sharp contrast to the Safe Motherhood Initiative's concern with harmful cultural practices that restrict pregnant women's intake of nutritious foods, none of the women I interviewed mentioned food taboos at all. I even specifically asked about cultural restrictions on food when women did not mention any themselves.[12] Although some women noted that pregnant women might have cravings for or aversions to particular foods, they characterized these as idiosyncrasies of the individual pregnant woman, rather than as cultural prohibitions. For example, a couple of women mentioned hating the smell of porridge during

TABLE 7.2.   Categories of Taboos Elicited by the Survey Question "Is There Anything that Women Are Forbidden to Do or Eat during Pregnancy?"

Taboo	Mentioned by Older Women	Mentioned by Younger Women
Can't cross river	yes	yes
Can't leave husband during pregnancy	yes	yes
Can't carry loads if moving to another residence	yes	yes
Can't apply mud plaster to walls or floor	yes	yes
Can't put stones together for cooking	no	yes
Can't carry stone on head	no	yes
Can't prepare place to beat sorghum/millet	no	yes
Can't go to graveyard	no	yes
Can't leave husband when child is small	no	yes
Must sleep at same level as guest	yes	yes
Some restrictions on frequency of sexual intercourse	yes	yes
Doesn't follow taboos because is a Christian	yes	yes

their pregnancies, while others told me they had experienced intense cravings for particular foods while pregnant, such as tomatoes or mangoes.

I do not mean to suggest that the absence of food taboos in Bulangwa is an indication that pregnant women no longer suffer from nutritional problems. Quite the contrary. Approximately 40 percent of the 104 younger women in my study also told me they craved dirt while pregnant, a craving the medical literature associates with severe iron deficiency (Berkow and Fletcher 1992).[13] Some women said they satisfied that particular craving by eating pieces of mud they had chipped off the walls of their homes. They noted that women who lived in cement houses in Shinyanga town could satisfy their cravings for dirt by purchasing sticks of preformed mud (*pemba*) that are sold in outdoor markets. When I asked if they thought dirt had any medicinal value, all acknowledged that it did not. They ate dirt while pregnant because that's what their "heart" or "soul" wanted (*moyo/roho inapenda tu*) or because "it just smelled good" (*inanukia vizuri tu*). One Arab woman, who used to eat dirt while pregnant, told me she stopped doing so because she heard it was against the tenets of Islam. Now when she is pregnant and has those intense cravings, she simply throws water on the mud wall of her outdoor kitchen and inhales the odor instead. According to the nurses who worked at the government clinic in Bulangwa, many of their pregnant clients were, in fact, anemic. Their claims are supported both by my survey data about women's cravings for dirt while pregnant, as well as by the fact that postpartum hemorrhage was a common occurrence in the area (see chap. 11).

It is possible that the apparent absence of food taboos in the community is itself a reflection of the success of previous health education efforts directed at abolishing such cultural practices. I am merely trying to point out that in terms of everyday practice in the contemporary context, food taboos, whether harmful or not, no longer appear to be *the* factor undermining the nutritional status of pregnant women in Bulangwa. Instead, policymakers and program planners would do better to target other factors that negatively affect pregnant women's nutritional status (such as insufficient economic resources to buy iron-rich foods), rather than focusing their efforts on changing cultural practices that are not relevant in the community.

CHAPTER 8

The Prenatal Period, Part 1:
The Risk of Infertility

Wiza w'ilaba, buti wa kisumo.
The beauty of the flower, but no fruit (referring to a beautiful girl who doesn't give birth).
—Sukuma proverb[1]

"I was so happy [during labor]. I couldn't believe I was finally having a baby. The whole time I was pushing, I kept asking myself: 'Is this really me giving birth?'"
—Comment made by a Tanzanian friend about her
first birth experience. She had four miscarriages
before finally carrying a pregnancy to term.

The provision of prenatal care was one of the four essential elements of the global Safe Motherhood strategy to improve maternal health outcomes (Mahler 1987). Prenatal care also figured significantly in national-level discussions in Tanzania. The result of those discussions, the *Safe Motherhood Strategy for Tanzania,* recognized, among other things, the benefits of prenatal care and the need for health education campaigns to encourage women to seek care during their pregnancies.

In the early 1990s it was estimated that 85 percent of pregnant women in Tanzania received prenatal care (United Republic of Tanzania 1992). But the Tanzanian government also acknowledged that this statistic was misleading and that in reality, the actual level of prenatal coverage for many women living in rural areas was often quite limited. Ministry of Health officials noted, for example, that the total number of prenatal visits per pregnant woman might be as few as one or two, or a woman's initial prenatal visit might occur very late in her pregnancy (United Republic of Tanzania 1992).

Why such an apparent lack of interest in prenatal care on the part of rural women? Is it possible that many do not consider pregnancy to be a particularly risky period of their reproductive lives, or could it be, as some of the Safe Motherhood literature suggests, that this "unwillingness" to participate in prenatal care is an indication that many of their pregnancies are, in fact, unwanted?

In this chapter and the next we examine these questions as they relate to women's prenatal experiences in Bulangwa. As we will see in the following pages, the women I spoke with in Bulangwa were very concerned about their pregnancy outcomes, so concerned that many sought biomedical and nonbiomedical sources of preventive and curative care throughout their pregnancies. For many of these women, prenatal care began quite early—even before conception had taken place—and continued up until the moment they gave birth. This broadening of the definition of *prenatal* to include the period before a woman's pregnancy even begins reveals, in turn, categories of prenatal risk not addressed in the Safe Motherhood Initiative. We will see, for example, that many women are also concerned about the physical and spiritual factors that may affect their ability to conceive or give birth in the future—that is, with the risk of unsuccessful fertility.

An identification of these unofficial categories of prenatal risk is important on several levels. In addition to providing insight into women's prenatal concerns as they themselves define them, an identification of these risks also provides an opportunity to explore the interrelatedness of fertility and infertility issues. As others have noted elsewhere, attention to both aspects of fertility can shed light on broader issues related to human reproduction, such as people's ideas regarding conception, their perception of risks to the reproductive process, the perceived dangers of contraception, and the social importance of being a parent (Inhorn 1994b:459; see also Browner and Sargent 1990).[2] Attention to these unofficial definitions of prenatal risk will also enable us to see how local discourses surrounding maternal health risk differ from those articulated at the international and national levels.

We begin with a brief review of the work of Per Brandström, an anthropologist who lived and worked for many years in northern Unyamwezi and southern Usukuma. Brandström's approach to fertility is quite different from mine in that he situates it within the context of what he calls "Sukuma-Nyamwezi thought and reality" (1990). I draw upon Brandström's analysis of Sukuma-Nyamwezi cosmology, in particular his attention to the core elements of fertility and parenthood, to help situate women's fertility-related experiences within a culturally heterogeneous,

albeit predominantly Sukuma, setting.[3] For example, the friend I refer to
in the second epigraph that opens this chapter was a Jaluo woman married
to a Sukuma man from northeastern Usukuma. She was born in the Mara
Region, which borders Kenya to the north, and had lived in Bulangwa for
less than five years. Her fertility concerns were similar to those described
by some Sukuma women in the community, and she, like many of them,
had spent several years seeking cures for her history of miscarriages.

In the second part of this chapter, we turn our attention to women's
fertility-related concerns in Bulangwa. In doing so, we will be paying
attention not only to women's descriptions of prenatal risks, but also to
how they acquire information about them.

Fertility and Parenthood in Sukuma-Nyamwezi Thought and Reality

> In the semi-arid and dry sub-humid areas of western Tanzania, where
> the agro-pastoral Bantu-speaking Sukuma-Nyamwezi live, disastrous
> droughts, epidemics and epizootics are not only hearsay and phantoms
> in the minds of the people, but well-known facts of life. Life is
> precarious. Threatened by destruction through famine, illness and
> death, life is always at risk.
> —Per Brandström, "Seeds and Soil"

According to Brandström (1990:167), although there is no single word in
the Sukuma language to express the notion of fertility, "the fact of life, its
generation, maintenance and regeneration, stands . . . at the core of
Sukuma-Nyamwezi thought and imagery." These themes of generation
and regeneration are present in a variety of contexts: in aspects of agricultural life and this group's relation to the land, in social and reproductive
relations between men and women, and in ritual life in the relationship
between the living and the dead. The fertility of women, the fecundity of
the land, and good relations between a person and his or her ancestors are
all the outcome of achieving *mhola,* a Sukuma-Nyamwezi word that
Brandström defines as a state of "wholeness and completeness" (168).[4] In
the passage below, he explores the interconnectedness between *mhola* and
human fertility:

> Fertility as potentiality is intrinsic in the very expressions for woman,
> *nkima,* and man, *ngosha.* In other words, these concepts convey a

message about male and female reproductive power. The words describing the state and quality of being female, *bukima,* and male, *bugosha,* both refer to femaleness and maleness and, most concretely to the genitals of the sexes. Women and men, provided that they find themselves in the state of *mhola,* represent human fecundity. A man who has fathered many children is a "true" man, *ngosha ng'hana,* and a woman of proven fecundity is a "true" woman, *nkima ng'hana.* They are *mhola.* But, and this must be underlined, the quality of human fertility, like all other aspects of *mhola,* is always under threat from non-*mhola* influences. Hence, there is a lot of preoccupation, both among women and men, to safeguard this aspect of *mhola* and, when there is a lack or loss of this quality, to restore it through various ritual and medical devices. (1990:170; cf. Bösch 1930:449; Blohm 1933:10–11; Cory 1949)

Given the absence of a single word to convey the concept of fertility, discussions of fertility or fecundity, according to Brandström, require the use of metaphor, analogy, or a series of descriptive phrases. Drawing from the body of ethnographic literature on the Sukuma and Nyamwezi peoples as well as from his own work, he explores how agricultural metaphors are invoked by Sukuma-Nyamwezi men to capture male and female roles in the reproductive process (Brandström 1990).

In Bösch's (n.d.)[5] analysis as summarized by Brandström, the woman's role in the reproductive process is a passive one; she is the land that man cultivates.[6] In Brandström's work, Sukuma-Nyamwezi men describe women's role as passive in similar ways. From the male point of view, women are the containers for men's seeds, and pregnant women merely "sacks filled with sorghum" (1990:170). Brandström points out, however, that men's perception of their role in reproduction as central is wittily contested by women who see themselves, not men, as the primary players in the reproductive process. It is this continuous and unresolved competition of words, he suggests, that highlights not only the differences between male and female roles in reproduction, but also their complementarity (170–71).

The women I spoke with in Bulangwa also referred to their central role in the reproductive process: it is they, not men, who conceive and give birth to children. Moreover, the fact that women conceive, give birth, and breast-feed children was the explanation many gave as to why a mother's "immoral" behavior (i.e., her promiscuity) could negatively affect the health of her unborn and living children. A father's promiscuity, I was told, could do so only in a very indirect way. When I asked why this was the case, one woman explained that it was because "men do not have much to do with children" (*wanaume hawana shuguli nyingi na watoto*).

Left-Sided Fathers and Right-Sided Mothers

Brandström's work also examines the core symbols associated with father-hood and motherhood and with all kin who are related through blood and womb. In brief, *buta,* or bow, represents male qualities and the "left-sided" paternal relatives, both living and dead, whereas *migongo,* or back, refers to female qualities and the "right-sided" maternal relatives, again, both the living and the dead (1991:122).[7] The preeminence of one hand, or side, over the other, according to Brandström, is contextual: each has its own strengths. The male hand is the left hand; it is the "strong" hand that holds the bow in the context of hunting.[8] The right hand is the female hand; it is the hand that a mother uses in placing a small child on her back (123). The male side is predominant in a general sense, as in "the superiority of male qualities" (131) as well as in the context of family: it is the father who has jural rights over the children through the payment of cattle as bridewealth. The female side, in contrast, is predominant in the context of succession to chiefship, that is, through the sister's son (see chap. 5), and as officiants in rituals connected to the births of twins.[9]

According to Brandström, these symbols of parenthood represent the individual strengths of each side, but when joined, they represent the two halves that make a person whole, illustrated in the concept of *budugu,* the collectivity of kin (1991:124). He expands on the two-sided nature of human beings:

Human beings are two-sided creatures. . . . Two-sided man is left and right, the father's side and the mother's side, man and woman. He is brought into physical being through the conjunction of the two dis-tinctive sides; that is, man according to the "natural order." But what makes man a social being is the disjunction of the male and female principles into father's side (*buta*) and mother's side (*migongo*); that is, man according to the "cultural order." A child without a socially recognized father, literally called "of the grass" (*wa mu maswa*), is a one-sided child, a child of the right. However, the child born on the cow hide, originating from the herd that made its mother its father's wife, is a two-sided child, a child of both the left and right side. (1991:122)

In other words, fatherhood and motherhood are each valued in their own right and for their collective value as well.

Fatherhood and motherhood were also important aspects of a person's social identity in Bulangwa, concepts that are invoked daily in the way people are greeted. An important component to greeting an adult in the Sukuma language is to include the term mother (*mayu*) or father (*baba*), regardless of whether that person has children. To say *ng'wadila* (good afternoon) instead of *ng'wadila mayu* (good afternoon mother) just wasn't done, unless, of course, it was by someone who was learning the language and hadn't caught on yet to the obligatory inclusion of the parental identifier. Even among members of the community who were not fluent in Kisukuma, most knew how to greet someone in the Sukuma language, and therefore it was not unusual to hear this form of greeting taking place between Sukuma- and non-Sukuma-speaking peoples.

The concept of parenthood was also drawn upon in the way that someone was directly or indirectly addressed. In general, men and women are referred to as the father or mother of a particular child, usually their firstborn. If the name of her firstborn is Masanja, a woman's social identity becomes that of Masanja's mother, "Mama Masanja." Her husband, the father of the child, would be known as "Baba Masanja," Masanja's father.[10] It is also the form a husband or wife might use when referring to his or her spouse in the context of a conversation with someone else. For example, a woman referring to the whereabouts of her husband might say "Baba Masanja went to Shinyanga" rather than using his first name. There are, of course, exceptions to this rule, as there are exceptions to many aspects of social life, but this form of address is seen by many as the proper way to do things. It is a form of address that occurs throughout Tanzania, within African and Arab communities (Beidelman 1993).[11]

The significance of being socially recognized as a parent became especially vivid to me during a funeral I attended for the eight-year-old child of a Haya woman and Sukuma man who lived in Bulangwa. Ali, the firstborn of their two children, had died suddenly after experiencing a severe headache. During the three-day Muslim funeral, the deceased's distraught mother repeatedly made heart-wrenching references to her changed social status. Sobbing, she would call out to no one in particular, "What will people call me now? I am Mama Ali! How will I now be called?" Throughout the course of my twenty months of residence in Bulangwa, I attended many funerals, but funerals of young children, regardless of their birth order, always seemed the saddest (cf. Scheper-Hughes 1992).[12]

Ancestors and Fertility

According to R. E. S. Tanner (1958:52), a district officer during the period of British colonial rule in Tanganyika who wrote extensively on the topic of ancestor worship and spirit mediumship among the Sukuma in northern Usukuma, when benevolent, ancestors can ensure "family health, plenty of children, good harvests and a large number of cattle." When malevolent, ancestors are seen as causing "the whole field of human suffering from sickness and death to everyday bad luck" (52). Tanner notes that ancestral power becomes particularly significant in the context of fertility in that the blessing of fertility or the misfortune of infertility is often linked directly to ancestral interventions. Citing Tanner's work, Brandström (1990:174) traces the chronology of events that occur once an "affliction of barrenness" has become apparent:

> The diviner, *mfumu*,[13] is called in as a mediating agent to unveil the hidden blockage in the flow of life between the ancestors and their descendants and to "arrange for the repair of disunity" (Tanner 1957:347) between the dead and the living. This work requires great exactitude; first, to identify whether the cause of the affliction is to be found within the *budugu* of the wife or that of the husband; second, to find out within the identified *budugu* whether *buta,* the patrilineal side, or *migongo,* the matrilineal side, is the party concerned; third to pinpoint the particular ancestor, or ancestors to be propitiated; and fourth, to prescribe the appropriate remedy, whether in the form of a libation, consecration or sacrifice.[14]

Mwana Nyanzanga once told me that although she believed ancestors can affect a woman's pregnancy outcome, she refused to treat her clients' health problems by prescribing ritual offerings to their ancestors as part of the cure. She won't, for example, tell her clients to keep a sheep or wear a copper bracelet, the offerings usually made to female ancestors. She believed that offerings to ancestors as a form of treatment were dangerous in two distinct ways. First, attention to ancestral spirits might result in a person's death, as in the case of a man she knew who was initiated into the

Bumanga society, a spirit possession cult, and who subsequently drowned while ritually bathing in the river.[15] Second, a healer might mistakenly identify an illness as ancestor-induced when in fact it was caused by sorcery. Such a misidentification of etiology, she explained, could result in a person's death due to the delay of proper treatment. In cases where a female client's ancestor appeared to be actively blocking a treatment, Mwana Nyanzanga would first symbolically tie the ancestor up (*kufunga mzimu* in Kiswahili) by placing a necklace with spiritual properties momentarily around the woman's neck. This caused the ancestor to "lie down" or "sleep" (*ilale kwanza*), after which she could begin her herbal treatment. She then recounted the case of one of her clients.

This particular woman had come to her several years ago for problems related to childbearing. Although the woman experienced no difficulty getting pregnant or giving birth, her children always died during their first year of life. The relatives who accompanied the woman told Mwana Nyanzanga that the problem was caused by an ancestor. Upon hearing this, Mwana Nyanzanga told them that she didn't treat illnesses by paying attention to ancestral spirits because she was a Christian (*Mimi ni Mkristo!*). Later that same night, after they had all gone to bed, the woman, or rather, her ancestor, began shouting "Bring me my sheep! Bring me my sheep!" (*Nileteni kondoo yangu! Nileteni kondoo yangu!*). Mwanza Nyanzanga refused. She recounted to me in Kiswahili what she told the woman's relatives in Kisukuma: "So I told them, 'Me, I don't want to bring someone her sheep. I don't want to, nor have I ever seen that when a person goes to a hospital for treatment, she goes with a sheep. I've never seen that! I don't like it at all that ancestral spirits say that they want to be brought a sheep!' " Nevertheless, she did tie the woman's ancestor up and continued with her herbal treatment. The woman now has two grown children, Elizabeth and David.[16]

Mwana Nyanzanga's version of this woman's story is interesting on several levels. First, her refusal to treat her Sukuma client's pregnancy-related problem in the manner the woman and her relatives were accustomed to and their apparent willingness to go along with the alternative treatment reveal a certain amount of give-and-take in people's health beliefs and practices. People, it appears, are not constrained by a particular "thought and reality" per se, but may draw instead upon values and beliefs held by others with whom they interact in the community (in this case, those of a non-Sukuma healer/midwife who prefers subduing troublesome ancestors to appeasing them). Second, in justifying her refusal to appease her client's disgruntled ancestor, she points out that hospital personnel do not heed ancestors' demands either. In other words, her method of treatment, like that prescribed in the hospital setting, is based upon legitimately recognized modern principles. In her case, that modern principle or authority is Christianity. In the hospital setting, the legitimate authority is biomedicine. Despite her proclaimed aversion to dealing with Sukuma ancestral spirits, however, she herself invokes the names of her female matrilineal ancestors when she uses particular spiritual medicines.

This woman's story is also interesting for what it reveals about the definition of certain prenatal conditions. In her case, the deaths of her previous children during their first year of life were characterized as an extension of a prenatal problem, a problem whose cause was tied to the pregnancy itself, rather than to health problems that developed after her children were born. As we will see later in this chapter and again in chapter 9, this reflects a general concern about the deferred power of certain factors, whether physical or spiritual in nature, to affect the quality of a person's fertility long after the initial contagion takes place.

In the remainder of this chapter, we stay with the concepts of parenthood and fertility as we examine women's concerns about their ability to conceive and bear children successfully. In doing so, we will be paying attention not only to beliefs and practices related to ensuring their own fertility and parenthood, but to ensuring the future fertility and parenthood of their children as well.

The Vocabulary of Fertility and Infertility

Female Fertility

A variety of descriptive phrases refer to the quality of women's fertility specifically.[17] For example, a woman's ability to conceive might be described as being "far away" (*uzazi wa mbali*), that is, she has difficulty conceiving, or "close" (*uzazi wa karibu*), meaning she experiences no such difficulty. *Mgongo,* which literally means the back or the back part of the body, is also used in the context of fertility. A woman who has difficulty getting pregnant or who experiences unwanted delays between pregnancies may be described as having a "hard" or "difficult" back (*mgongo ngumu*), while those who get pregnant without any difficulty, or perhaps even too quickly, might be referred to as having an "easy" or "light" back (*mgongo upesi*).[18]

A woman's fertility might also be expressed in terms of time in that she may describe herself, or may be described by others, as being late in getting pregnant (*amechelewa kupata mimba*) or in giving birth (*amechelewa kuzaa*). But what is considered late by one person may not be considered late by another. When, in the context of a group interview with twenty women, I asked for clarification of what *late* meant, they generally agreed that *late* could be defined as not getting pregnant within the first six months of marriage or relationship with a man. Mwana Nyanzanga, on the other hand, defined *late* as not getting pregnant within five months to a year of a relationship with a man, while an Arab woman in Bulangwa told me that she sought treatment for infertility when she failed to get pregnant within the first three months of her marriage. According to the doctor who ran a weekly fertility clinic at Kolondoto hospital, a woman was defined as clinically infertile if she experienced involuntary infertility for a consecutive period of three years.

Forty-three (28.5 percent) of the 151 women in my survey who were asked if they had been "late" in getting pregnant told me that they had, with the majority describing that lateness as a source of anxiety. Only one woman told me that her pregnancies were intentionally late: she had intercourse only during her safe days, that is, at the very beginning or the very end of her cycle. Thirteen women (30 percent of this subset of forty-three women) defined their lateness in terms similar to the doctor at the fertility clinic: they had been in a relationship with a man for three to five years but had not become pregnant. The responses of the remaining thirty women varied considerably. Two of those women told me they knew they were late because a neighbor who had been pregnant at the same time as them during a previous pregnancy had become pregnant again, although they had not. Two other women attributed their lateness in getting pregnant to a miscarriage and a death of an infant, while another woman attributed her delay in getting pregnant to having previously taken oral contraceptives. Although she stopped using them, she never got pregnant again.

That a concept of being late in becoming pregnant or in giving birth exists in the community raises the possibility that women may seek to prevent or counteract the risks associated with such an unwanted condition. Such preventive and curative measures do, in fact, exist. As we will see in the following section, many of the fertility-related conditions for which women sought treatment were spoken about as being closely linked to characteristics of their menstrual cycles.

The Menstrual Cycle

Physical and Spiritual Aspects

Women paid a lot of attention to the quality of their menstrual cycle—to its timing, duration, and flow, as well as to any physical discomfort associated with it. Any irregularity was seen as an indication that a woman's ability to bear children in the future was in jeopardy. The importance attached to a woman's menses was also reinforced in the divinations local healers conducted to diagnose the source of their clients' problems. Regardless of the life or health problem for which women initially sought treatment, healers usually started off their divinations with female clients by commenting on the current state of their menses. Menses that lasted more than three days, that occurred too early, too late, or that were characterized by a heavy flow were all cause for concern, and herbal remedies were usually prescribed to return menses to their normal state.[19]

The menstrual cycle was also associated with a spiritual reality. This spiritual aspect of a woman's menses was spoken about quite differently among the Muslim and non-Muslim women in the community. Muslim women tended to speak about dangers or risks during this time more often than non-Muslim women did, and in the former category, Arab women were more likely to mention specific purification rituals associated with their menstrual cycle than were African Muslim women. For Muslim women as a whole, the menses were generally spoken about as being a ritually unclean period of a woman's cycle (Delaney 1988; Good 1980). Because of their unclean state (*uchafu*), Muslim women could not pray, go to the mosque, touch religious books, or engage in sexual intercourse while they were experiencing their menstrual flow. Once a Muslim woman's menses ceased, she washed in water over which she had recited verses from the Koran. Afterward, she was once again ritually clean and could partake in activities associated with her religion, as well as resume sexual relations with her husband.[20]

Most of the non-Muslim women, in contrast, told me that there were no specific prohibitions or rituals associated with a woman's menstrual cycle. When I pursued this further, asking specifically if they were allowed to cook for other people or work in their fields while menstruating, they confirmed that no such prohibitions existed (Appell 1988; Gottlieb 1988). A few of the women I interviewed made the point that menstruation was not an illness, therefore they cooked and farmed as they usually did. If women did not mention it themselves, I also asked whether they could have sexual intercourse during their menses, to which all stated that no, they could not. Most, however, gave physical rather than spiritual explanations for not partaking in such a practice, such as the messiness of doing so (Gottlieb 1988).[21] Only seven non-Muslim women associated particular practices during menstruation with negative consequences. One woman told me that if a menstruating woman touched local medicine, the medicine would lose its effectiveness. Two women noted that sexual intercourse with a menstruating woman would lead to sickness in her male partner. Another told me that engaging in sexual intercourse during her period could ruin a woman's eggs (a concept discussed below), while another woman said that menstruating women should not bathe outside, although she gave no specific explanation as to why this particular behavior should be discouraged.

The Timing of the Menstrual Cycle

Women calculated the timing of their cycle in one of two ways. Some kept track of their menses by noting the position of the moon at the onset of bleeding. These women spoke of their menses as occurring when the moon was to the west, to the east, or directly above. This is how they knew if they were pregnant or if their menses were irregular.[22] Women who knew how to read, or who were familiar enough with numbers to calculate their menses by calendar dates, used a different method of keeping track of their cycle. These women told me that a normal cycle begins on the same date every month. If a woman's menses begin on the twelfth of every month, for example, they should begin on the twelfth of subsequent months, although a difference of one or two days is not a cause of great concern. When I asked the 154 women I interviewed how they kept track of their menstrual cycle, 95 women (61.6 percent of the sample) said they looked at the moon, and 57 (37 percent) said they looked at the date. One woman said she used both methods, while another told me she could not calculate because her menses were irregular.

Given the amount of attention that both women and healers paid to the menstrual cycle, I began wondering how women initially acquired that knowledge. Most of the women I interviewed spoke in terms of who first showed them how to use a menstrual cloth, or who first explained to them what the menstrual blood was. In table 8.1, I summarize their responses to my inquiries about how they initially acquired information about the menstrual cycle, as well as whether they had been told about the connection between their menstrual cycle and pregnancy. The table shows that neither older nor younger women acquired knowledge about menstruation in a uniform way. Although a woman's mother was the most often cited person responsible for teaching a young girl about menstruation for both the older and younger groups of women, we see that other women also provided this type of information. Further discussion revealed the additional information that the majority of the older and younger women had not heard about menstruation prior to the onset of their first menses.[23]

The percentage of women in all categories who said they taught themselves about the management of their menses is striking: 28 percent for the older women, 32.6 percent of the younger women with no formal education, 25 percent of the women with some, and 17.1 percent of young

TABLE 8.1. How Women Learned about Menarche and Its Connection to Their Reproductive Cycle (presented by age category and years of primary school education) (*N* = 154)

| | Older Women | | Younger Women | | | | | |
| | (0 years) | | (0 years) | | (< 7 yrs) | | (7 years) | |
Learned from . . .	*n*	%	*n*	%	*n*	%	*n*	%
Mother	27	54.0	17	39.5	5	25.0	15	36.6
Grandmother	4	8.0	7	16.3	3	15.0	6	14.6
Sister	—	—	2	4.7	1	5.0	5	12.2
Paternal aunt	—	—	1	2.3	2	10.0	2	4.9
Maternal aunt	—	—	—	—	—	—	2	4.9
Mother-in-law	—	—	1	2.3	—	—	—	—
Sister-in-law	—	—	—	—	3	15.0	1	2.4
Taught self	14	28.0	14	32.6	5	25.0	7	17.1
Neighbor	2	4.0	1	2.3	—	—	—	—
School teacher	—	—	—	—	—	—	2	4.9
Friend	3	6.0	—	—	1	5.0	1	2.4
Told how menstrual cycle is related to pregnancy?[a]								
Yes	25	50.0	19	44.2	11	55.0	21	51.2
No	21	42.0	18	41.9	8	40.0	19	46.3

[a]Numbers do not add up to 100% due to missing data for this question.

women who had completed primary school. Although the actual numbers are small, they may be suggestive of a larger trend. These women told me that they learned how to take care of themselves either by trial and error on their own, from general talk among peers, or from watching what female relatives living with them at home did.

The information presented in table 8.1 also reveals that while more than half of the older women I interviewed learned about the care of their menses from their mothers, this was not necessarily the case for younger women. Although the numbers in all groups of younger women for the category "mother" were relatively high, we see that the younger groups of women also looked to other female relatives not mentioned by the older women: sisters, maternal and paternal aunts, mothers-in-law, and sisters-in-law. Moreover, only two of the younger women who had completed primary school stated they learned about menstruation from a teacher.

When I asked these same women if they had been told about the connection between their menstrual cycle, sexual intercourse, and pregnancy, at least half of the older women, as well as half of the younger women with some level of formal education, had been told about the connection (50 percent, 55 percent, and 51 percent respectively), while a smaller percentage (44 percent) of the younger women without formal education had. Two of the younger women who had completed primary school said they had learned about the connection between their menses and pregnancy through their science classes in school. But instruction by a science teacher does not necessarily guarantee correct information. One of the women who learned about reproduction in school was also told that the most fertile period of a woman's cycle occurred during the days immediately following the cessation of menses. She told me she continues to use this information today: she waits one week after her menses have ceased before resuming sexual relations with her husband.

When I asked other women when they thought the most fertile part of a woman's cycle was (i.e., when she was most likely to conceive), they gave a variety of responses. Some thought that the most fertile time of the menstrual cycle was the last day of a woman's period, or just a few days after, because the menstrual blood was still "close." According to those women, if they wanted to avoid becoming pregnant, the safest time to have sex was halfway through their cycle when the menstrual blood was "farther" away (see Bledsoe et al. 1994). According to published methods of natural family planning, however, this is actually the most fertile period of a woman's cycle, and thus the time when she is most likely to conceive (WHO 1995b). Women who thought that the third or fourth week after a woman's cycle was the safest time to have sexual intercourse if they wanted to avoid pregnancy gave similar reasons (i.e., the menstrual blood was farther away). Unpublished results from the 1996 Tanzanian Demographic and Health Survey (DHS) reveal that misunderstanding regarding the fertile period exists in other parts of Tanzania as well. For example, only 16.4 percent of the women who took part in the DHS correctly identified the middle of the cycle as the most fertile period; 10.5 percent of the women said "right after her period," 2.2 percent said "just before," 22.4 percent said "at any time," and 47.6 percent said they didn't know (Westoff 2000).[24]

Given the variation in how women acquire knowledge about their menstrual cycle, it is not surprising that women held a variety of opinions about the factors that affected their ability to conceive and successfully give birth. As we will see in the following sections, these include both physical and spiritual risk factors.

Physical Risks to Fertility

Eggs

A woman's fertility was often referred to in terms of her having or not having eggs (*mayai* in Kiswahili, *magi* in Kisukuma). In terms of fertility problems, a woman's eggs were described as being cold, covered, cooked, few, far away, or completely finished. I first became aware of the connection women made between eggs and their fertility when, while driving to the home of Mwana Nyanzanga one day, I stopped to give a woman a lift to the next village. During the ride, the conversation drifted toward the topic of children, and after she asked me if I had any children, I asked her a similar question. She told me that she had had eleven pregnancies and had four living children. When I asked her how many more children she wanted, she told me that she had finished giving birth. "I don't have any more eggs," she said. "How do you know your eggs are finished?" I asked. "Because," she told me quite matter-of-factly, "I haven't had a pregnancy in many years." Her last-born child was five years old, and although she wasn't using any method of birth control, she hadn't had any more pregnancies since that birth.

When I mentioned this conversation later to Mwana Nyanzanga, she agreed that, yes, the woman's eggs were probably finished. "Well, how many eggs does each woman have?" I asked. "It depends on the woman," she told me. "For example, Luhende [her neighbor in the village], his wife gave birth fifteen times, fifteen times." "Fifteen times?" I repeated. "Eh," she responded in the affirmative. "Others give birth seven times, or nine, ten, four, five. It's different for every women," she explained. "Every woman has a different number of eggs?" I repeated, echoing her statement. "Eh," she confirmed. After a short pause she continued, "Others give birth only once." "Does that mean that they only have one egg?" I kept pressing for clarification, not sure if I was correctly grasping the concept. "I don't know," she said with a shrug of her shoulders. "So, the [fertility] medicine you give women, does it give them eggs?" I continued, not willing to drop the subject. "No, that's not possible," she said, shaking her head. "I don't have medicine that gives women eggs, nor have I ever heard of such a thing." In other words, as I eventually came to understand while observing her work, there is no such thing as a medicine that "gives" a woman eggs. Herbal medicine can only be used to enhance the quality of a woman's eggs or "repair" eggs that have been damaged. If a woman is unfortunate enough to be born without eggs, or with only a few, there is nothing of either a ritual or medicinal nature that can treat this specific kind of infertility.

Wombs

The position of a woman's womb might also be identified as the cause of her fertility problems. In terms of the cervix, which Mwana Nyanzanga referred to as the "door to the womb" (*mlango wa kizazi*), infertility can occur if the door is facing in the wrong direction. The proper position of the door, Mwana Nyanzanga told me, was directly in the middle, ready to receive the man's seed (*Ni lazima ikae kati-kati, tayari kupokea mbegu za mwanaume*). Conception was impossible if the door was facing straight up, straight down, or completely to the back. In response to my inquiries as to how the latter position prevented conception, Mwana Nyanzanga asked the rhetorical question "Could you eat *ugali* if your mouth was like this [turning her head to the back]?"[25] Fertility problems could also occur if the entire womb was "off to the side" (*kizazi cha upande*) or "missing" altogether (*hana kizazi*).

Itale

Itale, a Kisukuma word that refers to a condition in which the vagina is covered by an extremely thick membrane, was also mentioned as a possible cause of infertility. Although I never saw a case of *itale* myself, I learned about this condition in my interviews with women who were trained as traditional birth attendants (see chap. 7). *Itale* was linked to infertility not only because of the physical impossibility of sexual intercourse but also because this condition, when it occurred, was often accompanied by a very late onset of puberty. I was also told that many women who have this condition do not develop breasts. Although *itale* was not necessarily a condition that was talked about openly, if I asked people to describe the symptoms to me, the descriptions were always similar. Some people told me that in the past this condition was "cured" by piercing the thick membrane with an arrow, whereas nowadays parents took the child to the hospital. Tanner also makes reference to this condition in an article he wrote on marriage practices among the northern Sukuma in the 1950s: "A few women have their marriages delayed because there is some physical obstruction in the vagina which is usually dealt with surgically" (Tanner 1955:129). Three of the women who took part in my formal survey mentioned *itale* and "breasts that do not develop" as a cause of infertility.

Mchango

As noted already above, irregular menses are seen as an indication that a woman might experience problems with her fertility in the future. In most cases, this particular category of fertility-related problem was attributed to the illness *mchango. Mchango,* the Kiswahili word for a general category of health problems experienced by many in the community, is defined as "worms" in a Swahili dictionary, whereas in the Sukuma language this same condition is known as *nzoka,* or "snake" (Reid 1969; see also Renne 2001).[26] The concept in either language covers a range of health problems that can affect both male and female of any age. These health problems include, but are not limited to, colic in newborn infants, general digestive problems in the old and young, epileptic fits in young children, menstrual irregularities or discomfort in women, and impotence in men. A key characteristic of *mchango* in all its forms is that it is spoken about as having physical as well as spiritual origins and as not being very responsive to biomedicine. Instead, people consulted with local healers or friends and neighbors who knew the plants used to treat mchango, especially those involving illnesses among children or general digestive irregularities. In some cases, they might even self-treat for these conditions.

Mchango-related fertility problems were different in this regard. Women suffering from fertility problems do not usually self-treat for their condition. Instead, they seek treatment from local healers who are specialists in the treatment of infertility, or from vendors of herbal remedies who sell their wares in Shinyanga's herbal market. Herbal treatment of fertility problems caused by *mchango* is apparently quite common. Eighty-six of the 154 women I interviewed, or 55.8 percent of the sample, told me that they had, at some point in their lives, used an herbal remedy either to become pregnant or to ensure that they carried their pregnancy successfully to term. When I specifically asked whether they had ever used a medicine to become pregnant, fifty women, or approximately one-third of the 154 women I interviewed, told me they had.

Pain associated with the menstrual cycle was also seen as an indication that a woman was suffering from *mchango*. Several of the women I interviewed referred to this particular category of *mchango* by the Kisukuma word *buhale*. Women who had experienced *buhale* themselves, or knew women who had, characterized its defining features as sharp, stabbing pains in the lower abdomen, vagina, or rectum (*inachoma mbele; inachoma matakoni* in Kiswahili). Apparently, *buhale* is one of the most dreaded forms of *mchango* because of the risks it poses to a woman's fertility. *Buhale* is seen as able to cause miscarriage, turn a woman's uterus around, or burst a woman's eggs (*inapasuka mayai*). A woman suffering from *buhale* might also experience very light menses, a condition believed to decrease her chances of conceiving

When I asked a Tanzanian physician who worked at the regional hospital in Shinyanga town if he had ever heard of the illness *mchango,* he told me that he had, but in his opinion it was how women spoke about the symptoms of pelvic inflammatory disease, a condition that can develop if sexually transmitted diseases are not treated with appropriate biomedical interventions. He also suggested that *mchango* (pelvic infection) was a result of the unhygienic practices women followed during menstruation (see Dixon-Mueller and Wasserheit 1991). He told me that he had seen cases in which women had inserted a menstrual cloth into their vagina to absorb the menstrual flow, and then had left it there for several days. I spoke with this doctor toward the end of my fieldwork period, after I had already completed most of the interviews in my formal survey. Up until that time I had never heard of this form of menstrual management. Nevertheless, I subsequently asked some other women whether they managed their menses in this particular way. A few said they did, while others told me that they placed the menstrual cloth on the inside of their underwear and changed it periodically throughout the day. That practices associated with menstrual hygiene may, in fact, be associated with subsequent infections requires further investigation.

Spiritual Risks to Fertility

Women also expressed a concern with spiritual risks to their fertility. As we will see in the sections below, the resulting infertility has nothing to do with disease transmission as it is described in the biomedical literature. Instead, it is as if a spiritual, rather than physical form of disease transmission is taking place. And like physical forms of transmission, spiritual transmission can take place via a person's blood.

Blood Incompatibility

The incompatibility of a man and a woman's blood (*damu haipatani; damu inakosekana*) was seen as a source of impaired fertility (see Inhorn and Buss 1994).[27] As two different Sukuma men explained it to me, the blood of these two people is, in essence, engaged in warfare. One of these men, who made reference to the fact that Sukuma men and women have usually had several sexual partners before settling down and marrying, explained it to me this way: the woman's blood gets mixed up with the blood of every man she has slept with, and the man's blood gets mixed with the blood of every woman he has slept with. When these two people, in turn, sleep with each other, their separate "bloods" have to fight it out and come to terms. The illness *mchango,* he explained, is the result of their blood not making that necessary adjustment. The other Sukuma man, a vendor at the herbal market in Shinyanga town, gave me a slightly different version of the warfare metaphor: it is the man's blood that battles the blood of all the men the woman has ever slept with.

Although women also mentioned blood incompatibility in connection with fertility problems, I never heard them speak of it in terms of warfare, only in terms of general incompatibility. They noted that although a man and a woman may not be able to conceive a child together, they may each experience no difficulty having children if they try later with a different partner. They referred to this newfound fertility as the result of the compatibility of the new couple's blood. When I tried to press for clarification of the meaning of blood compatibility, a middle-aged Sukuma woman who had never attended school offered the explanation that finally helped me to understand the concept. She told me that the concept of blood compatibility between a man and woman or between people in general was similar to what happens when people are asked to give blood for family members or friends who are hospitalized. Hospital staff, she noted, have to examine the blood of lot of people before they find a person whose blood is compatible with the blood of the person needing a transfusion.

According to Renne (2001), blood incompatibility is also recognized as a factor that prevents conception among the Ekiti Yoruba people of southwestern Nigeria. The source of the incompatibility in that Yoruba community, however, is spoken about quite differently than it is in Bulangwa. Whereas Renne's data reveals that the incompatibility is traced to a bad mixing between the actual substances of menstrual blood and semen, my data from Bulangwa suggest that a different process is going on: a kind of metaphorical struggle between the essences of two individuals.[28]

Ancestral Spirits

Possession by disgruntled ancestors was also seen as a potential source of a woman's fertility problems. When I initially began asking women in the community about their experiences with possession, I didn't realize that spirits were spoken about in terms of having a specific ethnicity or gender. These ethnic and gender distinctions didn't occur to me until women themselves raised them in response to my inquiries about how they first knew they were possessed. For example, some Sukuma women told me they knew they were possessed because they started speaking Kimaasai or Kitaturu spontaneously. Given the history of intergroup relations in west central Tanzania (see chap. 5), in particular the long history of cattle raiding between the Sukuma, Maasai, and Taturu peoples, I find this cross-cultural aspect of possession in the contemporary setting of Bulangwa intriguing, a linking of the past to the present that people themselves acknowledge.

Other women I spoke with told me they knew they were possessed by an ancestor because they had asked for a sheep. When I asked about the significance of the sheep, they explained it was what ancestors from the mother's side of the family (*gu ng'ongo* in Kisukuma) asked for.[29] Some women expressed the belief that women could only be possessed by their female ancestors from their mothers' side, while others thought that women could also experience possession from patrilineal ancestors, *gu buta*, although in the latter case, a goat rather than sheep is demanded. In the context of my formal interviews with women, however, possession by an ancestral spirit, irrespective of its ethnicity or gender, did not emerge as significant in terms of actual experiences of fertility-related problems: only four women stated that a healer told them that their infertility was caused by an ancestor.[30]

Sorcery

Sorcery, in contrast, was seen as a likely cause of fertility problems. Of the 137 women whom I specifically asked about the link between sorcery and infertility, 72.4 percent (*n* = 106) agreed that sorcery could indeed cause infertility, while 9.5 percent (*n* = 13) said it wasn't possible, and 13.1 percent (*n* = 18) said they didn't know. I was told that sorcery could be used by blood relatives, disgruntled or jealous neighbors, cowives, past lovers, or former husbands (see Renne 2001 and Sargent 1982). Ten women specifically noted that care needed to be taken with regard to a woman's menstrual cloth. If a woman's menstrual cloth was stolen, it could be used in sorcery against her and result in her future infertility. Several women told me that after washing her menstrual cloth, a woman shouldn't leave it out in the open to dry, as anyone—male or female—could steal it. Another woman told me that a person could block a woman's menses, and thus fertility, by stealing a woman's menstrual cloth and burying it in a place where grass wouldn't grow. Sorcery-induced infertility was also believed to be the result of someone gaining access to a woman's postpartum blood, underwear, or the cloth used to clean the genitals after sexual intercourse. The use of any of these items in medicine could block a woman's future fertility, thus great care must be taken with regard to these items. A woman's fertility could also be placed in jeopardy if sorcery medicines were put in her food, placed at crossroads, or put on a chair on which she was likely to sit (Varkevisser 1973; see also Feldman-Savelsberg 1999). Of those women who agreed that sorcery was a possible cause of infertility, some specifically stated that it was a likely cause *only* if a woman had already given birth before. In other words, if a woman had never been pregnant in her life, sorcery was not the cause of her infertility. The source of the problem was instead attributed to either God's will (*kazi ya Mungu*) or to the fact that the woman had simply been born that way.

Immoral Behavior

Women also spoke about fertility problems as resulting from immoral behavior. Women who had previously tried to abort or young girls who started having sex at a very early age might find their future fertility in jeopardy. In the latter case, the wombs of sexually active young girls were described as either slipping out of place or being squeezed. The seed of older men who had already fathered children was identified as a particularly lethal source of risk for young girls who had not yet given birth because men's sperm was "hot" and could ruin a young girl's eggs, which had not yet matured. The seed of promiscuous men was also identified as dangerous to women's fertility. One woman stated that if a woman slept with a man who had had many sexual partners, her womb would dry up and disappear altogether.

Some people also associated some forms of *mchango* with immoral behavior. Although readers might assume, as I did, that this particular category of *mchango* was actually venereal disease in disguise, they would be mistaken. Venereal disease (*ugonjwa wa zinaa*), a source of infertility acknowledged by everyone I spoke to, is, apparently, an entirely different condition. One of the vendors I spoke with at the herbal market in Shinyanga town described the difference to me in the following manner: "Gonorrhea is gonorrhea. *Mchango* is *mchango* (*Kisonono ni kisonono. Mchango ni mchango*)."

Male Fertility

Although the focus of my inquiries was primarily on women's fertility concerns and practices, I did gain some insight into men's perspectives on fertility, either by speaking with men about such issues directly or by getting a sense of it secondhand as it was mediated through women's perspectives on what men thought or did. Men's fertility, like women's, was spoken about in terms of its quality, a quality that could be affected by both physical and spiritual factors.[31]

The Quality of Seed

Weak "seed" (*mbegu*) was the source of one type of fertility problem experienced by men. According to Mwana Nyanzanga, although the quantity of a man's ejaculate might be large, his seed was weak, that is, watery in color and consistency, and therefore not able to produce offspring. One of the male vendors I interviewed at the herbal market in Shinyanga town told me that a man's fertility problems might also be the result of his having "cold" as opposed to "hot" seed. We had been talking about infertility in general, and I had asked him how people knew if the source of the problem lay with the man or the woman. He told me that there were specific signs that indicated the man's fertility was the source of the problem. The first indication that a man might be infertile, he told me, was that quantity of his "water" (ejaculate) was large. Second, it wouldn't be hot. It would be cold and there would be a lot of it (*Itajulikana. Kwanza, maji ya mwanaume itakuwa mingi. Na ya pili, itakuwa siyo moto. Baridi baridi na tena mingi;* cf. Gottlieb 1990).[32] There appears to be no cure for this particular form of male infertility. It is simply the will of Almighty God (*Hamna dawa. Ni kazi ya Mwenyezi Mungu*).

Another form of male infertility women spoke about occurs in men who have only one testicle (*jibulunda* in Kisukuma). Although the man is able to get an erection, I was told, he will not have enough seed to father a child. Although the women who described *jibulunda* to me told me that there was no cure, I later spoke with a male healer who claimed that he had successfully treated this condition.

Impotence: Physical and Spiritual Causes

Male fertility problems were also spoken about in terms of the level of a man's virility. Impotence (*hanisi* in Kiswahili), according to women who participated in two group interviews I conducted in Mwana Nyanzanga's village, appears to be a common occurrence, an observation that was supported by my conversations with three male vendors in the herbal market in Shinyanga town, two male healers in Bulangwa, and Mwana Nyanzanga. All acknowledge four main causes of impotence, each with its own cure.

One source of impotence is said to be the illness schistosomiasis, a disease linked to the presence of snails in slow-moving or stagnant water. Infected snails release a parasite into the water, and when people bathe or come in contact with the water, they become infected and develop the disease. Impotence, I was told, is one of the disease's side effects. Schistosomiasis can be treated with modern medicine, and once a man is cured, his impotence is also usually cured.

Mchango and sorcery were two other recognized sources of impotence. Impotence caused by *mchango* is said to occur in degrees: a man might be rendered completely impotent, or he may experience difficulty maintaining an erection. Herbal treatments could cure either form. Sorcery-induced impotence was another matter. Women who suspected their husbands or lovers of having a mistress might use sorcery medicines to render their men impotent in any illicit encounter.

The cause of the fourth and most serious form of impotence was traced back to the first week of a male infant's life and was associated with the mother's care of the infant's umbilical cord. If the dried umbilical cord stump touched the infant's genitals as the cord fell off, the boy would be impotent for the rest of his life. Mothers apparently employ a variety of measures to ensure that such a catastrophic event does not take place. Some women tie a string or thread to the end of the dried umbilical cord and loop the thread or string around the child's neck to prevent the cord from falling onto the infant's genitals. Other women, I was told, simply cover the baby's genitals with a piece of cloth. This particular form of impotence was dreaded not just because of its consequences but also because of the drastic nature of its cure: the mother and son must engage in or reenact sexual intercourse.

I was actually told several versions of this cure. In one version, intercourse need not take place. Rather, a man's mother will go into a room and, unbeknownst to him, will disrobe completely. She then calls out to him. When he enters the room and sees his mother's nudity, I was told, he will receive such a shock that he will immediately get an erection and thus be cured. A male vendor I interviewed at the herbal market in Shinyanga town told me that the full act of sexual intercourse must take place, including ejaculation. Despite his claim, however, most people I spoke with stated emphatically that the cure could be activated by just a minimal insertion of the son's penis into his mother's vagina, with neither one having to disrobe (the point being that the son's penis, whether as an infant or adult, must once again come into contact with his mother's vagina).

This type of impotence was not talked about as being an exclusively Sukuma phenomenon. A neighbor of mine in Bulangwa, who was not Sukuma, told me it happened with her own son. When her son was only two weeks old, she noticed that his penis remained flaccid when he urinated. Her mother, who was staying with her at the time, saw this as an indication that the boy would be impotent in the future. She told her daughter what she must do to cure it. Although my neighbor told me that she had never heard of this cure prior to her mother's explanation, she took her son into the bedroom and inserted the tip of his penis into her vagina. She told me the whole process took only a few seconds. The treatment worked, she noted, because the next time her son urinated, his penis was erect.

I have no idea as to the prevalence of this category of impotence or its cure in the community. I only know that it was rumored to have occurred in one Sukuma man I knew in Bulangwa. He had been married several times, but his wives always left him because he could not get an erection and thus could not have intercourse. He eventually remarried and his wife did become pregnant. It was "general knowledge" that he had been "cured" by his mother.

When I asked the women who participated in the group interviews whether they would feel shame to have to enact this kind of cure with their own son, they all emphatically stressed that it wasn't sex, but, rather, a cure: "He is your child, he must be cured so that he can be married and have children!" (*Ni mtoto wako. Ni lazima. Aoe na apate watoto!*) When I later asked men and other women about this cure, they echoed similar sentiments: "It's a treatment. It must be done!" (*Ni uganga. Ni lazima!*). Everyone seemed to agree that there was no shame attached to it, but the best solution to avoid any potential embarrassment was to perform a symbolic reenactment of sexual intercourse while the child was still an infant.

But impotence isn't always detected in infancy, and thus in some cases the cure had to take place between a woman and her grown son. Some mothers, I was told, do refuse to enact this cure. Mwana Nyanzanga told me that she had seen this refusal with her own eyes: it happened with the wife of her maternal uncle. This woman had refused to "cure" her son and thus he never married or experienced fatherhood. The general sense I got from people with whom I spoke about this particular type of impotence was that it was a mother's duty to enact this cure if the need arose, as it was the only way to ensure her son's future parenthood.

Unwanted Fertility

Although women in the community spoke about their fertility as being susceptible to a variety of physical and spiritual dangers, their concerns with safeguarding their fertility did not necessarily mean they wanted to have as many children as possible. In fact, some of the younger women I interviewed also mentioned their concerns with having too many children. When I asked how many children they wanted, they gave a range of answers. In table 8.2 we see that the level of a woman's education does appear to be related to the total number of children a woman says she wants (see chaps. 3 and 4). Although 49 percent ($n = 51$) of the 104 younger women I interviewed told me they still wanted to have more children, 38 percent ($n = 40$) of the women did not want any more children at all. These data, however, could also be analyzed further in terms of how many children each woman already had at the time she was interviewed. One of the women who said she wanted twelve children had already given birth twelve times. Had I asked her this same question when she only had ten children, she might have said ten was all she wanted.

In table 8.3 I present women's reasons for not wanting any more children according to their level of education. Despite their small numbers, the variety of reasons women gave for not wanting more children are nevertheless important to note. As we see in the table, women's responses fall into five groups: those who believe they have had enough; those who cite physical reasons (tiredness, want to rest, getting old); those who had problems with previous births; those who mentioned specific life-related problems not directly associated with the physical act of giving birth (marital and economic); and those whose pregnancies just stopped on their own. Although these forty women stated that they did not want any more children, very few of them were using any form of contraception, either nonmodern or modern.

Nonmodern Methods of Preventing Conception

The women I spoke with described several nonmodern methods of preventing conception (Varkevisser 1973).[33] One, known as *pigi* in Kisukuma, consisted of a piece of root tied on a string and worn around the woman's hips. One Arab woman told me that she tried this method of birth control after giving birth to her ninth child, but it hadn't worked. She became pregnant within a month of wearing it. Other methods included the drinking of herbal remedies. One woman told me she had swallowed pieces of a particular root for the number of years she wanted to be infertile. Still others told me that some women tried to prevent unwanted pregnancies by burying their menstrual cloth themselves. This particular method had a dangerous side effect, however. If a woman forgot where she buried the cloth, she would never be able to conceive again. There was a similar danger attached to the wearing of a *pigi:* if the string that held it broke, the woman would remain infertile for the rest of her life. These local methods of birth control, however varied, do not appear to be widely used. Only eight out of the 104 younger women, or 7.7 percent, told me they had ever used a local means of preventing birth control in their life, while only two of the fifty older women had (4 percent). For the 154 women as a whole, 6.5 percent had ever used nonmodern methods of contraception, a figure considerably lower than the 15 percent reported by respondents in the 1996 Tanzanian Demographic Health Survey (DHS) (Bureau of Statistics [Tanzania] and Macro International Inc. 1997).

TABLE 8.2.   Responses to the Survey Question "How Many Children Would You Like to Have?" for the Subset of Younger Women by Years of Formal Education ($N = 104$)

Total Number of Children Wanted	0 years ($n = 43$)		<7 years ($n = 20$)		7 years ($n = 41$)	
	n	%	n	%	n	%
2	—	—	—	—	1	2.4
3	1	2.3	1	5.0	—	—
4	1	2.3	2	10.0	7	17.1
5	8	18.6	4	20.0	4	9.8
6	4	9.3	—	—	7	17.1
7	4	9.3	—	—	2	4.9
8	2	4.7	1	5.0	—	—
10	1	2.3	—	—	2	8.7
12	1	2.3	—	—	—	—
Depends on health	—	—	—	—	1	2.4
Until eggs finish	1	2.3	—	—	1	2.4
It's up to God	5	11.6	—	—	—	—
No specific number	3	7.0	—	—	2	4.9
Doesn't want to think about it	—	—	—	—	1	2.4
Doesn't know	2	4.7	—	—	1	2.4
Didn't ask	10	23.2	12	45.0	12	29.3
Average		6.2		4.8		5.4

Modern Methods of Preventing Conception

Modern methods of preventing pregnancy were not widely used in the community either, even though they were available at the local government clinic. Only twenty-three of the subset of 104 younger women, or 22.1 percent of the women who still experienced their menses, told me they had ever used a modern method of contraception, and of these, 30 percent ($n = 7$) were currently using a method. According to the 1996 DHS for Tanzania, these figures are 23 percent and 12 percent respectively for all women in Tanzania (Bureau of Statistics [Tanzania] and Macro International Inc. 1997).

Irregular periods, fears of getting *kansa* (cancer), and threats to their future fertility were common reasons women gave for their decision to discontinue the use of a chosen birth control method or for avoiding the use of modern methods of birth control altogether. Concerns about the harmful side effects of birth control methods also emerged in my formal interviews with women. Ten of the sixteen women (62.5 percent) who were no longer using a modern method of birth control told me they stopped using

TABLE 8.3. Responses to the Survey Question "Why Don't You Want Any More Children?" for the Subset of Younger Women by Years of Formal Education ($N = 40$)

Reasons for Not Wanting More Children	0 years ($n = 13$)		<7 years ($n = 13$)		7 years ($n = 16$)	
	n	%	n	%	n	%
Has enough	3	23.1	3	27.3	4	25.0
Is tired	1	7.7	2	18.2	2	12.5
Wants to rest	1	7.7	—	—	3	18.8
Is getting old	3	23.1	1	9.1	1	6.3
Has problem pregnancies	—	—	1	9.1	1	6.3
Last birth had complications	1	2.3	—	—	—	—
Has had 3 cesarean sections	—	—	—	—	1	6.3
Is afraid	1	2.3	—	—	—	—
Is having marital problems	—	—	1	9.1	—	—
Life is difficult (economic problems)	—	—	3	27.3	4	25.0
Pregnancies stopped on their own	3	23.1	—	—	—	—
Total	13	100.0	11	100.0	16	100.0

it because it was negatively affecting their health. Among the eighty-one younger women who had never used family planning, 14.9 percent ($n = 12$) told me they believed birth control caused health problems, 8.7 percent ($n = 7$) stated that they didn't want to use it, 8.7 percent ($n = 7$) said they still wanted to get pregnant, 3.7 percent ($n = 3$) said their husbands forbade it, and 48.1 percent ($n = 39$) stated that they "just didn't use it," without giving a specific reason. This last category of response, which accounted for nearly half of all responses, raises the possibility that something in addition to a woman's concerns about her health may be contributing to her decision not to use a method of family planning. The experience one woman had at the government clinic in Bulangwa offers insight into what that something else might be.

This particular woman had seven children and did not want to have any more. After her seventh birth, she went to the government clinic in Bulangwa with the intention of starting oral contraceptives. The nurse on duty, however, told her that before she could receive this method of birth control, she would first have to return to the clinic while menstruating and undergo a vaginal exam. Understandably, the woman never returned. She later told me that rather than subject herself to that humiliation, she decided it was just easier to have another child. She recounted her story to me while I was interviewing her for my study. She was breast-feeding a newborn infant as we spoke. It was her eighth child.

When I recounted her story later to a friend who was a nurse at the government clinic, she acknowledged that vaginal exams were conducted on some menstruating women. She explained that since many of the women who came to the clinic were illiterate, the only way to ensure they would start the pill at the right point in their cycle was to examine them when they were actually menstruating. The next time I traveled to Shinyanga town, I spoke with a nurse who worked in the regional Family Planning Unit and asked whether this was standard policy throughout Tanzania. She assured me that it was not. In other words, the policy as it was implemented at the government clinic in Bulangwa was an apparent aberration.

This woman's case illustrates some of the unofficial risks associated with illiteracy. Whereas the Safe Motherhood literature posits that illiteracy is linked to a woman's nonuse of family planning because it is also a reflection of her low social status and lack of autonomy in the context of marriage, in Bulangwa, only certain categories of rural women—illiterate ones—were subjected to unnecessary vaginal exams while menstruating. If the woman who recounted her story to me had been educated, it is quite possible that her experience at the clinic would have been very different. The "requirement" of a vaginal exam is problematic for several reasons. First, a vaginal exam while menstruating is not medically necessary, as evidenced by the fact that it is not required of all women who wish to use oral contraceptives. Second, given the symbolic power attributed to menstrual blood (that access to it may result in blocked fertility in the future), the fact that this woman was not willing to submit to a vaginal exam while menstruating, which would render her vulnerable to sorcery in the future, is hardly surprising. Her failure to obtain oral contraceptives and thus her subsequent birth underscore in a very striking way the complexity of the issue of access to health resources. As her experience illustrates quite vividly, the concept *access to family planning* covers more than just the physical existence of a family planning clinic.

Abortion

Cases in which women became pregnant and had then tried to abort also occurred in the community, although my knowledge surrounding women's experiences with self-induced abortion came from general conversation or observations in the community rather than questions asked in the formal interviews. During the course of my twenty months of residence in Bulangwa, several of the young girls at the local secondary school attempted abortion. Some of their attempts became public knowledge because the school's driver would transport the girl to one of the two private clinics located in the center of town. By the time the young girl arrived at the clinic she was often very sick. I became involved in a similar case when the young granddaughter of an elderly man I knew in town aborted using a combination of tetracycline and chloroquine. It was an incomplete abortion, and she acquired a serious infection and became quite ill. The medical aid who worked at the private clinic explained to the relatives who had accompanied her that she needed emergency care at a hospital. Her father and grandfather arrived at my house and asked for transportation, which I provided. When I had a chance to speak with her alone after she had returned from the hospital, she told me that she had been afraid of what her father would do if he learned about her pregnancy, and so she had aborted it. Although it is generally agreed that schoolgirls are the ones who are most likely to attempt abortion, I also heard stories of older women in the community who had tried to abort and succeeded.

Risk and Infertility

In contrast to the international and national emphasis on the risk of excessive fertility, in this chapter we have seen that the risk of unsuccessful fertility is also a predominant prenatal concern. Attention to this unofficial maternal health risk reveals an extensive vocabulary surrounding female and male fertility, as well as the various factors, both physical and spiritual, that may adversely affect it.

A recent analysis of primary and secondary infertility in Tanzania (Larsen 2001) indicates that women's concerns with safeguarding their fertility are not unfounded. Whereas the level of primary infertility (childlessness) in the Shinyanga Region was relatively low (2.6 percent), levels of secondary infertility (the inability to have another child among women who have already given birth) was 13 percent. Although this is lower than the level found for Tanzania as a whole (18 percent), it is still high and merits further attention (see also Boerma et al. 1996).

To what extent do the fertility-related concerns described in this chapter continue to be relevant once conception has taken place? To answer this, let us turn to chapter 9, where our focus will be on women's concerns and intentions during pregnancy and their experiences with prenatal care.

CHAPTER 9

The Prenatal Period, Part 2:
Risks during Pregnancy

> The antenatal clinic which [was] founded in the early nineteen fifties
> has radically modified the procedures which Sukuma women follow
> when they give birth. The success of its services for which there were
> no comparable traditional alternatives ingratiated the clinic to the
> population. According to the hospital staff, the clinic is the most
> popular and busiest ward of the hospital, frequented by Christians as
> well as by adherents of traditional religion. Those with traditional
> mentalities, however, often wait until they have suffered before they
> will seek modern treatment.
> —Corlien M. Varkevisser, *Socialization in a Changing Society*

> There is a local midwife who is practicing in a village about a 15
> minute drive from my fieldsite. She is well-known not only as a
> midwife but as a "traditional" healer. She has even built a special
> house for her prenatal consultations that includes a birthing room as
> well as a postpartum room for women to stay after giving birth. It is
> quite an incredible set-up, and although it is a mud house with mud
> floors, it's considerably cleaner than the regional hospital. At times her
> home seems to serve as a home for women waiting to give birth, with
> many arriving a few days to a few weeks before birthing. A very nice
> set-up, with everyone pitching in with the work. So, for example, you
> may find women who are waiting for their "prenatal appointments"
> going to fetch water, pounding corn, preparing food, or helping with
> the preparation of the herbal remedies.
> —Letter from the field, April 7, 1993, Bulangwa, Tanzania

Although many women in Bulangwa place a positive value on fertility and
motherhood, in this chapter we will see that pregnancy also appears to be
a period of increased stress for women, as evidenced by the negative emotions many admit to feeling while pregnant, their concerns with preventing
or counteracting a variety of physical and spiritual prenatal risks, and the
hassles many encounter while trying to obtain care in clinic and hospital

settings. In the epigraph that opens this chapter, Corlien Varkevisser suggests that some Sukuma women's reluctance to seek modern prenatal care in the mid-1960s was a result of their having "traditional mentalities." My research during the early 1990s in Bulangwa, in contrast, indicates that some women's reluctance to seek prenatal care in the clinic or hospital setting is a result of their past experiences of being *labeled* as having a traditional mentality once they arrive seeking treatment. This labeling, in turn, negatively affects the quality of care they receive (Wood 1985).

Our examination of women's pregnancy-related experiences in this chapter is divided into three parts. We begin by exploring women's actual experiences of being pregnant, from their initial self-diagnosis to the emotions many associate with this phase of the reproductive cycle. Next, we turn our attention to women's experiences with clinic-based prenatal care, paying particular attention to two components of the government's prenatal-care program: the risk referral system and the home-based maternal health record. We then move to the community of Bulangwa to explore what happens when these core aspects of Tanzania's maternal health policy are implemented at the local level. What, for example, constitutes a necessary referral from the perspective of health-care personnel at the local level, and what happens to a pregnant woman once a referral has been made? Do she and the relatives who accompany her actually travel to a health facility better equipped to handle her specific case? And if not, why not?

In the last part of this chapter we explore local cultural options for prenatal care, with particular emphasis on Mwana Nyanzanga's work, the local midwife referred to in the second epigraph above. We will examine some of the categories of prenatal risk her herbal remedies address and meet some of her clients.

Women's Experiences of Being Pregnant

The Initial Diagnosis

Previous anthropological and sociological studies of the Sukuma and Nyamwezi peoples provide some insight into past beliefs and practices associated with the prenatal period. According to Varkevisser's study in the Mwanza Region in the mid-1960s, "the newly-married [Sukuma] woman knows for certain she has conceived when she has missed her period for the second time" (1973:109). Citing Blohm's work among the Nyamwezi in 1933, Swantz notes that Nyamwezi women living in southern Sukumaland had a similar way of calculating the onset of pregnancy. She offers the additional information that "Nyamwezi believed that pregnancy lasted seven months for a girl and eight months for a boy" (1969:230). Cory (n.d.) makes a similar observation regarding the gender of gestation among the Sukuma. Although I didn't specifically ask women about the length of the gestation period in my formal survey, many of the informal conversations I had with women indicated that nine months was generally considered to be the normal period of gestation. It is quite possible that women's exposure to information about pregnancy through their participation in clinic-based prenatal care has contributed to a change in local perceptions about gestational length over time.

My insight into Mwana Nyanzanga's perceptions of the gestational period was shaped to a very large extent by my observations of the prenatal consultations she conducted at her home. Her calculation of gestational age was similar in some ways to my own, which, in turn, was based on what I had learned as a lay midwifery trainee in El Paso: that is, every four centimeters of the fundal measurement is equivalent to one month of pregnancy.[1] If, for example, Mwana Nyanzanga told me that a particular woman was seven months pregnant and I measured the woman's fundus with a tape measure, it was usually twenty-eight centimeters, give or take a centimeter. Although she was also of the opinion that nine months was the normal period of gestation, Mwana Nyanzanga measured the age of the fetus differently than I did. From five to seven months of gestational age, she estimated the age of the fetus by gauging the top of the fundus in relation to the woman's navel with her hand. A woman was five months pregnant (i.e., twenty centimeters) when the top of the fundus was at or slightly above the navel. After seven months she measured the bottom of the fundus. It was in this manner, she told me, she could begin to measure the age of the fetus in relation to its descent into the birth canal.

When I asked women both informally and in my formal interviews how they initially knew they were pregnant, they gave a variety of responses, from describing particular physical symptoms, such as nausea, lack of strength, drowsiness, breast changes, and fetal movements, to statements that they knew they were pregnant because their menses had stopped. This latter concept was expressed in different ways. Some women simply said that the blood "closed up" or was "sealed" (*kufunga damu*), that the "days closed" (*kufunga siku*), or that the moon or month passed without signs of their menses (*kupitisha mwezi*). Five older women noted that they hadn't even known they were pregnant the first time until they actually gave birth. Several of the others I interviewed told me they were married even before their first menses had begun, a finding that suggests an earlier age at marriage for women in the past.

Emotions and Pregnancy

Varkevisser describes a much more active role for the Sukuma husband during his wife's pregnancy than I found. She notes that from the fifth month of pregnancy until a woman gives birth, the "traditional" Sukuma husband is expected to "watch the womb" (*kulela nda*), meaning that he is expected to continue sexual relations with his pregnant wife so that the fetus will mature in the womb (1973:112). According to Varkevisser, this aspect of the father's role is so crucial to the survival of the fetus that if he has other wives, he will temporarily cease having sexual relations with them until his pregnant wife gives birth.

Varkevisser's description of the husband's role during his wife's pregnancy is in sharp contrast to how both Sukuma and non-Sukuma women in my study talked about their husbands' behavior during their pregnancies. Although I didn't ask specifically about the practice of watching the womb because it didn't emerge as a concept in the context of either my informal conversations or formal interviews, several women I knew spoke about this period as a time when their husbands had taken lovers or cohabited with their other wives. When I asked Sukuma women taking part in a group interview whether a man's sexual relations with other women during his wife's pregnancy could harm the child in his wife's womb, they uniformly agreed that that was just not possible; only the promiscuity of the pregnant woman could cause harm to the unborn child.[2]

Although I never heard women speak about husbands watching their wives' wombs, husbands did emerge as an issue within the context of my informal conversations with women about their experiences of *being* pregnant. Despite women's positive statements about motherhood and the value of children, some of their comments indicated that pregnancy was not a particularly blissful period of their lives. Several women mentioned general feelings of anger and uncharacteristic irritability, with much of that anger and dislike directed toward relatives and often toward the husband specifically. One woman I knew quite well in the community told me that during her second pregnancy, the first with her current husband, she just couldn't stand the sight of him. They were usually quite compatible, she told me, but during that particular pregnancy her feelings of dislike were so strong that she almost told him she wanted a divorce. After receiving counseling from family members who told her that her negative feelings toward her husband were directly related to her pregnancy, she decided to live out the final months of her pregnancy at her mother's home in a nearby town. As predicted, her dislike was fleeting; her husband showed up the week after she gave birth and she was no longer irritated. In fact, she told me, she was very happy to see him. Another woman, an Arab friend whose husband had traveled during the latter months of her pregnancy, told me that she was actually relieved he was gone. When I expressed my surprise, she told me that during some of her pregnancies, she just couldn't stand his smell. He only smelled when she was pregnant, and she would become nauseated every time he drew near. She said that the smell of him left her feeling so nauseated during one particular pregnancy that, rather than risk hurting his feelings, she told him her back hurt and so she preferred to sleep on the floor. She slept on the floor during the remainder of that pregnancy.

After hearing these and similar stories, I decided to include a question about emotional and behavioral changes during pregnancy in my formal interviews with women (see table 9.1). Not surprisingly, those women also mentioned similar negative changes during their pregnancies. One Arab woman told me that she had felt a strong aversion toward a sister-in-law during one of her pregnancies, while her own middle child became the object of her scorn during the next. An older Sukuma woman I interviewed told me that she had always felt intense dislike for her husband and all of her male children during her pregnancies. Her daughters' presence didn't provoke any negative reactions at all.

Table 9.1 shows that women's responses to this question differed according to their age category. Of the forty-five older women whose answers were recorded, twenty-seven, or 59 percent said they experienced no emotional or behavioral changes during their pregnancies, compared to forty-five of the one hundred younger women who did not, or 45 percent of the recorded answers. Among those women who did experience changes, a larger proportion of younger women reported negative feelings toward family members and people in general (42 percent) than did the older subset of women (26 percent). Among the subset of younger women who answered this question, a higher percentage of women who had some level of education said they had experienced negative feelings during pregnancy than the younger women who had never attended school (data not shown). Of the thirty-nine women who had finished primary school and answered this question, 69.2 percent ($n = 27$) said they experienced emotional or behavioral changes during pregnancy. With only one exception, they described these changes as negative feelings directed primarily at family members. This is similar to what was reported by the women who had begun primary school but had not completed it: 65 percent ($n = 13$) of the twenty women in this subset reported emotional or behavioral changes during pregnancy, and again with only one exception all of these women described the feelings as negative. Only 39 percent ($n = 16$) of the younger

TABLE 9.1. Responses to the Survey Question "During Your Pregnancies, Do You Experience Any Emotional or Behavioral Changes?" for the Subsets of Older and Younger Women ($N = 146$)

Categories of Changes	Older Women ($n = 46$)		Younger Women ($n = 100$)	
	n	%	n	%
No changes	27	58.7	45	45.0
Negative emotions				
Dislikes or is angry with husband	4	8.7	10	10.0
Husband smells	1	2.2	3	3.0
Dislikes mother-in-law	2	4.3	1	1.0
Dislikes a family member	1	2.2	4	4.0
Dislikes one of her children	—	—	1	1.0
Dislike of men in general	—	—	1	1.0
General feelings of anger/irritableness	2	4.3	13	13.0
Dislikes or refuses to greet certain people	2	4.3	9	9.0
Positive emotions				
Loves husband a lot	—	—	1	1.0
Likes people a lot	—	—	1	1.0
Physical symptoms				
Dislikes certain foods	1	2.2	5	5.0
Likes certain foods	5	10.9	2	2.0
Doesn't want to do work	—	—	1	1.0
Keeps quiet/doesn't talk much	—	—	3	3.0
Feels tired	1	2.2	—	—
No change total	27	58.7	45	45.0
Negative change total	12	26.0	42	42.0
Positive change total	—	—	2	2.0
Physical change total	7	15.3	11	11.0
Total	46	100.0	100.0	100.0

women who had never attended school said they had experienced these kinds of negative feelings during pregnancy.

Given the small sample size, the question remains as to whether there is any value in this type of data. I would argue that there is and that the insight to be gained is contextual. First, in looking at how women themselves define "negative" emotional or behavioral changes, we can learn a bit more about what constitutes the cultural norm. For example, several women mentioned "not wanting to greet people," "passing people without greeting them," or simply "keeping quiet, not responding when spoken to" as a negative change in their behavior when they were pregnant. They did not usually behave that way, nor did they usually feel such intense dislike for their husbands, mothers-in-law, particular children, or other relatives.

The other value of this data is the light it sheds on women's experience of negative emotions or behaviors during pregnancy compared to their experiences of similar changes during other phases of their reproductive cycles, such as during the menstrual cycle or after giving birth. In the United States, emotional and behavioral changes during these latter phases of the reproductive cycle are often portrayed as an inherent part of being female, changes the medical literature describes in terms of fluctuating hormonal levels (Martin 1988; Martinez et al. 2000). According to women in Bulangwa, however, the menstrual cycle and the postpartum period were relatively unmarked in terms of emotional or behavioral changes (Roth 1996: 288–90). It was during pregnancy, rather than after giving birth or during particular points in a woman's menstrual cycle, that the women noticed negative changes in their emotions or behavior.

Changes in pregnant women's behavior is apparently also noticed by men. Prior to beginning my formal interviews, I asked a Sukuma man I knew if men generally believed that women's behavior changed in any way during the different stages of a woman's reproductive cycle, for example, during their menstrual cycle or in the months following childbirth. When he said no, I continued my questions, trying to be more specific. Was there a general belief circulating among men, for example, that men needed to be careful what they said to women during certain periods of the menstrual cycle because women were known to be especially irritable or susceptible to emotional changes during that time? Again he said no. Men only say that, he continued, about a woman's behavior during pregnancy. A woman's irritability during pregnancy was expected, and thus a man is supposed to take that into consideration if disputes between him and his wife occur while she is pregnant. A wife's argumentativeness, he told me, is tolerated only when she is pregnant. He noted that a man will be admonished by family members and neighbors alike if he beats his wife for her argumentativeness during pregnancy because such behavior is attributed to the changes brought on by pregnancy and not to any specific flaw in the woman's character per se.

Although both younger and older women were overall more likely to mention negative changes during pregnancy and less likely to acknowledge similar changes during a woman's menstrual cycle or the postpartum period, there was, as already noted above, a difference between their respective responses. Older women on the whole appear to be less likely than younger women to mention emotional changes, and within the younger group of women, women without any formal education are less likely than women with some formal education to mention emotional changes.

What does this mean? These results could be interpreted in several ways, although given the small size of my sample, such interpretations would require further investigation. One could, for example, suggest that the tendency of younger women to mention negative emotional feelings during pregnancy more often than older women is a reflection that rituals associated with the reproductive cycle are on the decline. Although this may be true to some extent, we also learned in chapter 8 that rituals associated with puberty are not common in this part of the country. The older and younger women I interviewed acquired information about their bodies and about reproduction in a nonuniform, nonstructured way. Another explanation for the difference in older and younger women's emotions during pregnancy might be that women nowadays live under harsher economic conditions than women did in the past, which may account for different levels of stress experienced during pregnancy by these two groups of women. Since I do not have any specific information on these women's economic resources, this latter possibility is harder to prove. Nevertheless, I think that it is at least a credible interpretation of this data. It is also possible that the answer to this question lies in a combination of these two possibilities: perhaps women nowadays receive less social and economic support during their pregnancies. The differences that emerge within the younger group of women, that is, between those who had attended primary school and those who had not, are more difficult to explain, as it is education beyond primary school that is associated with expanding women's ways of thinking about the world as well as their opportunities (Dixon-Mueller 1993:121; see also Puja and Kassimoto 1994). Only two of the women I interviewed had attended secondary school: an Arab woman who lived in Bulangwa and a Sukuma woman who lived in Mwana Nyanzanga's village.

In addition to exploring women's emotions during pregnancy and their experiences of being pregnant, I also spoke with them about their participation in prenatal care. In the section below, we turn our attention to their experiences of prenatal care within the biomedical setting.

Prenatal Care in the Biomedical Setting

The Risk Approach to Maternal Health Care

According to the *Safe Motherhood Strategy for Tanzania,* prenatal care is an important source of preventive and curative treatment for women during their pregnancies. By participating in prenatal care on a regular basis, pregnant women gain access to health information, iron supplements to prevent anemia, and chloroquine tablets to prevent malaria (United Republic of Tanzania 1992). Prenatal visits also involve the regular monitoring of women's pregnancies, a monitoring that enables health-care personnel to detect and respond to potential obstetrical problems early on. In the event that such complications do arise, women are then referred out to a higher-level medical facility to receive the appropriate medical attention.

During the early 1990s, the Tanzanian government's policy regarding prenatal care centered around the risk approach to maternal health care and the risk-referral system (de Groot et al. 1993). This approach, which has as its goal the efficient allocation of scarce health resources, involves the classification of pregnant women according to their risk of experiencing obstetric complications. Those who are classified as being "at risk" for experiencing a complication may, in turn, be referred out to a health facility better equipped to handle difficult births. In theory, the purpose of the risk approach to maternal health is to ensure that pregnant women receive appropriate and timely care (see also Backett et al. 1984; WHO 1977; cf. Hayes 1991).[3]

The *Safe Motherhood Strategy for Tanzania* was quite candid in its assessment of the risk-referral system in Tanzania. Staffing problems, shortages in supplies and equipment, and problems with transportation were identified as key factors that negatively affected the quality of routine care and referral available to pregnant women (United Republic of Tanzania 1992:9). Having defined the problem for the Tanzanian context specifically, and following the recommendations laid out in the Safe Motherhood Initiative (Kaisi 1989; Starrs 1987), the *Safe Motherhood Strategy for Tanzania* proposed a variety of measures to strengthen prenatal health services in general and the risk-referral system in particular. These included: (1) improving the skills of government health-care personnel so that they will be able to quickly identify and manage medical conditions that pose risks to the survival of pregnant women; (2) improving the referral system so that it guarantees a woman's timely arrival at medical facilities better equipped to handle obstetric complications; and (3) strengthening the community-based pregnancy monitoring system by improving and promoting the use of a home-based maternal health record (United Republic of Tanzania 1992).

This latter solution, also known as the prenatal card, is a key component of Tanzania's risk-referral system. The card, which is used in government and nongovernment prenatal clinics throughout the country, is meant to function as a tool for the efficient evaluation of a pregnant woman's health status, a kind of mobile hospital record that facilitates and ensures consistent prenatal care. In theory, a pregnant woman is supposed to keep the card at home and bring it with her to each of her prenatal visits. Updated information about her health and her pregnancy—blood pressure, weight, hemoglobin, and the measurement of the growth of the fetus and its heart rate—is recorded on the card by the clinic nurse. Regardless of where her prenatal visits take place or where she ultimately decides to give birth, her card provides health-care personnel working in prenatal clinics and on maternity wards with an instant record of her prenatal care. This includes a history of her previous pregnancies and births, where she is currently receiving prenatal care, and reference to any health problems she may have experienced during her most recent pregnancy.

The prenatal card also functions as a screening device. Nurses mark the appropriate boxes on the front of the card to indicate whether the woman is considered to be at risk for experiencing obstetric complications. If she is classified as being at high risk and her visits take place at a clinic that provides only a minimum level of care, her birth is supposed to be referred out to a higher-level medical facility. A star is also drawn in the upper corner on the front of the card as a warning sign to nonliterate traditional birth attendants that this particular woman is not a candidate for home birth. Once a woman is referred out of the smaller clinic or out of the village setting, it is expected that she will travel to a higher-level health facility, taking her mobile medical record, the prenatal card, with her.

But the risk-referral system also functions in ways not intended by health-care planners and policymakers in that it can, ironically, also be used to restrict a pregnant woman's access to care. I first became aware of this unintended consequence of the government's risk-referral system through my observations of how some health-care providers interacted with their pregnant clients. Some of the unofficial risks women associated with participating in clinic-based prenatal care also emerged as a theme in my observations in the community and in the conversations I had with women about their experiences of being pregnant.

Clinic-Based Prenatal Care

The government clinic in Bulangwa was staffed by six nurse assistants, one maternal and child health (MCH) aid, and one rural medical aid (RMA) who also served as the head of the clinic.[4] In addition to providing health services for the general public, the clinic provided a variety of services for pregnant women and young children in a separate maternal and child health clinic within the same compound. These included health education sessions, family planning, growth monitoring for children up to the age of five years, a monthly outreach maternal and child clinic to surrounding villages, and a two-bed maternity room for birthing women.

As noted in the previous chapter, the Tanzanian Ministry of Health estimates that approximately 85 percent of all Tanzanian women receive some level of clinic-based prenatal care. The results of my formal interviews with women revealed an even higher level of participation. Ninety-eight percent ($n = 101$) of the 103 younger women who were asked this question said they visited a prenatal clinic during their pregnancies.

Many of the younger women who took part in my formal interviews acknowledged the benefits of attending prenatal care. "Getting medicine" (*kupata dawa*) was one benefit. Eighty-eight percent ($n = 89$) of the younger women said that the nurses at the clinic gave them medicine to use during their pregnancies. At the same time, however, six women told me they never received anything at all, while another six women noted that although they had been given prenatal supplements and malaria prophylaxes in the past, they had not received anything from nurses during their most recent pregnancy. These latter responses are similar to the results of my informal conversations with women in the community, in that many of them told me that although they might be given some medicine by nurses at the clinic during the course of their prenatal care, overall it was less than they had received in the past, with some remarking that nowadays they didn't receive anything at all (*Siku hizi hatupati cho chote!*). The scarcity or complete lack of medicines at the government clinic was actually a common complaint expressed by many in the community. Despite the monthly supply of medicines the government clinic received as part of a European-funded "Essential Drug Program," people often arrived at the clinic only to learn that the medicines had run out. Throughout my two-year stay in Tanzania I often heard people referring to this chronic shortage of medicines at government hospitals and clinics alike, and even at some mission facilities. Community members often blamed the shortage of medicines on clinic and hospital personnel who, many believed, sold the medicines to augment their meager monthly salaries.

Although very few women were able to identify the medications or supplements they received during pregnancy specifically by name, many mentioned a medicine either in terms of its preventive qualities or its specific health benefits. Table 9.2 presents the categories of prenatal "medicines" elicited in my formal interviews with women. Only four of the prenatal medicines women received were mentioned by name. The largest cat-

TABLE 9.2.   Categories Elicited When Women Were Asked What Kind of Prenatal Medicine They Received at the Prenatal Clinic

Categories of Prenatal Medicines

1.   Mentioned by name of medicine
     Aspirin
     Perratin
     Tetanus vaccine
     Vitamins

2.   Mentioned by type of preventive benefit
     Pills to prevent malaria
     Pills or tonic to increase the strength of their blood
     For the health of the fetus
     For the general health of the mother
     To increase their appetite
     To reduce pain

3.   Mentioned by side effect of medicine
     Causes drowsiness

4.   Mentioned by form of medicine, benefit not specified
     Pill by color
     Tonic

5.   Received medicine during pregnancy but didn't ask why or wasn't told what is was for.

egory, "Mentioned by type of preventive benefit," is interesting: pills to prevent malaria, for the health of the fetus and the mother, and to increase the strength of the blood are included here. This mostly likely reflects how nurses at the prenatal clinic described these medicines to their clients.

Given that 98 percent of the younger women in my formal survey stated that they participated in prenatal care and that many women acknowledged the health benefits of prenatal supplements and medicines they sometimes received, it would seem safe to assume that many rural women view prenatal care in a positive light, as a means of ensuring their well-being during pregnancy. When we begin to look closer at these assumptions, however, it becomes clear that a woman's attendance at a prenatal clinic has unacknowledged benefits as well. To understand the nature of these additional benefits we need to ask different kinds of questions; for example, *who* begins prenatal care *when,* and *why* do they do so?

As we already saw in chapter 3, the Safe Motherhood Initiative notes that the less educated a woman is, the less likely it is that she will be aware of the benefits of prenatal care and thus attend a prenatal clinic when she is pregnant. This scenario, however, was not particularly true for the women I interviewed, as can be seen by the results presented in table 9.3.

Given the associations the Safe Motherhood literature makes between literacy and women's participation in maternal health care, I find it striking that 95 percent of the younger women who never attended primary school had, nevertheless, participated in the government's prenatal-care program. This suggests that education may not be an adequate predictor of whether a woman will attend a prenatal clinic in Tanzania, a finding that has been reported in other parts of the country as well (Kaisi

TABLE 9.3.   Responses to the Survey Question "Do You Attend the Prenatal Clinic When You Are Pregnant?" among the Subset of Younger Women by Years of Formal Education ($N = 103$)

Response	0 years[a] ($n = 42$)		<7 years ($n = 20$)		7 years ($n = 41$)	
	n	(%)	n	(%)	n	(%)
Yes	40	95	20	100	41	100
No	2	5	—	—	—	—
Total	42	100	20	100	41	100

[a]Although 43 of the younger women fall into this category, 1 woman's responses were not recorded for this question.

1989:18). Since the level of a woman's education does not appear to be a significant factor in her decision to participate in prenatal care, does it appear to be a factor in her decision about *when* to seek care? In table 9.4 I present data regarding the timing of women's initial prenatal visits according to their level of education. Once again, the difference in the history of prenatal care between women who have finished primary school and those women who never attended school at all varies from what is suggested by the Safe Motherhood literature. Although some of the women who had attended primary school began their prenatal care earlier than did women without any education, that is, during the first or second month of their pregnancies, when we look at the number of women who said they begin their prenatal visits by their third month of pregnancy, the results are surprising. Among the subset of women who had never attended primary school, 25 percent stated that they had begun their prenatal care by their third month of pregnancy. This is similar to what was reported by the women who had had some level of primary school education (25 percent). When the subset of women who had finished primary school was asked a similar question, however, only 17 percent of them reported that they usually began prenatal care by their third month of pregnancy.

TABLE 9.4.   Responses to the Survey Question "During Which Month of Your Pregnancy Do You Usually Begin Attending the Prenatal Clinic?" for the Subset of Younger Women by Years of Formal Education ($N = 101$)

Response	0 years[a] ($n = 40$)		<7 years ($n = 20$)		7 years ($n = 41$)	
	n	(%)	n	(%)	n	(%)
1	—	—	1	5.0	1	2.4
2	—	—	1	5.0	1	2.4
3	10	25.0	3	15.0	5	12.4
4	10	25.0	9	45.0	24	58.5
5	15	37.5	3	15.0	3	7.3
6	3	7.5	3	15.0	4	9.8
7	1	2.5	—	—	2	4.9
8	1	2.5	—	—	1	2.4
Total	40	100.0	20	100.0	41	100.0

[a]Two of the 42 women's responses were not recorded.

When we look at the number of women who reported beginning prenatal care by their fourth month of pregnancy, these numbers begin to change again. Fifty percent of the women who had never attended primary school stated that they had begun prenatal care by their fourth month of pregnancy, as compared to 70 percent of women with some years of formal education and 76 percent of women who had completed primary school.

When we look at the proportion of women who waited to begin prenatal care until quite late in their pregnancies (during their sixth, seventh, or eighth month), we see that these numbers, while more similar than those reported above, are still surprising. Among women with no formal education, those with some, and those with at least seven years, 12 percent, 15 percent, and 17 percent respectively waited until at least their sixth month of pregnancy to begin prenatal care. Since illiteracy is clearly not a factor accounting for these latter women's decisions to delay their prenatal care, we need to look for alternative explanations.

Barriers to Prenatal Care: Alternative Explanations

Previous researchers suggest that women's reluctance to participate in prenatal care, or at least their willingness to delay it, may be a result of their belief in the supernatural. In her study among Sukuma women living in the Mwanza Region in the 1960s, for example, Varkevisser noted that "traditionally," prenatal care among the Sukuma was heavily influenced by a belief in the supernatural (Varkevisser 1973; see also Lang and Lang 1973; Reid 1969). She also found that both literate and nonliterate Sukuma women were apt to keep their pregnancies a secret "in order not to attract the attention of malevolent sorcerers towards their vulnerable foetus" (Varkevisser 1973:109). Although I also found that an aura of secrecy surrounded women's pregnancies in Bulangwa and that many identified "supernatural forces" such as sorcery or the displeasure of ancestors as potential prenatal risks, a belief in the supernatural was not the *only* explanation for women's reluctance to begin prenatal care. As we see below, other factors influence women's decisions about whether to seek clinic-based care.

Codes of Public Modesty

Through my conversations with four Arab women who became pregnant during the course of my fieldwork I learned that Arab women were also reluctant to declare their pregnancies publicly. Although many in the Arab community acknowledge that sorcery may be used to harm a woman's pregnancy, fear was not the only reason these women preferred to keep their pregnancies secret. In addition to their stated happiness about being pregnant, all four of the pregnant women I spoke with expressed a sense of embarrassment as well, as if their pregnancies were public proof of their most recent sexual activity. Their embarrassment seemed to be related, in turn, to the understood codes of public modesty imposed by the Arab community on its women.

Even when they are not pregnant, Arab women as a whole were less likely to be seen outside of their homes in Bulangwa than were African women. It wasn't that they were overtly forbidden to be outside; the control was much more subtle. Most of the Arab women I knew well in the community claimed to feel more comfortable staying inside: that is how women show respect for themselves and for their families (*Ni heshima*). A woman would be talked about if she didn't adhere to these norms.[5] As noted already in chapter 6, the Arab population lived in the center of Bulangwa, and it was quite rare to see an Arab woman walking by herself outside of that central location. When they did walk about in the community, they were usually on their way to visit relatives four or five houses away or to morning or afternoon coffee with nearby Arab neighbors.

One young Arab woman who was pregnant for the second time told me she put off going to prenatal care because she felt embarrassed to walk to the clinic. The clinic was on the other side of the community, and to get there she had to walk down the main road in town, past several shops and many houses. Her concern was justified; an Arab woman walking alone through the middle of town would undoubtedly provoke a lot of speculation by people as to her final destination. Another woman, a friend who was seven and a half months pregnant with her eleventh pregnancy, cautioned me not to mention her pregnancy to her brother, my neighbor. "But he can see you are pregnant just by looking at you!" I responded in surprise. "Just don't tell him," she repeated. I later learned from her sister that this was typical of her behavior when pregnant in that she didn't tell certain family members. She hadn't, in fact, even mentioned this latest pregnancy to her sister.[6]

Quality of Care

In addition to codes of modesty, some women's unwillingness to begin prenatal care was an outcome of their negative expectations as to what those visits entailed. Some women complained about the treatment they received once they arrived at the government clinic in Bulangwa, with several mentioning the behavior of the MCH aid in particular. She was rude, they told me, and had often insulted them either when they arrived for their prenatal appointments or while they were giving birth. One woman, who had recently given birth, told me that she had been so worried that the MCH aid would be on duty when she went into labor that she avoided the clinic altogether and gave birth at home instead. On one occasion, I witnessed for myself this MCH aid's interaction with a woman who had just given birth. She was abusive to the woman, insulting her for crying out during labor and refusing to bring her water when the woman said she was thirsty.

When I mentioned women's comments about the MCH aid's behavior later to a friend who was a nurse assistant at the clinic, she told me that she and some of the other nurses had received similar complaints about her. They informed the head of the clinic, who, in turn, made some general comments at a staff meeting about treating patients better, but the MCH aid in question was never confronted directly.

Some men in the community also expressed dissatisfaction with the way pregnant women were treated at the clinic. One day while I was visiting a local healer, an older man who lived nearby saw me and came over to express his concerns about the care women received at the clinic. He wanted me to do something about some of the nurses who, he told me, often ignored women in labor, sometimes leaving them to give birth "even outside!" (*Hata nje!*). I had been living in the community for over a year by that time, and everyone knew that I was interested in women's experiences during pregnancy and childbirth. I told him that although I had no power to change things in the community, my interviews with women had uncovered similar problems. Perhaps after I had written my "book," I told him, the Ministry of Health would do something about it.

Another woman who recounted her experience at a clinic in a different community told me that women who obtained their prenatal care in nongovernment clinics risked being insulted by nurses if they later showed up at a government clinic to give birth. She had given birth at a government clinic in the middle of the night. When a different nurse came on duty in the morning and saw from her prenatal card that she had received her prenatal care at Kolondoto hospital, the nurse informed her that had she been on duty when the woman arrived in labor, she would have refused to assist with the birth and told her to go back to the mission hospital instead.

When I asked other women in my formal survey why they waited so long to begin prenatal care, they gave a variety of reasons. Some characterized their own delay in seeking prenatal care as "just laziness" (*Ni uvivu tu*). Others said they delayed their initial visit because they never experienced problems during their pregnancies (*Sipati matatizo*).

Then why bother to go to prenatal care at all? The sense I gained from my interviews as well as my observations of interactions between clinic staff and pregnant women is that many of those who delay starting prenatal care eventually do make a visit to a prenatal clinic. Their decision to finally begin prenatal care does not necessarily stem from any firm conviction that prenatal care in and of itself is in their best interests healthwise. Rather, their goal is getting a prenatal card. For some women, possession of the card appears to be an end in itself; it is the entry ticket to the maternity ward that ensures their admittance should complications arise during birth. In other words, women eventually register for prenatal care even if quite late in their pregnancies because of the risks they face if they do not—they may be insulted or hassled by nurses for not having a prenatal card or be turned away completely. We've already seen reference to this in chapter 7, in the case of the "traditional" birth attendant who delivered her grandchild at home. When her pregnant daughter arrived at a clinic in labor, she was turned away because she did not have a prenatal card in hand.

The Risk-Referral System in Bulangwa

In addition to eliciting women's perspectives on prenatal care, I was also interested in getting a sense of how the risk-referral system actually worked at the local level, and so during one of my first visits to the government clinic in Bulangwa, I asked the head of the clinic about the types of births clinic staff referred out of the clinic to higher-level medical facilities. Two days later he gave me a handwritten list in English that identified the kinds of births the clinic was not equipped to handle, as well as categories of pregnant women who are referred out of their clinic prior to beginning labor (see table 9.5). Theoretically, women who came to the clinic and were diagnosed with any of the conditions that appear in table 9.5 were then referred out to medical facilities better equipped to handle obstetric complications. Two hospitals served that function for pregnant women in Bulangwa: Kolondoto hospital, located about an hour's drive away, and the regional hospital in Shinyanga town, located about half an hour's drive beyond that.

Over the course of my stay in Bulangwa, I gradually learned that there were different levels of urgency in these referrals. Some referrals were not immediate, in that they were made in terms of a woman's future labor. For example, although a woman might be told that she could not give birth at the clinic because she fell within a particular risk category (e.g., more than six previous pregnancies, or shorter than 150 cm), she could nevertheless continue her prenatal care at the clinic until she went into labor. Other referrals had a more urgent quality. These were characterized by more immediate concerns, for example, vaginal bleeding during pregnancy, the absence of a fetal heartbeat, or signs of preeclampsia (swelling, proteinuria, or high blood pressure). Women who arrived at the government clinic with such symptoms were immediately referred out to one of the two hospitals mentioned above. This referring out requires that the woman, or her relatives who accompanied her to the clinic, find transportation.

But what actually happens once a referral is made? The action taken depends on several factors, including the urgency of the referral (is it a life-or-death situation?), the character of the relationship between the health-care provider and the person seeking treatment, and the extent to which the pregnant women and/or her family members believe she is indeed at risk. Some of these referrals work as they are intended, that is, a woman is

TABLE 9.5. List of Conditions for which Pregnant Women Were Referred Out of the Government Clinic in Bulangwa

1. Intrauterine fetal death[a]
2. Grand multipara (women who have already given birth six times)[b]
3. Malpresentation of the fetus[c]
4. Antepartum hemorrhage
5. Postpartum hemorrhage
6. Presence of operational scar[d]
7. Short stature (less than 150 cm)
8. Chronic illness (TB, asthma)
9. Swelling, proteinuria, and high blood pressure (indications of preeclampsia)
10. Early primigravida (first-time pregnancy in young girls less than 16 years of age)
11. Old primigravida (first-time pregnancy in women older than 30 years of age)
12. Retained placenta

[a]Death of the fetus in the womb. This is diagnosed primarily by an absence of fetal heartbeat during a prenatal examination. If no fetal heartbeats are detected, a women might be referred out to a hospital for a sonogram.

[b]The prenatal card distributed by the Ministry of Health sets this limit higher: eight rather than six previous pregnancies.

[c]Malpresentation in this case meant a transverse lie of the fetus in the womb. Breech births were not referred out of this clinic.

[d]This could be an indication of a previous cesarean section.

referred to a higher-level medical facility, travels there, and receives immediate treatment. My concern here, however, is with the opposite case: why
do some referrals go awry?

In some of the cases I was familiar with, referrals out of the clinic
worked contrary to the intentions stated in the *Safe Motherhood Strategy
for Tanzania*. With regard to the less urgent referrals—those made in terms
of a woman's future labor—many times this type of referral resulted in the
pregnant woman deciding to give birth at home or at the home of a local
midwife. There were a variety of reasons women gave for not heeding the
advice of clinic nurses that they birth in a hospital. Some women cited the
cost involved in hospital-based births. In relative terms, these costs were
often quite high, including the cost of transportation to the regional or
mission hospital, the cost of medicines or supplies needed during the
woman's hospital stay, as well as the cost of food for the woman and those
family members who accompanied her. Other women told me that they
birthed at home because they simply wanted to avoid the hassle that giving birth far from home entailed. Still others stated that they didn't believe
that they were really at any particular risk for complications. One such
woman noted that she had already given birth six times without any problems. She expected a similar outcome for her seventh birth.

I also gained insight into how the more urgent categories of referrals
can go awry. This latter category of referrals required immediate transport
to a higher-level medical facility and included women who had been
referred out of the local government clinic, those who had been referred
out of either of the two private clinics in the center of town, or those
women who experienced pregnancy or birth complications in the village
setting.[7] Sometimes I was directly involved in that I drove the woman and
her family members to the hospital. In some of those cases, the head of the
government clinic arrived at my home and asked me to drive women to the
hospital. Other times he or the clinic staff sent the woman's family members to ask for my help. And still other times people showed up on their
own and asked me for transportation to the hospital. There were times
when I was not involved directly at all; either I was present when an emergency unfolded, and others in the community provided the transportation,
or I heard about an emergency secondhand.

Although nurses sometimes tried to find transportation for women
they had referred out, at other times the risk-referral system resulted in
their simply washing their hands of a pregnant woman's case. In other
words, she was referred out of the clinic but left to deal with the problem,

that is, to find transportation, on her own or with the help of relatives. The story of one woman's experience in Bulangwa is illustrative of this latter type of referral.

Anna's Story: Miscarriage in the Marketplace

One morning toward the end of my stay in Bulangwa, as I was preparing to drive to Mwana Nyanzanga's village to finish up the last of my formal interviews with women, the owner of a local food establishment came to my home to tell me that a woman was in labor in the marketplace. I arrived there a couple of minutes later and found a young woman who looked vaguely familiar sitting on the ground behind the man's place of business. Initially, I saw no indication there was cause for concern. Since I had not been told otherwise, I assumed that she was in the early stages of normal labor and that her birth could be handled at the government clinic about a five-minute drive away. I told her relatives who were standing nearby that I could give them a ride to the clinic, but that I couldn't drive to Kolondoto hospital because of my prior commitments in a nearby village. They accepted my offer, and I walked back to my house to get my car.

When I returned about five minutes later, the young woman's relatives informed me they didn't want to go to the clinic after all. They had been there earlier, they explained, but the nurses told them to go to the hospital instead because the clinic was out of medicine. Apparently, while I had been off getting my car, someone else had agreed to drive them to the hospital, and they were just waiting for him to return with his car. Since the young woman didn't appear to be in hard labor and her relatives had assured me that transport was on its way, I decided to continue on to my prior commitment. But as I drove away, I wanted to be sure she was indeed okay. I stopped by one of the two private clinics located nearby and asked the medical aid on duty if he would come to the marketplace and check on the young woman himself. Although the clinic was packed with people and he was working alone, he agreed to come and assess the situation.

When we arrived back at the marketplace about fifteen minutes later, there was still no sign of the promised car. The young woman now looked in pain and was experiencing strong contractions. It was at that point that we learned she was only seven months pregnant. The medical aid told the woman's relatives to bring her to his clinic so he could examine her there. As he turned to walk back to work and I turned to bring my car closer to her, one of the three women standing near the pregnant woman called out "*Tayari!*" (It's finished!), indicating she had just given birth.

I felt horrified and frightened at the same time; I had never seen a miscarriage before and didn't know what to expect. I quickly ran to my car and grabbed a disposable birth kit.[8] In the meantime, the three women held up pieces of cloth (*khanga*) to block the view of curious onlookers.[9] I returned and handed the medical aid a pair of gloves (which he donned), a razor blade, and clamps for the umbilical cord. He cut the cord, but the placenta didn't come out immediately. After waiting about ten minutes, he inserted his hand into her uterus to remove the placenta manually. His manual removal of the placenta was followed a few minutes later by a large dried blood clot. He told the woman's family that she needed to be put on antibiotics, and so we transported her to his clinic where she could get the medicine and lie down to rest.

Anna's miscarriage filled me with a variety of conflicting emotions. To begin with, I felt horrible that she had suffered the indignity of miscarrying in the public arena of the marketplace. I also felt responsible because I had been quick to assume her labor was normal and so had left her sitting in the marketplace waiting for a ride that didn't come. But I also felt a sense of frustration that she had been referred out of the government clinic in the first place. Why had the nurses on duty refused to let her stay at the clinic and miscarry there? If they had first done a vaginal exam before referring her out of the clinic, they would have known she was very close to miscarrying and would have done so before reaching the hospital an hour's drive away.

I later learned that the young woman looked vaguely familiar because she had been one of the respondents in my formal survey the previous month. Her name was Anna, she was twenty years old, married, pregnant for the first time, and had started her prenatal care at the clinic during the third month of her pregnancy. She had also finished primary school and was a member of the Seventh-Day Adventist Church in the community. When I had interviewed her a month prior to her miscarriage, she had not been experiencing any problems with her pregnancy. Despite the fact that she had all the makings of what Varkevisser (1973) might refer to as a "modern mentality"—education, participation in an organized religion, stable marriage, appropriate age for a first pregnancy, early prenatal care—these indicators of her modernity did not prevent her from miscarrying in the public arena of the marketplace.

Anna's story raises other important questions. Had she really even arrived at the clinic, or had her family members decided not to take her because they expected that she would be told to go elsewhere? I don't know the answer to these questions as I didn't interview her or her family members afterward. The entire incident depressed me, and I couldn't bring myself to pursue it with them further.

When I discussed it with the medical aid later, he told me there were two main reasons he preferred not to handle emergency obstetric cases. First, in addition to being overworked, there wasn't enough space in the clinic to deliver babies.[10] Second, from his prior experience with medical emergencies, he has observed that once the emergency has been taken care of, people often do not return to pay for the services rendered. He only agreed to help with this particular woman's case, he told me, because he knew me and I had asked for his help.

Anna's story highlights another issue about pregnancy: the very real risk of miscarriage. As discussed in chapter 3, miscarriage can be caused by a variety of factors, such as episodes of high fever or malaria during pregnancy, or sexually transmitted infections that are left untreated. Miscarriage also emerged as the predominant prenatal concern in my formal interviews and informal conversations with women as well as in my observations of Mwana Nyanzanga's consultations with pregnant women.

Prenatal Care outside of the Biomedical Context

The Risk of Miscarriage

Women's descriptions of the causes and prevention of miscarriage were similar to their perspectives on fertility-related conditions discussed in chapter 8. That is, threatened or failed pregnancies, like infertility or impaired fertility, were spoken about in terms of physical and spiritual risks. *Mchango,* the displeasure of ancestral and nonancestral spirits, as well as the jealousy of disgruntled relatives, friends, and neighbors, were all seen as posing potential risks to a woman's pregnancy. As with the treatment of infertility, the prevention of miscarriage might involve the use of herbal or spiritual remedies, or both.

When I asked women in the formal survey whether they had ever used herbal remedies during their pregnancies, 57.3 percent ($n = 86$) of the 150 women whose answers were recorded stated that they had, with an almost equal representation of younger and older women (Mbura et al. 1985).[11] When I asked why they used such remedies, they gave a variety of responses (see table 9.6). "To prevent miscarriage" and "for *mchango*" account for at least half of all responses for younger and older women. The third most common response, "for stomach problems," accounted for an additional ten responses among younger women and five among the older women. Although I did not ask women who gave this particular response to clarify it further, it is quite possible that some were using it as euphemism for miscarriage, as this is also how some women refer to their labor pains.[12] "Stomach problems" is also how some women refer to their menstrual cramps, which are a symptom of *mchango*. A similar percentage of the older and younger women mentioned using herbal remedies for the first three categories combined: 69.2 and 70.7 percent, respectively. In other words, the primary use of herbal remedies during pregnancy among this particular group of women appears to be that of ensuring their pregnancy is successfully carried to term.

Two notable differences between the older and younger women's use of herbal remedies emerge for the categories listed as "Protection of mother/fetus" and "Had used fertility medicine." Although the data show that a larger percentage of older women (19.2 percent) than younger

TABLE 9.6.   Responses to the Survey Question "Why Did You Use Herbal Medicines during Pregnancy?" for the Subsets of Older and Younger Women (*N* = 84)

Reason	Older Women (*n* = 26)[a]		Younger Women (*n* = 58)	
	n	%	*n*	%
To prevent miscarriage[b]	7	26.9	16	27.6
For *mchango*[c]	6	23.1	15	25.9
For "stomach" problems	5	19.2	10	17.2
For protection of mother/fetus	5	19.2	7	12.1
Had used fertility medicine	—	—	6	10.3
For nausea	1	3.8	2	3.4
For general health	—	—	1	1.7
Pain medicine	1	3.8	1	1.7
To prevent spoilage of breastmilk	1	3.8	—	—
Total	26	100.0	58	100.0

[a]Although 28 older women stated that they had used herbal medicines during pregnancy, 1 of these women didn't know what it was for, while another wasn't asked.
[b]This includes women who had a history of miscarriage and those who did not.
[c]This includes the prevention and treatment of *mchango*.

women (12.1 percent) mentioned using herbal medicines to protect the health of the mother and fetus, none of the older women specifically tied their use of herbal medicines to their previous use of fertility medicines, as compared to six of the younger women who did.

Why such a discrepancy for this latter category of medicine? Through my observations of the work of local healers I learned that these two categories of medicines (those used for infertility and those used for the protection of the mother and fetus during a woman's pregnancy) are, in fact, related. Women who have used an herbal remedy to become pregnant must continue using it during their subsequent pregnancy to protect the health of the mother and fetus. It could be that the older women I interviewed were simply referring to the same type of medicine in a different way.

There also appears to be a generational difference in terms of women's personal experience with miscarriage: 46.8 percent ($n = 22$) of the forty-seven older women whose answers were recorded stated that they had experienced at least one miscarriage compared to 37.9 percent ($n = 39$) of 103 younger women. This difference makes sense as older women would have had a longer time to experience pregnancy. Older women did, in fact, report more total pregnancies than the younger women, 7.1 versus 5.6.

A brief discussion of the concept of miscarriage is warranted here. The Kiswahili term that conveys the concept of miscarriage is *kuharibika mimba*. The verb *kuharibika* literally means "to be ruined, to suffer loss of." *Mimba* is the Kiswahili word for pregnancy. My inquiries into women's experience of miscarriage were preceded by a series of questions about their pregnancy histories. I first asked women how many pregnancies they had had in their lifetime (*Umeshabeba mimba ngapi?*). Next I asked, "Of these pregnancies, how many did you birth well?" (*Mimba ngapi umezaa salama?*). This was followed by the question "*Mimba ngapi zimeharibika?*" which literally means "How many of these pregnancies were ruined?" Thus, rather than just listing the pregnancies they miscarried, some women also included stillbirths they had experienced. In other words, local definitions of miscarriage include any pregnancy that did not result in a live birth, regardless of the length of time a woman carried that particular pregnancy.

Nda Ya Gupinda Ngongo: Pregnancies That "Turn to the Back"

Women spoke about another risk during pregnancy whereby pregnancies are said to "turn to the back" or disappear, only to be returned, if at all, through the use of herbal or spiritual remedies. The sign that a pregnancy had indeed turned to the back was similar to that of a miscarriage, in that a woman may be several months pregnant and then experience vaginal bleeding. A change in a woman's menstrual flow might also be considered as a sign that her pregnancy had turned to the back. Ninety-nine percent ($n = 152$) of the 154 women in the formal survey said that they had heard of this condition—referred to in the Kisukuma dialect spoken in Shinyanga as *nda ya gupinda ngongo* and in Kiswahili as *mimba kurudi mgongoni*.[13] Several older women told me that this condition, which they characterized as being concocted by sorcerers, was more common in the past when there was no known cure. They noted that it has been on the decline in recent years because local healers had finally learned how to treat it successfully.[14]

I initially learned that pregnancies can turn to the back during my observations of Mwana Nyanzanga's healing practice. Out of sixty consultations I observed and recorded, five women were receiving treatment for pregnancies that had turned to the back. Three of these women had had four previous pregnancies, one had been pregnant seven times and had three living children, while another woman had had one previous pregnancy and one living child. One of the women with four previous pregnancies had been "carrying" her fifth pregnancy for the last three years. Of her four previous pregnancies, one ended in miscarriage, one child died, and two were still living.

Mwana Nyanzanga herself made distinctions between pregnancies that turned to the back and those that simply miscarried during the early months of pregnancy. She told me that although these two conditions may appear similar in that both involve vaginal bleeding, they are very different. Proof that a miscarriage had actually occurred, she patiently explained to me, was the presence of the expelled fetus. Although very small, it is quite distinguishable because it looks like a "small white bug" (*kadudu cheupe*); if the expelled fetus is a boy, this "small white bug" is long, and if the expelled fetus is a girl, the "bug" is short. When I asked how she could be certain that the fetus had not been expelled prior to her client's arrival at her home, she told me that there were other ways to verify whether a miscarriage had taken place. Sometimes she did a vaginal exam. If the door to the uterus (i.e., the cervix) was wide open, the woman had miscarried. If Mwana Nyanzanga could not insert even one finger into the door, the pregnancy was still inside. Additional proof that a woman had not miscarried, she told me, could be verified by using a hollowed-out gourd. She used it as one does a fetoscope by placing one end of the gourd on the woman's abdomen while at the same time listening through the small opening on the opposite end. If she could "hear the baby breathing inside" she knew that the woman was still pregnant.

Pregnancies were also said to move to the back in the absence of vaginal bleeding—that is, in the absence of menstruation. In such cases, women might not experience their menses for several months, and then all of a sudden begin menstruating again. Another sign that a woman's pregnancy had turned to the back, I was told, was a change in the duration of her menses. One older woman told me she had been diagnosed with a pregnancy that had turned to the back when her period, which normally lasted three days, suddenly changed to a duration of just one day.

But what makes pregnancies turn to the back in the first place? According to Varkevisser, women are active participants in bringing this condition upon themselves in that they make unwanted pregnancies "disappear" by using herbal remedies to "bring (the child) to the back" (*bugota kupindya ku ngongo*) (1973:103).[15] Kisseka (1973:55, cited in Kilbride and Kilbride 1990:110) acknowledges a similar concept in Uganda, whereby Baganda women "tie up" their unwanted pregnancies to make them "disappear on the back."

Women in Bulangwa, however, spoke about pregnancies that turned to the back or "disappeared" quite differently: as an unwanted condition women tried to rectify by visiting herbal or ritual specialists or both. Women experiencing this type of "pregnancy" were not spoken about as taking charge of an unwanted pregnancy, but as victims acted upon by jealous persons using sorcery or by displeased ancestral or nonancestral spirits. They were active participants in a different way in that they were actively seeking treatment to "return" this type of pregnancy to its proper place (Kleiner-Bossaller 1993).[16]

Only three of the 154 women I interviewed linked this condition to unwanted pregnancy specifically. One woman gave a definition similar to that described by Varkevisser and Kisseka above. She told me that in addition to being caused by sorcery, she had heard that pregnancies can be made to turn to the back by women who become pregnant while their husbands are away. She gave the specific example of women who become pregnant while their husbands are in jail. These women first drink a medicine to make the pregnancy disappear, she told me, and then another to make it "reappear" only after their husbands have returned home. The woman recounting this version to me, however, wasn't a permanent resident of the community. She came only occasionally to visit her husband who held a government position in the community. Furthermore, she wasn't Sukuma; she came from the southern part of Singida Region, which is southeast of Shinyanga.

The two other women who linked this condition to unwanted pregnancy were Sukuma women and permanent residents in the community. Both spoke about pregnancies that turn to the back as a consequence of an abortion gone awry, rather than as an abortion itself. One of these women gave me the specific example of her own mother who, upon learning that she was pregnant for the eighth time, tried to abort her one-month-old pregnancy. She told me that her mother had first mixed ashes with water in a gourd. After letting the concoction stand for a short period of time, she strained it and then drank the contents. Two days later, the woman told me, her mother started bleeding vaginally and thus assumed she had successfully aborted. She experienced a lot of pain for a month following the abortion. She finally went to a local healer, hoping he would be able to identify the specific cause of her pain. The healer diagnosed the pain as the result of her attempted abortion. Rather than aborting completely, he told her, the pregnancy had turned to the back instead. When I interviewed her daughter in 1994, it had been seven years since her mother's attempted abortion. She told me her mother had never menstruated again and was still experiencing a lot of pain. Moreover, she had spent the last seven years trying to find a healer whose medicine would successfully return her pregnancy to its proper place. Once it had returned, she would abort it using better medicine. Only then would her seven years of recurring health problems come to an end.

Two of the nurses I knew in Bulangwa also referred to *nda ya gupinda ngongo* as an unwanted condition. Although neither were Sukuma, they had worked in the area for many years and had either heard of or witnessed this condition themselves.[17] Both told me that the concept of pregnancies disappearing or turning to the back did not exist in either of their own ethnic groups. Instead, they perceived it to be a Sukuma phenomenon, or at least a phenomenon that existed in areas populated predominantly by Sukuma people.[18]

When I asked a Sukuma man who owned one of the two private clinics in Bulangwa if he had ever been approached by a woman or her family members to treat such a case, he told me that he had. In his analysis, however, a pregnancy that turned to the back was a sociopsychological condition that reflected the societal pressure exerted on women to bear children.

In his experience, women who had never given birth before, or those who had histories of miscarriages, seemed quicker than women with no prior history of fertility problems to define their missed menses as pregnancies. He had also noticed that this type of "pregnancy" was usually a woman's first or second pregnancy. According to his analysis, the stigma of infertility diminishes somewhat, or at least initially, if the woman is instead diagnosed with a pregnancy that had temporarily disappeared or turned to the back. He suggested that when I talk to women who had experienced this condition, I should specifically ask them *which* pregnancy had turned to the back. I thought his analysis was quite plausible, so I incorporated his suggestions into my formal questionnaire.

Overall, pregnancies that turn to the back were not a very common occurrence among the sample of women I interviewed. Only four of the younger women and five of the older women had experienced it themselves. One woman told me that she had been diagnosed with the condition but she had not believed the healer, while another woman thought she might have it, although she was not sure.[19] And contrary to what was suggested by the Sukuma man above, pregnancies that turned to the back were not necessarily a woman's first or second pregnancy. Three of the younger women who had had *nda ya gupinda ngongo* told me it had been their fourth, sixth, and eighth pregnancy, while four of the older women noted that it had been their fifth, seventh, and tenth pregnancy. There was also a variation in the length of time women carried these pregnancies. Two of the younger women told me they had carried the pregnancy for one to two years before finally giving birth, while four women (one younger woman and three older women) said they had been pregnant for a period of three to five years. One older woman, who appeared to be in her late sixties, told me that she had been pregnant for the last five years and from time to time she felt the pregnancy trying to return to its proper place. When it moves to the front, she told me, it sometimes stays there for a few weeks or even a few months, after which time she feels it returning ever so slowly to the small of her back again.

In May 1994, I decided to interview a few of the women who were currently receiving treatment at Mwana Nyanzanga's home. I used the same questionnaire that I had used in my formal interviews with 154 women. Over the course of the next few days I interviewed ten of her clients. Out of these ten women, two had been diagnosed with pregnancies that had turned to the back. Both were Sukuma women who lived in villages quite far away. One woman appeared to be in her early fifties. She told me it was her ninth pregnancy and that she had been carrying it for the past two years. It had turned to the back when she was five months pregnant. Prior to arriving at Mwana Nyanzanga's home, she had consulted with seven other healers, all of whom told her she had been bewitched. She had also sought treatment at a hospital for her condition, where she was told that her symptoms were related to the onset of menopause. Not quite convinced of this diagnosis, she decided to seek another opinion and ended up at Mwana Nyanzanga's home. I interviewed her the day she arrived. Mwana Nyanzanga had already seen her and had told her that she did, in fact, have a pregnancy that had turned to the back and that she should begin taking medicine to return it to its proper place. At the time of our interview, the woman still hadn't made a decision as to what she would do next.

The other person who had been diagnosed with this condition was a woman named Njile. She was twenty-two years of age, had completed primary school, and defined her religious affiliation as Roman Catholic. She had been pregnant twice before and both of these children, ages three and a half and two and a half years, were living. Her first child had been born at Kolondoto hospital, the second at a government clinic. She told me she eventually wanted a total of seven children. She also told me she been carrying this most recent pregnancy for a total of seventeen months. When she was eight months pregnant, she woke up one morning to find that her pregnancy had completely disappeared, leaving no trace at all: no blood, no miscarried fetus, nothing. She consulted two different healers, and both told her that she had been bewitched, although neither had identified the culprit. She used both of their medicines, but to no avail.

She sought treatment for her condition at Mwana Nyanzanga's home for the first time in December 1993. Both she and Mwana Nyanzanga told me that when she arrived for the first time there were no outward signs she was pregnant. I remembered having seen her at different times during the months preceding our May interview when she came for refills of her herbal medicine. She gave birth on May 4, 1994, two days after I interviewed her and five months after her initial consultation with Mwana Nyanzanga. When I visited her the day after the birth she appeared quite happy and told me that the birth had gone well. The baby appeared to be full term.

Two weeks later Njile's relatives brought her and the baby back to Mwana Nyanzanga's home. By coincidence I was also there when they arrived. Although the baby was fine, I was shocked by the dramatic change Njile had undergone in that short period. Something was definitely wrong. Whereas she had been happy and talkative two days after giving birth, when I saw her again fourteen days later, she was unable to communicate verbally at all. From time to time she would glance wild-eyed around her, and if asked a question, she would widen her eyes and raise her eyebrows to indicate that she had understood. Sometimes she would also make high-pitched short noises from the back of her throat, as if responding to the question put to her, but she couldn't speak. For want of a better description, she looked as if she were experiencing some type of severe postpartum psychosis. Everyone agreed her behavior was evidence of sorcery, most likely from the same person who had caused her pregnancy to turn to the back in the first place. No one thought her present condition had been caused by an ancestral spirit, because she had already carried out the required offerings. She stayed at Mwana Nyanzanga's home for three days, but when she didn't seem to be getting any better, her family members took her to another healer's home about a day's walk away. I later heard that her condition had improved slightly and that she would most likely stay at that healer's home with her now three-week-old child until she recovered.

When I asked women in the formal survey what caused pregnancies to turn to the back, they gave a variety of responses (see table 9.7). Most causes appear to be of a spiritual nature: sorcery, ancestral or nonancestral spirits, or even God. Only five women mentioned a physical cause, *mchango*. In addition, an equal and significant proportion of the younger and older women said that they didn't know the cause, 38.5 and 38.8 percent respectively. From these figures, it also appears that younger women are more likely to believe that sorcery figures significantly in pregnancies that turn to the back. But this statistic is misleading. It simply represents the percentage of women who told me that they had heard that it is caused by sorcery. They may not necessarily believe so themselves.

Although pregnancies that turn to the back appear to be rare among women in the community, the few cases discussed above suggest that this condition is not easily explained away simply by saying it is how infertile women account for their fertility problems in a society in which a woman's ability to bear children is highly valued. This type of analysis appears to be applicable in only some, but not all, of the cases we reviewed. In terms of Mwana Nyanzanga's clients who had been diagnosed with this condition, some had histories of miscarriage or had successfully carried a pregnancy to term but then had experienced the death of a child later on. But some had experienced several successful pregnancies. Even older women well beyond their reproductive years might be diagnosed with the condition. Some women who are diagnosed with this condition did not want to be pregnant at all, as in the case of the woman who had tried to abort, but found that her pregnancy had turned to the back instead. Which pregnancy turns to the back also appears to vary, as does the length of time a woman carries it. In other words, this particular prenatal condition does not occur in a uniform way. Whatever their manifestations, pregnancies that turn to the back, like miscarriages, are generally spoken about in terms of being a risk to a woman's successful pregnancy outcome.

Referrals Out of the Village Setting

Mwana Nyanzanga was not averse to referring pregnant women out to the hospital if she felt she was not able to treat their health problems. One such case involved a nineteen-year-old woman who had completed primary school several years earlier and who lived in the same village. She stopped at Mwana Nyanzanga's home one day with the intention of beginning prenatal care; she had felt something growing in her lower abdomen and had taken this as an indication she was pregnant. Upon examining her, however, Mwana Nyanzanga had serious doubts. Although something was

TABLE 9.7. Responses to the Survey Question "Why Do Pregnancies 'Turn to the Back'?" for the Subsets of of Older and Younger Women (*N* = 151)

Cause	Older Women (*n* = 49)		Younger Women (*n* = 102)	
	n	%	*n*	%
Sorcery	14	28.6	46	45.0
Ancestral or nonancestral spirit	3	6.1	10	9.8
Sorcery or ancestral spirit	4	8.2	—	—
God	2	4.1	2	2.0
Sorcery or God	1	2.0	—	—
Mchango	3	6.1	1	1.0
Sorcery, spirits, or *mchango*	—	—	1	1.0
Bad luck	—	—	1	1.0
Tried to abort	1	2.0	—	—
Doesn't believe it is possible	2	4.1	1	1.0
Doesn't know cause	19	38.8	40	39.2
Total	49	100.0	102	100.0

definitely there, she didn't think it was a pregnancy. It was too hard and it remained fixed when she palpated it, she explained to me, and then asked me for my opinion.[20] I agreed that the growth didn't seem to be a pregnancy and suggested that it might be a tumor of some kind instead.

Not knowing just how serious it could be, I offered to drive the woman to the hospital so she could be examined by someone there. Mwana Nyanzanga agreed, and all three of us drove to the hospital, about an hour and a half away. When we arrived at the hospital, the doctor verified Mwana Nyanzanga's initial suspicions: the woman wasn't pregnant at all. The growth was a fibroid tumor that would have to be removed by surgery. The young woman told him she couldn't afford the cost of an operation, so he agreed to try medication first. When I spoke to her a couple of months later, the tumor had already disappeared.

But not all of the women Mwana Nyanzanga referred to the hospital were treated well upon their arrival. I conclude this chapter with a case study of one of her pregnant clients who experienced a complication and for whom I provided emergency transportation to a hospital.

Milembe's Story: Intrauterine Fetal Death

I first met Milembe in January 1993 during my observations of prenatal consultations at Mwana Nyanzanga's home. During Milembe's prenatal visit, I learned she was five months pregnant, and that this particular pregnancy, her seventh, had turned to the back in September 1992, a condition for which she was currently receiving treatment. I subsequently learned that Milembe had never attended primary school and that she had three living children.

I met Milembe again a month and a half later during another of my visits to Mwana Nyanzanga's home. Mwana Nyanzanga was concerned as she had not heard the baby's heartbeat during Milembe's prenatal examination.[21] She asked to listen with the fetoscope I had brought along, which she did, and then I tried, but I couldn't hear a heartbeat either. After consulting with Milembe's husband, who had accompanied her that morning, we decided to drive her to Kolondoto hospital located an hour and a half away. Milembe's husband told us he would follow on his bike, as he would need it later to travel to his relatives and inform them that Milembe was in the hospital and ask for some financial assistance.

By the time we arrived at the hospital, I was feeling a bit panicked. Because of the urgency of the problem, I drove directly to the maternity ward, where I quickly explained the problem to the nurses on duty. I told them that although Milembe was approximately six and a half months pregnant, neither Mwana Nyanzanga, whom I introduced to them as a traditional birth attendant, nor I had been able to hear a fetal heartbeat when we examined her in the village. The nurses informed me that we had brought Milembe to the wrong place: all women with pregnancies less than twenty-eight weeks must first be seen at the maternal and child health (MCH) clinic located at the opposite end of the hospital.

One of the nurses then asked Milembe for her prenatal card. When Milembe told her she didn't have one, the nurse began scolding her, first for not having the card and then for wearing dirty clothes to the hospital. As Milembe seemed quite embarrassed by this latter comment, I explained that when she set out from her home that morning she hadn't known she would be coming to the hospital. She had only done so at our insistence; because of the urgency of the problem, we had left the village in a hurry. Would they at least listen for the baby's heartbeat, I asked, before we set off for the MCH clinic?

The nurses' reaction seemed to be a combination of amusement at my panicked state and irritation with my insistence, as if I should know better than to bring a woman without a prenatal card to them, and a woman in dirty clothes at that. Eventually the heartbeats were listened for; one nurse heard them, while another did not. The nurse in charge told us that Milembe must still go to the MCH clinic. If the nurses there didn't hear a fetal heartbeat, she told us, Milembe would then need to be examined by the doctor. If he also couldn't hear a heartbeat, he would refer her back to the maternity ward, where labor would be induced. Nothing could be done, we were told, until we went through the proper procedures. As we left the maternity ward, one of the nurses reminded Milembe that the next time she came to the hospital, she must bathe first.

When we arrived at the MCH clinic, one of the nurses on duty asked Milembe for her prenatal card. Milembe told her she didn't have one yet; her current problem arose before her first appointment.[22] Another nurse then began criticizing Milembe for arriving at the hospital in dirty clothes, telling her that the next time, she should wash before coming. She then asked Milembe how many months she was pregnant. Milembe explained to her that in total she was really eleven months pregnant because her pregnancy had disappeared for a short period during the previous year.

At this point Mwana Nyanzanga spoke up. Patiently she related the history of Milembe's pregnancy to the nurses, how Milembe had first become pregnant in April 1992, but the pregnancy had disappeared five months later in September. She told the nurses she began treating Milembe, and the pregnancy had reappeared almost immediately. One of the nurses regarded Mwana Nyanzanga with skepticism as she spoke, while another smirked at her version of the events. I found this entire inter-action quite painful to watch, as I was accustomed to observing Mwana Nyanzanga's work in the village setting where she was accorded much authority and respect for her skills as a healer. In the hospital setting, how-ever, surrounded by nurses wearing white uniforms and nurses' caps, Mwana Nyanzanga's status was reduced simply to that of "illiterate tradi-tional midwife." The nurses tried but neither heard a heartbeat. They informed Milembe that she would have to be seen by the doctor.

Upon examining Milembe about an hour later, the doctor told us he was almost certain that the fetus had died in utero, and labor would have to be induced. He wanted to be absolutely sure, however, and so he needed to do a sonogram first. Unfortunately, the person who had the key to the room in which the machine was kept had traveled to a town located a six-hour bus ride away and wouldn't return until the next day. He suggested that Milembe stay at the hospital for the night. He assured us that her sonogram would be done the next day. Milembe's husband then accom-panied her to the laboratory to have her blood drawn, a standard hospital procedure that would identify her blood type and whether she was anemic.

Mwana Nyanzanga and I met up with Milembe an hour later in the maternity ward, where she had just finished taking a shower. As we walked onto the ward, a nurse was accusing her of not washing well. In our absence Milembe had started having contractions, and the nurse told us that she thought Milembe would give birth during the night. We left her at the hospital, promising to return the next day. Her husband told us he planned to spend the night with relatives in Shinyanga town and would return the next morning also.

I stopped by the hospital the next day and learned that Milembe had given birth during the night. As expected, it was a stillbirth. She told me that she had had a lot of problems. The baby had been born in the breech position after many hours of labor. Although her husband had not yet returned, she expected him sometime that day.

Three days later, when I went to visit Mwana Nyanzanga at her home, I was surprised to find Milembe's husband there. He told me that Milembe was still in the hospital; the nurses had refused to discharge her because no one had paid her bill. Although her health was fine, she could-n't leave until her bill was paid, and he was having trouble finding money.

Moreover, the longer she stayed there, the more money she would have to pay. I offered to drive with him to the hospital and pay the bill.

As we approached the hospital a little over an hour later, we saw Milembe walking in the middle of a field, far away from the side of the road. She had "escaped" and was on her way home. She looked upset and told us that when the nurses refused to discharge her, she decided to leave when no one was looking. I told her we were actually on our way to pay the bill. She got in the car, and we continued on to the hospital together.

When we arrived back at the maternity ward, I asked one of the nurses for the bill. She wanted to know why I was paying it. Milembe's husband didn't have enough money at that moment, I explained, and so I was lending him some. She looked quite skeptical and asked, "Are you *sure* he really doesn't have the money?" I replied that he tried to get some financial assistance from several relatives, but to no avail. She then turned to him and asked him why he didn't have any money. He should plant crops, she told him, and harvest them so he could sell them and get money. He responded that he had planted crops that year, but if she knew how one could farm and get a good harvest without any rain, please tell him how and he would follow her advice.

I left to pay the bill. The total charges for four days at the hospital came to 3,900 shillings (U.S.$9.50). Upon my return to the ward, Milembe told me that she had never been given any of the medicine for which she had been charged, so I went back to the accountant and made him deduct 400 shillings from the remaining charges. I returned to the maternity ward again and asked the nurses if Milembe could have the results of the blood test for which she had been charged, but they told me that the results had been lost. By this time Milembe was quite anxious to leave; she told me she didn't want to wait to have more blood drawn, and so we just left.

During the twenty-two months of my fieldwork I had ample opportunity to observe interactions between patients, their family members, and hospital staff. It soon became clear that different categories of people were treated differently. People who appeared educated, or those who were assumed to have wealth, such as the Arab members of the community or myself, received better treatment. Those without these symbols of modernity or who didn't know the proper way to behave in the modern setting of the hospital or clinic encountered many problems. Even though they had physically arrived at the hospital, they still did not have access to its resources (or to a limited extent only). They often had no negotiating power at all and, as illustrated so vividly in Milembe's story, were often scolded and assumed to be ignorant. Nurses, on the other hand, garbed in their white uniforms and nurses' caps, served as the representatives of modernity and functioned as gatekeepers who decided who would be admitted hassle-free to the maternity ward.

Risk and Prenatal Care

Our examination of women's prenatal concerns indicates that many pregnant women seek biomedical and nonbiomedical forms of prenatal care simultaneously. A closer look at the reasons why reveals that these various options are responding to different perspectives on maternal health risk. In the biomedical approach to prenatal care the risks *of* motherhood are stressed. This approach, also known as the risk approach to maternal health, is geared toward identifying and responding to a host of very real life-threatening complications that can arise once a woman becomes pregnant. In contrast, the nonbiomedical forms of prenatal care that women sought in Bulangwa were addressing women's concerns with risks *to* motherhood, that is, with conditions that prevented them from carrying a pregnancy successfully to term, such as secondary infertility and miscarriage. Although some of the health development literature suggests that women's use of traditional medicine is a direct result of their belief in the supernatural, our examination of women's concerns with the risk of unsuccessful fertility reveals that most of those locally recognized conditions are spoken about in terms of physical rather than supernatural causes.

Our examination of women's prenatal concerns also highlights some of the unofficial risks associated with biomedical care: the harsh treatment some women are subjected to in clinic and hospital settings. Although not everyone I spoke with complained about the treatment they received—some women, in fact, told me they were treated very well—complaints were, nevertheless, common. In other words, Varkevisser's statement at the beginning of this chapter that "the success of [the clinic's] services . . . ingratiated the clinic to the population" does not appear to hold true thirty years later in another rural setting to the south.

CHAPTER 10

Risks during Childbirth

Kaya nogu, ng'wana nambu.
It is easy to marry, but difficult to give birth.
—Sukuma proverb[1]

The meaning conveyed in the Sukuma proverb above is ambiguous. Should it be understood in a general sense, as in it is "difficult to give birth" due to the risk of infertility and miscarriage, or that it is literally "difficult to give birth," due to the dangers inherent in the actual experience of childbirth itself? In this chapter we address the latter of these two interpretations and, in doing so, focus our attention on births that take place on the labor ward in the hospital setting and at Mwana Nyanzanga's home in the village setting. Three aspects of childbirth will be examined: how labor and birth are managed, what happens when complications arise, and how the birthing woman is treated throughout the whole process.

The Proper Way to Give Birth

One of the things that struck me most about the majority of births I observed in Tanzania was the overall stoicism of the birthing women. Although childbirth in no way appeared to be pain-free, it nevertheless was not characterized by a lot of noise. Very rarely did a woman yell out loudly in pain, and if she did, she was quickly admonished either by midwives or nurse assistants on the labor ward or by Mwana Nyanzanga in the village setting.

When, upon finishing my fieldwork and returning to the States, I discussed the stoic nature of the births I had observed with a Tanzanian woman I knew, she spoke about such stoicism as if it were an inherent quality of rural women. She admired those women, she told me, because even in the face of their harsh living conditions, they persevered, especially during childbirth. These were qualities she felt she wouldn't be able to exhibit were she to live in a similar environment. Another Tanzanian woman I knew, who lived in Australia but was visiting relatives in Dar es Salaam when I met her in 1992, also spoke about women's stoicism during birth as a trait to be admired. She recounted her own experience of giving birth in an Australian hospital: "I gave birth like an *African* woman!" she told me, her voice filled with pride. She noted that her ability to remain relatively quiet throughout labor and during the actual birth was met with surprise, but admiration, by the Australian nurses attending her.

Women living in Bulangwa were also of the opinion that a woman should be stoic during childbirth—it was the proper way to behave. Never having given birth myself, many of my first conversations with women about childbirth focused on whether the whole process was painful. All assured me that it definitely was. Well, then, how were they able to keep from crying out? I would ask, adding in the same breath that were I to give birth some day, I didn't think I would be able to keep quiet. In fact, I often told them, I would probably yell rather loudly. After assuring me that "of course" I would give birth some day, and then joking they would enjoy seeing the spectacle of my giving birth and "threatening" to chastise and hit me if I cried out, they gave several reasons why a woman must remain calm during labor (see Sargent 1982). Some women explained that crying during labor was *aibu,* a shameful way to behave. One older woman noted that it was bad to call out and cry during labor because if people heard you, they would think you were having problems. Another common explanation was that a calm demeanor during labor prevented harm to the baby. Still other women would scoff at the idea of yelling out during labor, noting that the woman had "enjoyed" herself during the baby's conception, so why should she cry about it now?

The Proper Way to Manage Birth

My experience as a lay midwifery trainee in El Paso, Texas, initially constituted for me the norm against which I evaluated the births I observed in Tanzania. As a result of that five-month training, I had come to view certain features of labor and birth management as essential: regular monitoring of the pregnant woman's vital signs during and after labor and of the baby's before and after birth, combined with positive reinforcement and encouragement of the birthing woman's efforts throughout. These latter aspects of birth management were not always evident during the births I observed in Tanzania, which became the major reason many of my initial reactions were negative.

Although there were some differences between the births I observed in El Paso and Tanzania, there were also similarities. Births in both contexts were managed almost exclusively by women. In the El Paso clinic, the midwives and the midwifery trainees were all female. The only men present were the few who had accompanied their wives or girlfriends. In the hospital setting in Tanzania, female midwives, nurses, and nurse assistants were the ones primarily responsible for managing births. Obstetricians, all of whom were male, were called only if complications arose and some type of intervention was needed, such as to turn the child manually in the womb or to assess whether a cesarean section was warranted. The only other men who entered the labor ward were hospital personnel;[2] husbands were not allowed.[3] Nor were any men present at the births I observed in the village setting, as Mwana Nyanzanga strictly forbade men to enter her "hospital" during a woman's labor.

But births that are managed exclusively by women are not necessarily devoid of tensions and power struggles. In this chapter, we examine some of the reasons why they are not. In the next section, we turn our attention to births that take place on a hospital labor ward.[4]

Childbirth in the Hospital Setting

Overall there appears to be a consistent lack of attention to the laboring women on the maternity ward of the government hospital. And it isn't always because the nurses are overworked. I've observed births where at least five nurses are sitting around a table laughing and joking and virtually ignoring the laboring woman, maybe once or twice calling out to her to quit crying and making so much noise.

There is also a lot of delay in treatment. . . . One day a woman who was seven months pregnant was brought in with eclampsia. Her face, hands, and feet were incredibly swollen. She was unconscious and having seizures due to an elevated blood pressure 240/140. (Normal is around 120/80.) No one seemed to know what to do and it took the doctor forever to arrive. They kept injecting her with Valium and then later at night tried to induce labor, which due to the heavy doses of Valium, never started. She died 12 hours after arriving at the hospital.

One young woman, who had a very small pelvis and had been staying in the prenatal ward for a month prior to her expected due date to await a cesarean section, finally went into labor. Her family, however, had not bought the required two liters of a saline solution needed to set up an intravenous drip (IV). As a result, the doctor couldn't perform the operation. The hospital supposedly has no supplies and patients have to come with everything, including IV drips if surgery is required. In the case of this particular young woman, her relatives had come a week before and had been told to bring the needed supplies. They never returned, so she was stranded without any family members to help her. The cost of the IV is 3,000 shillings (minimum wage is 5,000 shillings per month) so it is quite expensive. She was in hard labor but there wasn't going to be any operation. They were just going to let her go through it, which might have meant her death or the baby's. I kept thinking that the doctors would do something, but nobody did. I finally offered to pay for the drip. But even after getting that, there was still a delay because there was only one stretcher in the entire hospital and it was being used. I was so frustrated and kept asking the nurses what was going to happen, until finally someone went and got a wheelchair.

—Letter from the field, October 26, 1992, Shinyanga, Tanzania

The maternity ward of the regional hospital in Shinyanga town was a U-shaped building consisting of four smaller wards: the prenatal ward, the labor ward, the intensive care unit, and the postlabor ward. The prenatal ward and the postlabor ward formed the two sides of the U. The labor ward and the intensive care unit joined both sides at the middle.

The Prenatal Ward.   Women who experienced complications after their twenty-eighth week of pregnancy were hospitalized in the prenatal ward (seventeen beds). Reasons for prelabor hospitalization might include bleeding during the third trimester of pregnancy, a previous cesarean section, an anticipated difficult labor due to a woman's short stature or contracted pelvis, or the expected birth of twins. Some of the women pregnant with twins were admitted after their thirty-second week of pregnancy and stayed there until they delivered.

Labor Ward.   A total of six nurse-midwives were employed on the labor ward (three beds). Two worked on the day shift, two on the evening shift, and one at night. Nurse assistants and the occasional nursing student also made up the labor ward staff. An overall in-charge nurse was also assigned to each shift.

Intensive Care Unit. Women with severe pregnancy or birth complications were hospitalized in this small unit (three beds). Women who had cesarean sections also stayed here for three to five days before moving to the postlabor ward. The average hospital stay for women who birthed by cesarean section was two weeks.

Postlabor Ward. After giving birth, women walked through the intensive care unit to the postlabor ward (sixteen beds). Women who gave birth before midnight were discharged out of the postlabor ward the next morning. Those giving birth after midnight were not discharged until the morning of the following day, although if no complications arose, they might be discharged earlier. Two small rooms for premature infants were located at the far end of the postlabor ward. Nurses assigned to the postlabor ward were also responsible for keeping bottles of hot water wrapped in cloth next to the premature infants in the bassinets to keep them warm.

Labor and Birth Observations

When I first began observing births at the regional hospital in September 1992, I was struck by its overall appearance. Although the nurses mopped the floors every morning, it never appeared to be very clean. Most of the mattresses and stretchers in all four wards were bloodstained. Screens were missing from most of the windows, a factor that accounted for the large number of flies and mosquitoes seen in the ward at any given time. Toilet facilities were also limited. Although the actual toilets were located in an adjacent building, there was a small room just off the labor ward that served as a combination toilet/shower. Basically this "facility" was a small room with a concrete floor. A small drainage hole in the corner of the room allowed the water to flow outside. During the three-week period that I observed in the maternity ward, I occasionally saw some of the patients use it as a shower facility. There were no curtains on the windows, so anyone walking by might see a woman bathing or squatting to urinate. The nurses also used this combination shower/toilet to discard bloody water after cleaning the utensils used during the births. In short, the risk of acquiring an infection on the maternity ward seemed ever-present.

From September to October 1992 I observed twenty-one births on the labor ward, after which I decided not to observe any more. Several factors contributed to my decision. First, I was quite disturbed by the hostility some of the nursing staff directed toward the birthing women and by what appeared to be a high level of mismanagement. Although I felt that it wasn't my place to intervene, sitting and observing such births was nevertheless upsetting. A few of the midwives were particularly abusive to women during labor, often yelling at them to stop crying and sometimes slapping them on the legs if they tried to sit in an upright position or raise their hips off the birthing table. Labor coaching as such did not exist. When a woman was coached, it was often from a seated position several feet away and consisted of the midwife or nurse assistants telling her to lie flat on her back, or to quit crying and making so much noise. I also did not see much consistent monitoring of either the woman's blood pressure during labor, cervical dilation, or fetal heart tones, all which I had come to expect as essential aspects of labor and birth management during my brief lay midwifery training in El Paso. Second, I didn't know how to write about it other than negatively. Scattered throughout the notes I took during those births are repeated references to how disturbed I felt observing the harsh treatment women were subjected to and notes to myself wondering if the births attended by traditional midwives in the village setting would be any different.

Although many of the women whose births I observed were treated in a hostile manner, I was not. I was the guest (*mgeni*), and guests, whether African, European, or American, are generally treated with respect in Tanzania. Most of the nursing staff were very nice to me and incredibly patient with my endless questions. But I was also an oddity. Although there were other "Europeans" (*wazungu*) living in Shinyanga town, I suspected that many of the nurses did not have many opportunities to ask a "European" woman personal questions.[5] The attention directed toward me while I was observing on the labor ward actually posed quite a dilemma, as sometimes the nurses on duty seemed more interested in me than the woman in labor, often ignoring her pleas for help because they were busy asking me questions about myself and my life in America.[6]

The period immediately following birth was also quite different from my experience in El Paso, in that neither the woman nor her newborn infant received much attention from the nurses. Immediately after the umbilical cord was cut, the baby was wrapped in a piece of cloth (*khanga*) and placed on a nearby bed. No postpartum assessments of its heartbeat or respiration were conducted.[7] As soon as the placenta was delivered, the new mother would climb down off the birthing table (oftentimes unassisted), secure a piece of *khanga* between her legs to stanch the blood flow, and walk to the postpartum ward unaided.

In the following passage I present an excerpt from the notes I made while observing the last hour of a young woman's labor. She was eighteen years old, giving birth for the second time. Her first child had died.

10:25   The woman is standing and pushing. She is alone and leaning on the bed.

10:45   Sitting on top of the metal bed in a squatting position. At one point the nurse tells her to lie correctly. No one has monitored her blood pressure or the fetal heartbeats in the past hour.

10:50   Lying on her side and wanting to push. Five nurses are sitting at a table twenty feet away. One of them calls over to her not to push and to lie right (*Kaa vizuri!*)

10:51   Another nurse calls out instructions to her on how she should lie on the table.

10:52   A nurse goes over to bed and listens to the fetal heartbeat for a few seconds. The woman is lying flat on her back, holding her ankles and pushing.

10:53   Flat on her back, legs down.

10:55   Alone and pushing while lying on her back. A nurse calls out to her: "Lie right! You, young girl, lie right!" (*Lala vizuri! Wewe msichana, lala vizuri!*)

10:58   [Still calling out from the table] "Grab your ankles. Don't push!" (*Shika miguu. Usisukume!*) A different nurse walks by and says in English "Who is crying here?" as the young girl lies whimpering on the bed. She seems to want to give birth while lying on her side, holding her right leg up.

11:02   A nurse brings her tea to "give her strength."

11:07   She sits up to push and is told to lie down.

11:10   Nurse from the table points her finger and scolds her, "You!" (*Wewe!*)

11:11   A small bit of the baby's head begins to show. A nurse looks around for gloves and then walks over to the birthing table. The head comes out, doesn't rotate and turns blue. The nurse rotates the head herself. Another nurse hits the young woman on the legs because she is lifting her bottom off the table.

11:12   Baby born and cries immediately. The young mother is whimpering and is scolded not to cry.

11:15   Cord cut and tied. A nurse suctions mucus out of baby's mouth using a machine operated by a footpedal.

11:16   Baby is weighed: 3.550 kilograms.

11:17   Baby is wrapped in a *khanga* and set on a nearby bed.

11:20   Woman is given an injection of ergometrine as the placenta begins to come out.

11:21   Placenta is out and is immediately dropped into a nearby bucket without being checked to see if any pieces are missing.[8]

11:23   A nurse is wiping the blood off of the woman's legs with a dirty cloth and water. Another *khanga* is folded and placed between the woman's legs.

11:26   The new mother is up off the bed.

11:28   She is having a hard time walking. Bent over in pain. Having to carry own bags at first. It looks like she might faint. Nurse sees blood trickling down her leg and scolds her for not tying the cloth right. One nurse takes her bag, another takes the baby, and they walk ahead of her into the post-natal ward.

Throughout the last hour of this woman's labor, the nurses rarely approached her, and verbal interaction consisted mainly of commands given in harsh tones. During the last thirty-five minutes of her labor, she was pushing but no nurse checked to see if she was actually close to birthing. Ten minutes before she gave birth, a nurse scolded her, telling her not to push. The birth happened "unexpectedly," and the baby's head started to come out before the nurse had even put her gloves on. Unexpected births were actually quite common. Due to the shortage of gloves, nurses do not conduct many vaginal exams to assess how close an impending birth is. On one of the days that I observed, four births happened "suddenly," within a period of eighteen minutes, two taking place on the floor. Both of these women had told the nurses they felt the urge to push, but their own analyses were not taken seriously, and no vaginal exams were done.

Not everyone on the nursing staff exhibited hostility toward the birthing women. In fact, some of the nurses or nurse assistants appeared to be just as upset as I was by how women were treated or how a birth was mismanaged. One such case involved a woman who had given birth to the first of her twins at 7:30 in the morning. The second, however, couldn't be delivered vaginally because it was lying crosswise in her uterus. The obstetrician on duty had examined her a half hour after she gave birth to the first twin. Due to a power outage in town, there was no electricity at the hospital. She was kept in the ward for two more hours, waiting to be taken to the operating room for a cesarean section. During that entire time she was moaning and calling out to the nurses to help her. Some simply ignored her, while others tried to explain that the doctor couldn't perform a cesarean because there was no electricity. One of the nurse assistants became quite concerned about the woman's slow but continuous blood loss, and so she went to look for the doctor again to inform him the woman was still bleeding. When she arrived at his office (she recounted to us upon her return), he became angry and yelled at her, "How am I supposed to do it [the surgery]?" (*Nitafanyaje?*). Apparently, he was as stressed as everyone else about the delay.

On a different day, this same nurse assistant appeared quite disturbed by how one of the midwives was handling another woman's birth of twins. The first twin was born breech at 1:04 in the afternoon. It came feetfirst, and the head was finally delivered four minutes later. The second twin was still high up in the womb. The woman was quite weak, and a nurse brought her a cup of tea to "give her strength." After nearly twenty minutes had passed, the midwife attending the birth became irritated with the woman for "taking so long" to birth the second twin, as we can see in the following excerpt from my fieldnotes:

1:23   "Are you pushing or are you playing?" (*Unasukuma au unacheza?*) She begins mocking how the woman is pushing.

1:24   It looks like the woman has a bad tear. The midwife does a vaginal exam and states the head is close. [I make a note that she has inserted her whole hand into the woman's vagina, which means the head couldn't be *that* close.]

1:32   The woman is bleeding.

1:34   The woman looks exhausted. Another nurse goes to her side and talks to her.

1:36   The midwife attending the birth walks away to check the first twin who is lying on a nearby bed. The nurse assistant sitting next to me at the table looks visibly upset, looks over at me and shakes her head. She then suggests to the midwife that the woman be given more tea.

1:38   The midwife instructs the nurse assistant to listen for the baby's heartbeat. The midwife then turns to the woman and says, "And me, I'm tired of standing!" (*Na mimi, nimechoka kusimama!*)

1:40   The midwife sits down at a nearby table. The nurse assistant tells the midwife that she can hear the baby's heartbeat.

1:44   The midwife begins scolding the woman for not drinking tea, and tells her again that she is tired of standing.

1:46   Woman is lying on her side and drinking tea.

1:56   Woman begins pushing again.

2:04   Second twin is born.

Fifteen months later, in January 1994, I accompanied an Arab friend of mine who was pregnant and who lived in Shinyanga town to that same maternity ward when her labor started. I hadn't observed a birth there for over a year and was pleasantly surprised at the maternity ward's new appearance: a fresh coat of paint and new screens on the windows. Hadija (my friend) and I arrived at the maternity ward at 1:30 P.M. Two and a half hours later she gave birth to a baby girl weighing 3.7 kilograms. When I returned three hours later with some of her family members, another woman was in labor. The nurses were sitting around a nearby table just talking to each other and ignoring the woman who was lying on the birthing table.

On my return to the hospital with Hadija's family, I had brought a video camera to videotape Hadija and her newborn baby. I hoped to shoot some video footage of the maternity ward, so I asked the nurses for permission to videotape the labor room. When I returned with my camera, they immediately stood up and began attaching their nurses' caps to their heads. One made the comment that she didn't want people "in Europe" to think she wasn't doing her job. She walked over to the pregnant woman lying on the birthing table and began diligently listening to the fetal heartbeats, pressing the aluminum fetoscope to the woman's belly. She also began rubbing the laboring woman's back, as I had done during Hadija's labor several hours earlier, although I had never seen this particular nurse do this during my observations on the ward a year earlier. Another nurse took a bag of IV solution over to the woman and began acting as if she were inserting the needle into the laboring woman's arm, as a third nurse brought the metal IV stand over. As soon as I finished videotaping and turned the camera off, they went back to the table and sat down, leaving the woman in labor alone once again.

The next morning when I drove Hadija home, I asked her how she had been treated during the night. Although she had been treated fine, she told me, some of the other women on the postlabor ward cried out all night and had been largely ignored by the nurse on duty. One woman had called out repeatedly to the nurse that her baby's umbilical cord was bleeding. According to Hadija, the nurse scolded her for making so much noise. Hadija asked the nurse why she wasn't helping the woman; the nurse eventually did.

As Hadija's experience suggests, not all of the births that take place in a hospital maternity ward are characterized by harsh treatment and mismanagement. One factor accounting for the difference in how birthing women are treated is the social or economic class of the birthing woman. For example, I observed two Arab women's births during my fieldwork, and neither woman was treated harshly by nurses. African women of high social standing or economic class were also treated better. The atmosphere on the labor ward was less hostile when nurses knew the birthing woman personally, either as friend, neighbor or relative. There also appeared to be a difference in how some of the newer nursing staff treated the birthing women. Overall, nursing students and the newly employed nurse assistants treated women more kindly.

Other evaluations of women's birth experiences in African settings have noted similar tensions between health-care providers and their clients, tensions that some attribute to local factors such as poor working conditions and low salaries (Fonn et al. 1998; Laakso and Agnarsson 1997; Okafor and Rizzuto 1994; see also Ruck 1996), as well as to internationally imposed economic policies that have had a negative impact on the health sector (Bassett et al. 1997; Harrison 1996; Turshen 1999). Although some might argue that poor working conditions do not justify the harsh treatment some nurses mete out to their birthing clients, it should be recognized that health-care workers themselves are experiencing stress. As Sargent and Rawlins (1991:186) have noted regarding factors that influence the quality of prenatal care in a Jamaican setting: "Until such time as nurses receive adequate remuneration and are supplied with necessary working materials . . . strained relations between staff and clients will prevail."

Childbirth in the Village Setting

In November 1992, I moved to the community of Bulangwa. During my first week there, one of the local government officials told me about Mwana Nyanzanga, a traditional birth attendant who lived in a nearby village and assisted with a lot of births in the area. A week later, I drove to her home and met her for the first time. After introducing myself and explaining that I had come to Tanzania to learn about women's birthing experiences, I asked if I could observe her work. She readily agreed. By the time I observed my first birth at her home three weeks later, I had already spent much time observing her prenatal appointments and talking to her about her work.

Once I began observing births at her home, I soon realized that there were some general similarities in how births were managed on the labor ward in Shinyanga town and her own style of birth management: (1) women were expected to bring their prenatal cards with them; (2) most of the women gave birth lying flat on their backs; (3) women who called out or cried during labor were admonished to keep quiet; and (4) the baby was separated from the mother immediately after birth. Let us look at each of these in more detail.

The Prenatal Card

Similar to what I had observed in the hospital setting, many of Mwana Nyanzanga's clients showed up with their prenatal card in hand. I first became aware of this during my observations of her prenatal consultations. Sometimes her clients would enter her consultation room and hand their prenatal card to me, although I hadn't asked to see it. (I later realized that she was telling them to do this.) Although Mwana Nyanzanga didn't demand to see the prenatal card of every woman she examined, I once saw her turn away a woman who arrived without one. Although the woman looked to be around nine months pregnant, Mwana Nyanzanga refused to examine her, telling her to go to the clinic instead. When I asked her about this later, she explained the reason for her refusal: she hadn't met the woman before, nor did she know anything about her previous birth history. She also didn't know anything about the woman's family members and so couldn't attest to their "character." Most of her clients were women who had been recommended through previous clients, either their immediate family members, in-laws, friends, or neighbors. In this particular woman's case, there were no such connections. As a result, Mwana Nyanzanga had no way of knowing whether she or her relatives would pay for the services rendered. Nor did she know how they would react if complications arose during the woman's birth.

The Birth Position

As with the births that took place on the labor ward, most of Mwana Nyanzanga's clients gave birth lying flat on their backs, a position she jokingly referred to as "giving birth the European way" (*kuzaa kizungu*). She contrasted this with how women gave birth "a long time ago": sitting upright on an animal skin, their back against the wall.[9]

Several of the older women I met during my fieldwork offered similar descriptions, usually without any prompting on my part. One such occasion occurred during a group interview I was conducting with women who lived in Mwana Nyanzanga's village. We had been talking about pregnancy-related issues, when an older woman who appeared to be in her early seventies suddenly stood up and asked if I wanted to see how women gave birth "a long time ago." Accompanied by peals of laughter and encouragement from the other women present, she proceeded to show me. She sat on the ground, put her back against the wall of the house we were sitting next to, and with her knees bent halfway to her chest, began "pushing."

Labor Coaching

There were similar expectations as to how women should behave when giving birth in the hospital or village settings. In both contexts, women were admonished if they made "too much noise" or if they moved around when it was time to push. Although the births I observed at Mwana Nyanzanga's home took place in a significantly less hostile environment, she nevertheless insisted that her clients remain calm during labor.

One day, after observing a birth in which she had scolded the woman throughout and had threatened to hit her at one point, I asked if she had been angry. "Eh," she replied, "You saw what she was doing with her legs [the young woman had tried to close her legs when it came time to push], so I told her 'I'm going to hit you!'" "But why?" I asked. "She could have hurt the child!" she explained, in a tone that implied the danger inherent in that type of behavior was obvious. "Have you ever actually hit a woman during birth?" I asked. "Yes, I hit them," she replied, and then gave her reasons for doing so.

Women came to her in order to be helped during labor, she explained. If she allowed them to cry and move around, the birth might turn out badly and could result in the death of the infant. And if that happened, she asked me, who would be willing to pay a cow? (She was paid a cow if an infertile woman used her medicine, became pregnant, and birthed successfully.) Although she had a reputation for being stern during a woman's birth, she continued, people came anyway because they knew they would birth successfully. When she threatened to hit a woman, she explained, the woman usually quieted down, which allowed the birth to proceed without further problems.

She then chuckled and recounted the story of one of her clients, a woman who lived in a different village and who had already had four stillbirths before Mwana Nyanzanga met her for the first time. People attributed the cause of those stillbirths to the woman herself: she apparently always cried out during labor and never lay still when it came time to push. When she became pregnant a fifth time, a neighbor suggested to the woman's mother that she take her daughter to Mwana Nyanzanga, who had a reputation for being able to handle such cases.

The woman took her neighbor's advice and brought her daughter to Mwana Nyanzanga's home when the time for delivery drew near. Sure enough, according to Mwana Nyanzanga, when her labor began, the woman cried out a lot and wouldn't push when she was supposed to. The woman's mother—whom Mwana Nyanzanga described as a fool (*Mama yake, alikuwa mjinga, kweli!*)—was also in the room and became distressed at her daughter's cries. When Mwana Nyanzanga saw that birth was imminent, she sent the mother on an errand to get rid of her. As soon as the mother left, Mwana Nyanzanga picked up a heavy stick she had placed earlier in a corner, held it over her head, and threatened to "kill" the woman if she didn't shut up and concentrate on pushing. "It's only you and me now," she supposedly told the woman. "When your mother returns, she will simply think that you died while giving birth." Her strategy apparently worked. By the time her mother returned, the woman had given birth to a boy. Mwana Nyanzanga proudly noted that the boy is still alive today, and the woman has become a regular client.

Care of the Newborn

Babies born at Mwana Nyanzanga's home were immediately wrapped in a *khanga,* placed apart from the mother, and not monitored for vital signs. Once wrapped, the infant was placed on a bed in a separate room and left alone until its mother joined it later.

The Management of Labor and Birth

Heat figured significantly in Mwana Nyanzanga's management of a woman's labor. During the early stages of labor, she often sent her pregnant clients to sit outside in the sun. When I asked why, she explained that the sun's heat stimulated a woman's contractions and kept them coming at regular intervals. She gave similar reasons for giving women hot herbal remedies to drink during labor: the combination of hot water and ground herbs ensured the progression of labor. Cool liquids, in contrast, were avoided at all costs because they would cool the contractions and stall the labor unnecessarily.

The hot herbal remedies Mwana Nyanzanga gave her clients to drink during labor fell into three main categories and were administered depending on the specifics of a particular case. She might, for example, give a woman something to change the position of the child in the womb. She explained that this remedy brought on contractions, the strength of which changed the position of the child in the womb. In cases where she felt the labor was progressing too slowly, she might give the woman something to speed it up. A third category of remedy ensured the normal progression of labor. This latter category of herbal remedy was differentiated further depending on whether she suspected a woman had taken a lover while pregnant, a point we will return to below.

I do not know whether the herbal remedies Mwana Nyanzanga gave her clients during labor actually affected the outcome of their births. I only know that on two separate occasions my presence appeared to influence the type of remedy she gave and when she gave it. On one occasion, I had been sitting with a woman whose contractions had begun around nine o'clock in the morning. Due to a previously scheduled appointment in Shinyanga town, I had to leave while she was still in the early stages of labor. I told her and Mwana Nyanzanga that I didn't think the appointment would take long and that I expected to return in the early afternoon, hopefully before she gave birth. My appointment took longer than anticipated, however, and I didn't return until seven o'clock in the evening. Upon my arrival, I was surprised to find that the woman had not yet given birth. Mwana Nyanzanga explained that she had purposely delayed the birth by withholding the woman's "medicine." When I hadn't returned by four o'clock in the afternoon, she felt it she couldn't wait any longer, and so she finally administered it.

This was not the first time I suspected my presence was affecting the way she managed births, nor was it the last. The birth I describe below provides another example. It also highlights some of the ethical dilemmas I encountered when Mwana Nyanzanga's style of birth management involved practices I had been taught were dangerous during my brief tenure as a lay midwifery trainee in El Paso.

Nkamba's Birth

A week and a half after I began observing Mwana Nyanzanga's work, two pregnant women arrived at her home to await their impending births. Both lived in villages far from Mwana Nyanzanga's home. One made the two-hour journey on the back of her husband's bicycle. He returned to pick her up about three weeks later, visiting once in the interim. The other woman traveled to Mwana Nyanzanga's home alone on foot. She lived in a village located about a three-hour walk away. Neither was in labor at the time of their arrival, but both expected to give birth "soon." The first woman gave birth in the middle of the night on December 4, 1992, nearly a week and a half after she arrived. As I had spent that particular evening at my home in Bulangwa, I missed the birth.

Nkamba, the second woman, gave birth six days later, in the early morning hours of December 10. Anticipating her labor, I had spent the previous two nights at Mwana Nyanzanga's home. I was present throughout the early hours of her labor and during the actual birth. On the morning of December 9 her lower back began to hurt. By nine o'clock in the morning she began experiencing light and very irregular contractions. An hour and a half later, Mwana Nyanzanga began preparing for the birth. She placed her birthing instruments in a small pan of water and boiled them on a charcoal stove in front of her "hospital" for about thirty minutes.[10] She then put another small bowl over the fire and began boiling water. Once the water boiled, she added a finely ground herbal mixture. She poured the hot mixture into a plastic cup, brought it into the birthing room, and gave it to Nkamba, who was sitting on the side of the bed.

As soon as Nkamba finished drinking the mixture, Mwana Nyanzanga took the empty cup and held it up to Nkamba's breastbone, anchoring it in place with the stick she had used to stir the herbal mixture. She then let go of the cup, which tumbled straight down the length of Nkamba's pregnant belly onto the floor. Mwana Nyanzanga picked up the cup and tapped it three times on each side of Nkamba's belly, held it once more up to her breastbone, and again let it drop straight down onto the floor. When I asked her later what all the "tapping and dropping" meant, she explained that the medicine wouldn't work without it. The cup falling in a straight line down the length of Nkamba's belly symbolized how the child should be born: straight out of the womb without any problems (*moja kwa moja*). Nkamba then went outside to sit in the sun.

Earlier in the day, I had asked Mwana Nyanzanga how she assessed a woman's progress during labor. She told me she measured the opening of the door to the womb (*mlango wa kizazi*) with her fingers. This was similar to how I had been taught to measure cervical dilation during my lay midwifery training in El Paso. A fully dilated cervix has a measurement of ten centimeters, a measurement roughly equivalent to the distance between the index and middle finger when they are stretched far apart. Pushing before full dilation can be dangerous as it can lead to swelling or tears in the cervix (Davis 1987).

Over the course of the day, both Mwana Nyanzanga and I intermittently monitored the dilation of Nkamba's cervix, first putting on latex gloves I had brought along.[11] By 9:00 in the evening Nkamba's contractions were coming more frequently, although the measurement of her cervical dilation indicated that the time for the actual birth was still far off. Her cervix was dilated to about five centimeters, which, in terms of cervical dilation, meant she was only halfway there.[12] Because her contractions were neither very strong nor closely spaced, I was convinced she wouldn't give birth until much later. Anticipating a long night ahead, I wanted to catch a few hours of sleep, so I asked Mwana Nyanzanga to wake me when Nkamba's contractions became stronger. I went to lie down in a room about thirty yards away in a different building on her compound.

At 11:30 P.M. she woke me up to tell me that Nkamba was close to giving birth. When I entered the birthing room (now lit by a lantern), Nkamba was lying flat on her back and pushing. She pushed hard for forty-five minutes. I was uneasy throughout because it didn't seem to me that it was really time for her to push. Although her contractions were coming at regular intervals and were closely spaced, they weren't very strong. I asked Mwana Nyanzanga if she would check her. Upon inserting her fingers into the woman's vagina, she told me that the baby was "right there" (*Yuko karibu tu*).

Another ten minutes of pushing went by. I was still uneasy yet hesitant about intervening. After all, Mwana Nyanzanga was not an inexperienced midwife—she had been attending births for many years. Worried that my intervening might be seen as an attempt to undermine her authority, I nevertheless asked if I could also check. She said okay, but gave me an odd look. I checked Nkamba's cervical dilation and found it to be about seven centimeters. I told Mwana Nyanzanga that I thought it was too early for Nkamba to push.

Nkamba got up off the bed, and both she and Mwana Nyanzanga walked outside. I stayed behind for a few minutes, wondering what I should do next. I felt bad at what just happened and wished I could just disappear. When I walked outside they were both sitting next to the charcoal stove; Mwana Nyanzanga was heating up what appeared to be more medicine. She suggested I go rest; she'd call me when it was time. Feeling a bit sheepish, I went back to my room and after a while fell asleep again. Three hours later I was woken up by a loud banging on my door. I opened it and saw Mwana Nyanzanga rushing back to her hospital. When I entered the birthing room, Nkamba was pushing and the baby's head was showing a little bit with each push. The baby was born about twenty minutes later, at 3:35 in the morning.

Before cutting the cord, Mwana Nyanzanga said a prayer, thanking God for the safe birth and asking him to bless the child. She cut the umbilical cord about ten minutes later, wrapped the baby in a *khanga,* and took it to the postpartum room. She returned, collected the placenta, took it outside, and threw it into the nearby latrine. Nkamba got up off the bed and began wiping it with her *khanga,* as if embarrassed by the mess she had just made. Upon her return, Mwana Nyanzanga helped Nkamba secure a cloth between her legs. Nkamba then wrapped another *khanga* around her body and went to lay down in the room with the baby.

Despite the false start, this birth actually went quite well. Although I was initially worried that my unsolicited intervention would jeopardize the friendship that had begun to develop between Mwana Nyanzanga and myself, my fears turned out to be unfounded. It is important to note that my role in this birth was not typical, in that I never again intervened so drastically, although I did on occasion check a woman's cervical dilation. I believe Mwana Nyanzanga's potential mismanagement of Nkamba's birth had more to do with the fact that she knew I had been disappointed at missing the first woman's birth, and so in her eagerness to accommodate her guest, she miscalculated.

The Management of Prolonged Labor: *Usangalija*

As mentioned in the first part of this chapter, a woman's behavior during labor was seen as having a direct bearing on the birth outcome. If she "misbehaved" by calling out or crying loudly, she might not concentrate on pushing and, as a result, might cause harm to the baby. A woman's misbehavior during pregnancy was also associated with birth complications later on. Prolonged or stalled labor (*usangalija*) was one such complication.

Usangalija, a Kisukuma word that conveys the meaning of "mixing" or "coming together," was attributed to a woman's "mixing" of men while pregnant. Although the source of this particular complication, its etiology, is attributed to the presence of "foreign" sperm, that is, sperm from a man who had not fathered the child already in the womb, the woman is seen as primarily responsible for bringing on the complication because she should have refused the man's amorous advances in the first place. Her mixing of men is perceived as life-threatening in two regards: it can result in the death of the child in the womb or of the mother herself. I was often told that cases of *usangalija* are easily diagnosed because its symptoms are unique and always the same. Instead of descending down the birth canal, the child moves up in the uterus instead (*mtoto anapanda juu*).

I first learned about *usangalija* during a conversation I had with Agnes and Mhindi, two of the traditional birth attendants who attended the TBA training in October 1992. After explaining the cause of this particular obstetric complication, they described some of its cures. One such cure consisted of taking a pinch of sand from the exact spot where a dog had previously given birth and mixing it with water. The concoction was then drunk by the laboring woman. The value of this particular medicine was symbolic: just as a dog in heat mates with many males, so too had the woman taken more than one lover during the course of her pregnancy. Another cure involved taking a piece of any root found growing in the middle of a road, grinding it, and mixing it with water. The inclusion of this root, over which many people have passed on their way to other places, symbolized the fact the woman had more than one lover during her pregnancy, that is, many men had passed through. Over the course of my fieldwork women recounted different versions of this cure, all of which were taken to cancel out the effects of a pregnant woman's "promiscuous" behavior. I was also told that some pregnant women might even take such a remedy prior to the onset of labor so as to prevent the possibility of experiencing birth complications later on.

In December 1992, Agnes's husband Samweli stopped by my house on his way to visit family members in a nearby village. As we sat drinking coffee, he told me about a woman in their village who had recently died after a very difficult labor. According to his version of the events, both Agnes (his wife) and Mhindi (the other traditional birth attendant in the village) had been called to the woman's house at eleven o'clock in the morning. They stayed with her until eight o'clock in the evening, at which point they told the woman's husband they were unable to help her and recommended that she be transported to the government hospital. The husband refused, saying the cost of transport was too expensive. By nine o'clock the next morning, when his wife had still not given birth, he finally agreed. She was transported by oxcart to the government hospital in Shinyanga town, a journey of approximately two hours. Although a doctor performed a cesarean section, the baby was born in a very weak state and died a few hours later. The woman died later that same day.

Samweli then asked me if it were true that a woman could die during childbirth if she slept with a man other than her husband while pregnant. I told him that although I had heard of this before, I didn't think it was true. What did he think? He told me he didn't believe it either, but was puzzled because the woman whose story he had just recounted had admitted it herself. When I asked if her confession was the reason her husband had initially refused to take her to the hospital, he said no; the husband's refusal had occurred long before she confessed. He also noted that the woman who died was the first of two wives, and that the husband had been neglecting her for quite some time. Although the nurses at the prenatal clinic had apparently told her she needed medicine to strengthen her blood, her husband never bought it. The nurses had also told her she must give birth in the hospital. Although some of the man's neighbors condemned him for refusing to transport his wife to the hospital early on, others were convinced the birth complications were a result of the wife's promiscuity.

Mwana Nyanzanga also treated cases of *usangalija,* although she told me she did so without making the woman confess. She recounted the story of one woman whose birth she had assisted almost twenty years previously. During labor, the woman's abdomen began rising up toward her breasts, the defining feature of *usangalija.* As soon as Mwana Nyanzanga saw this, she told me, she wanted to administer the appropriate medicine. She asked the woman if her pregnancy was really the pregnancy of one person (*Kweli hii mimba ni ya mtu moja?*). The woman told her it was, and she stuck to her story throughout her entire labor. When the child was finally born (he had a very big head, Mwana Nyanzanga remarked), the woman lifted her head off the bed, looked at the child, and died. It was as a result of this particular case, Mwana Nyanzanga explained, that she no longer asks women if they have slept with more than one man while pregnant. If she sees the symptoms of *usangalija,* she simply administers the appropriate cure without asking because they might just deny it. The woman whose story she had just recounted had apparently denied it ten times. "But maybe she really hadn't slept with more than one man," I suggested. She assured me the woman had, because all of the symptoms were there. In her opinion, the woman was probably just too ashamed to admit it.

I then asked if she thought it possible that some women might just say they had slept with more than one man when complications arose just so she would give them medicine. No woman would do this, she patiently explained, because symptoms of *usangalija* wouldn't present themselves if she had only slept with one man, an opinion shared by other women I spoke with. No woman would admit to it, they all claimed, unless she had, in fact, mixed men. Their reasoning was twofold. First, the symptoms indicating *usangalija* wouldn't appear, and second, the medicine only worked if a woman had indeed slept with more than one man.

Despite their claims, I interviewed one woman who told me that she had been unjustly accused of having mixed men when she encountered difficulties during her last birth at the government clinic. The nurses attending her birth accused her of having slept with more than one man while pregnant. Although she steadfastly denied their claims throughout her labor, the nurses accused her of lying.

When I later asked nurses who worked at the clinic about *usangalija,* they described it as a psychological rather than a physical condition. They noted that some women who experience an extended labor might even offer the information that they have slept with more than one man during pregnancy. Upon hearing such confessions, the nurses told me, they usually gave the women a placebo such as an iron supplement. Apparently, convinced that they had been cured, the women give birth soon after.

I was present at Mwana Nyanzanga's home when one of her clients, a fifteen-year-old girl who was pregnant for the first time, confessed to having slept with more than one man during her pregnancy. Her confession was unsolicited and took place several hours after the onset of her labor. I present the details of her case below.

Sayi's Story

When I arrived at Mwana Nyanzanga's home at eleven o'clock one morning, she told me that a young girl had arrived earlier that morning in labor. The girl, whose name was Sayi, lived in that same village and had been accompanied by a sister and another female relative; her mother arrived later. At that point in time, her contractions were not coming at regular intervals. Her cervix was dilated to four centimeters, and the baby's heartbeat was fine. Since it was her first birth, I assumed her labor would be long.

Sayi's demeanor throughout her labor was in sharp contrast to what I had observed at other births since my arrival in Tanzania in that she cried throughout her labor, during both the early and later stages. Her relatives and Mwana Nyanzanga repeatedly admonished her to keep quiet so as not to "hurt the baby." Like them, I too was concerned that she would exhaust herself with her cries and not have any energy when it eventually came time to push. Since this was her first birth, it was quite possible her labor would be a long one, and so it was important that she conserve her energy. Initially, I stayed with her to try to calm her down, but I noticed that my presence seemed to have the opposite effect. As she didn't seem to be getting much sympathy from anyone else, whenever I walked in the room her cries and pleas for help would either start up again or get louder. Once I realized the effect that my presence was having, I limited the time I spent with her, only coming occasionally to make sure that her vital signs and those of the baby were okay.

During one of the periods I sat with her she told me that she had mixed men. When I asked why, she said when she had taken a new lover during the first month of her pregnancy, she hadn't known she was already pregnant. (Mwana Nyanzanga had pointed out the signs of *usangalija* to me earlier and had already begun administering the appropriate herbal remedy.) Despite her admission, no one appeared to be openly castigating her for it.

By one o'clock in the morning, Sayi's cervix was almost fully dilated, and I could feel the baby's head when I checked her dilation. The baby's heartbeat was still normal. Both Mwana Nyanzanga and I kept thinking she would birth soon, and we kept urging her to calm down so that she would have energy to push when it came time to do so. Our pleas went unheeded. By two o'clock in the morning her cervix was fully dilated: it was time to push. Again Mwana Nyanzanga and I told her that she needed to calm down and focus on pushing. Realizing our pleas were useless and starting to feel frustrated with her myself, I left the room, thinking that she would quiet down and birth if left alone with Mwana Nyanzanga. When she still hadn't birthed by three o'clock, I became alarmed. It was at that point that the baby's heartbeat had also begun to slow down. Although I considered driving her to the hospital, I had recently been having problems with my car and felt it dangerous to transport her in the middle of the night lest it break down on the way, stranding us in the middle of nowhere. Mwana Nyanzanga and I decided it was best to wait until it was light outside.

At 5:30 in the morning I told Sayi's mother that I wanted to drive her daughter to the hospital. She refused. She couldn't make that decision, she told me, without the approval of her husband, and he was visiting relatives in a different village. She explained that the previous evening she had sent a daughter to tell him that Sayi had gone into labor, so she expected he would arrive shortly. When he arrived, they would find transport and take Sayi to the hospital then. When I expressed my surprise to Mwana Nyanzanga that the woman failed to see the urgency of her daughter's predicament (now that it was light outside and I felt I could do something about it), she explained that the husband was well-known for having a bad temper (*Mume yake ni mkali sana*). In other words, the woman's concern that her husband would be angry if she made a decision without consulting him first was well-founded. Despite my repeated pleas, she refused to give permission. Frustrated and angry, I drove back to my home in Bulangwa. Once I arrived, however, I couldn't put Sayi out of my mind. What if she died? After about an hour of these haunting thoughts, I decided to return to Mwana Nyanzanga's home and demand that Sayi's mother allow me to drive her daughter to the hospital. Upon my return, however, I found Sayi's father sitting outside. No one appeared to be making any preparations to transport her to the hospital. In fact, he seemed quite unconcerned, as did Mwana Nyanzanga.

Without asking anyone what was going on, I lost my temper and demanded to know why no one was preparing to take Sayi to the hospital. Sayi's father seemed surprised at my anger and agreed that yes, I could drive his daughter to the hospital. Two of Sayi's sisters helped her into the car, and all four of us (Sayi, her two sisters, and myself) drove off to the hospital. On the way there, one of Sayi's sisters told me that when their father arrived, Mwana Nyanzanga assured him that Sayi would give birth without any problem and didn't need to be transported to the hospital.

When we arrived at Kolondoto, the nurses responded immediately. One nurse quickly brought a wheelchair and whisked Sayi into the labor room, while another sent for the doctor. The nurses pointed to Sayi's bladder, noting that it was full; I hadn't noticed it myself. The midwife tried to insert a catheter into Sayi's urethra, but the position of the baby's head prevented any drainage of urine. When the doctor arrived, he also remarked on Sayi's distended bladder. After giving her a local anesthetic, he then proceeded to deliver the baby with a combination of deep cuts on both sides of her vagina and the use of vacuum extraction. This was actually quite a frightening procedure to watch. A suctionlike cup was placed onto the baby's head, then it was literally pulled out of the birth canal.

Sayi was conscious throughout. After being admonished once by the doctor to quiet down, she never made another sound, despite all the cutting and pulling that was being done to her body. The baby was finally delivered. Although its heart was beating when it was born, it never started breathing and was declared dead an hour later.

On the surface, Sayi's story shares similarities with the story I presented in the preface to this book. Like the girl I saw lying on the hospital bed in Dar es Salaam in 1990, Sayi was young, unmarried, and under the care of a parent. But in contrast to what had been suggested by the nurse in Dar es Salaam, a belief in the supernatural was not the reason for Sayi's delayed arrival at the hospital. Nor did the traditional belief that a woman's misbehavior during pregnancy could lead to birth complications later have any bearing on her case. Instead, Sayi's mother's fear of the real reprisals she might experience if she made a decision without the approval of her husband seemed to be a major factor in the decisions made. My role in the whole ordeal is also problematic, and it continues to haunt me to this day. What if I had noticed Sayi's bladder was full and impeding the descent of the child's head into the birth canal? Would it have changed the outcome? Or if I had ignored the mother's refusal and Mwana Nyanzanga's advice and insisted on transporting Sayi to the hospital at 5:30 in the morning anyway?

But Sayi's story is revealing for another reason as well: how it relates to Mary Douglas's observation that anger, hope, and fear are part of most risky situations and that a decision that involves costs also involves consultations with neighbors, family, and friends (1992:12). It was after observing Sayi's ordeal that I began to understand why women might be admonished to keep quiet during labor and childbirth. In addition to the effects the experience has on the birthing woman herself, others around her are affected as well. In situations where the solutions are limited, especially in the village setting in the middle of the night, a woman's cries only serve to distress those around her. I certainly remember my own distress during Sayi's labor, especially when her complications took place in the middle of the night and I felt it was too risky to try to transport her to the hospital. We saw other examples of distress at the government hospital in

Shinyanga town, when, as the result of a power outage, a doctor was unable to perform the emergency cesarean section.

Do some of the physical, spiritual, and economic risks women encounter in the context of childbirth carry over into the period immediately following birth? To answer this question, let us turn now to chapter 11, where we examine some of the unofficial risks women face during the postpartum period.

CHAPTER 11

Risks during the Postpartum Period

The majority of maternal deaths (61 percent in developing countries) occur after delivery. Most of these (78 percent) take place during the first 24–48 hours after delivery, largely due to postpartum haemorrhage or hypertensive disorder, but also later, due primarily to sepsis. Women, families, and even health professionals are often not aware of the risks to women during this period.

—Ann Starrs, *The Safe Motherhood Action Agenda*

Women in Bulangwa spoke about the hours and days immediately following birth as a period fraught with danger. In some cases, the dangers associated with this final stage of the birth process were directly attributed to the physical act of giving birth. In other cases, the risks were described as being spiritual in nature and associated with the by-products of birth. As we will see in the following pages, the concept of risk during the postpartum period applies not only to the dangers posed to the new mother, but to people within her wider social network as well.

Rituals of Prevention: Muslim and Non-Muslim Distinctions

Muslim women were more likely than non-Muslim women in Bulangwa to state that they followed certain practices during the postpartum period, and within the community of Muslim women, Arab women were more likely than non-Arab Muslim women to adhere strictly to those rules. For Muslim women in general, the postpartum period was spoken about as a distinctly dangerous period of time for the mother and child, a forty-day period in which the graves of each were considered to be wide open.[1] The postpartum period was also referred to as a period of ritual uncleanliness. Like a menstruating woman, a new mother could not pray, touch religious books, or visit the mosque. If the forty-day postpartum period fell during the holy month of Ramadan, the new mother did not fast either (Delaney 1988; Good 1980).

All fourteen of the Arab women who took part in my formal survey told me they slept with a knife, lime, salt, and incense under their pillows during this forty-day period as protection against evil spirits. If they needed to urinate during the middle of the night, they carried the knife (and sometimes the salt and lime) outside with them as further protection against evil spirits that dwelled in latrines. When I asked African Muslim women if they also kept such items nearby during the period following birth, all said they did not. In other words, sleeping with knives, limes, salt, and incense during the postpartum period was not seen as a Muslim custom per se, but, rather, an idiosyncrasy of Arab culture (cf. Riesman 1992).[2]

There were also differences within the Muslim community in how the end of the forty-day postpartum period was marked. Arab families in Bulangwa usually celebrated the end of the postpartum period with a religious ceremony (*maulidi*) that included prayers to bless the infant and a communal feast. The feast, to which many in the community were invited (and others simply showed up), could be rather expensive. The more economic resources a family had, the more elaborate the feast. Those without sufficient economic resources marked the end of the forty-day postpartum period in a less public manner.

Although these beliefs and practices were not followed by all women in the community, other practices associated with the postpartum period were. Some of these addressed dangers attributed to the placenta and postpartum blood, as discussed below.

Placental Risks

> Normally the placenta is expelled within 30 minutes of the birth of the
> baby, and uterine contractions continue so that bleeding soon stops.
> For a variety of reasons, the placenta may fail to separate, and
> bleeding will not stop altogether for as long as the placenta, or part of
> it, remains in the uterus.
> —Erica Royston and Sue Armstrong, *Preventing Maternal Deaths*

Although my interviews with women trained as traditional birth attendants in Shinyanga indicate that there was no long-established tradition of midwifery among the Sukuma, some women were called upon if the placenta was not expelled after birth. Retained placenta is apparently a common phenomenon, and a variety of methods are used to aid in its expulsion. According to an American nurse who had trained traditional birth attendants near the Kolondoto mission hospital in the late 1980s and early 1990s, those methods varied from village to village, and even from household to household.[3]

One method described by the women who attended her TBA training seminars involved obtaining a pair of the husband's sandals and hitting the woman on the back with it. This worked, the women told her, because hitting the woman on the back would cause her body to jerk, a movement that aided in the expulsion of the placenta. In other cases, a woman might be given an herbal remedy to drink, or the woman assisting her might push on her abdomen.

Mwana Nyanzanga used similar methods to treat retained placentas. At one of the births I observed, she hit the woman hard in the middle of her back with her hand when the woman's placenta did not come out immediately. Other times, I saw her push on a woman's abdomen to aid in the placenta's expulsion. She also told me that in very delayed cases, she would give the woman an herbal remedy to drink, although I never saw her do this myself.

There were no specific rituals associated with the disposal of the placenta; Mwana Nyanzanga simply dropped it in a nearby latrine, a method of disposal that some of the other traditional birth attendants I interviewed told me they employed as well. This was in sharp contrast to how the placenta was disposed of in the past. According to many of the older women I spoke with, the placenta used to be buried in the same room where the woman had given birth. Their descriptions of this past practice were similar: a hole was dug, the placenta was placed in it, and dirt was pushed back over the hole to cover it. The new mother then bathed over that exact spot; it was believed this practice would ensure her fertility in the future. Much care was apparently taken with regard to the depth of the hole. If it was dug too deeply, the woman might experience difficulty conceiving later on. One of the women who explained the reason behind this particular practice noted jokingly that women who wanted to delay their next pregnancy might dig a deep hole on purpose.

Although many of the younger women I spoke with had also heard that the placenta was buried inside the house "a long time ago," most did not know the reason why. Some speculated that it was buried and then bathed over in order to prevent the smell of the decaying placenta from permeating the room in which it was buried. Others hypothesized that it was buried inside to prevent people from gaining access to it and using it in sorcery medicine that would then be used to block the woman's ability to conceive in the future. All noted that nowadays placentas are simply thrown into the latrine. In addition to the sanitary benefits of pit latrines, there were preventive benefits as well: the depth of the hole (as well as its contents) discouraged anyone from attempting to steal the placenta later (Lindenbaum 1979).[4]

Some of the men I spoke with also attributed a supernatural power to placentas. One man, who was the leader of one of the Sukuma dance societies in a different community, told me that placentas from twin or breech births were important ingredients in medicines used to ensure success in the dance competitions (Bessire 2001; Hall 1936).[5] When I asked how such medicines were prepared, he explained that the placenta is first hung in a tree for several days to dry, after which it is ground into a powder. A small portion is then added to the medicine's other ingredients. When I asked how he gained access to placentas in the first place, he said he bought them either from people who had access to them in the village setting or from nurses who worked on the labor wards of hospitals or clinics.[6]

Mwana Nyanzanga told me that some people had also tried to buy placentas from her in the past. They eventually gave up because, due to her Christianity, she always refused. The only people she gave placentas to, she told me, were *wakango* (*mkango,* sing.), the officiants at *ukango* ceremonies, the cleansing ritual performed after the birth of twins or breech births (see chap. 7, n. 9). According to Mwana Nyanzanga, one important component of the *ukango* ritual involved placing the placenta in a ceramic pot and then burying it at the edge of a river or in a dry river bed (Cory 1944).[7] She noted, however, that nowadays she didn't receive many of these requests, because *ukango* rituals were no longer performed as frequently as they had been in the past.

When I asked an older healer I knew in Bulangwa why placentas were an essential ingredient in some sorcery medicines, he gave four reasons why: (1) a placenta comes from a place where it can't be seen; (2) placentas are unclean (*uchafu*), and unclean substances are important ingredients of medicines used to bewitch people; (3) a placenta is powerful because it feeds a human being; and (4) the sac attached to the placenta held life itself (a child). When I asked if only the placentas from twin or breech births were used in such medicines, he told me that any placenta would do, but especially those from young girls' first births.

As we were on the topic of sorcery, I then asked him who were most likely to be witches, women or men. Most witches are women, he told me, because women were the ones who had access to placentas, and placentas were one of the most important ingredients in sorcery medicines. I was struck by his analysis, that women gain access to supernatural power through the by-products of childbirth, because it was the first time in my fieldwork that I had heard such an explanation. I was additionally intrigued by his statements regarding the connection between placentas, sorcery, and women because he was the same healer who told me about past female chiefs, and that succession to chiefship changed from one based on matriliny to one based on patriliny precisely because of female intrigue (see chap. 5).

Although this was the only time I heard someone link negative aspects of female power to reproduction specifically, another male healer in the community invoked women's primary role in biological reproduction as an explanation for the predominance of women in rituals of possession. Women were more likely than men to experience possession, he noted, because a woman was, in effect, like a second god (*Mwanamke ni kama Mungu ya pili*). Although the feminist in me was pleasantly surprised at his analogy, I wanted to know *why* he thought women had godlike qualities. Women are like a second god, he explained, because of their ability to bear children and their important social role of feeding and raising their children once they were born. In other words, just as God is responsible for bestowing life, so, too, are women.

I include these healers' remarks in my analysis because I think their conflicting statements capture the ambiguous nature of local perceptions regarding women's role in society. In the latter healer's view, women's reproductive power is positive and derived from their ability to bear children. From the perspective of the former healer, however, women's ability to procreate, thus their access to power through the by-products of birth, is precisely the reason they should be feared. Although each of these healers offered different perspectives regarding the nature and essence of women's social power, their place in the community as healers (and male healers at that) and thus their own power to shape, support, or propagate local discourses about the nature of female power is a very strong social position to be in (Keesing 1987). It is also important to point out that women as well as men create and support some of these same local discourses about women's role in society. We have already seen many examples of how some women do this, whether they be nurses, female healers, or simply women living in the community.

Risks Associated with Postpartum Blood

> Postpartum haemorrhage refers to excessive bleeding through the birth
> canal after birth of the baby. The action of the uterus during labour is
> directed not only towards expelling the baby and the placenta but also
> closing down the blood vessels afterwards. . . . Apart from retained
> placenta, other causes of postpartum haemorrhage include prolonged
> labor, all forms of operative vaginal delivery, the action of anaesthetic
> agents, and uterine tumours such as fibroids.
> —Erica Royston and Sue Armstrong, *Preventing Maternal Deaths*

Postpartum blood was also spoken about in terms of physical and spiritual risks. Nearly all of the women who took part in my formal interviews noted that serious risks to a woman's health, including death, could occur if the postpartum blood was not completely expelled from her body within the first week after giving birth. In order to prevent, or at least minimize, such risks, women submitted to hot sponge baths for several days following the birth of a child. Six benefits of the hot bath were commonly cited: (1) it gets rid of excess blood; (2) it gives the woman energy and strength; (3) it helps reduce pain; (4) it stimulates healing inside; (5) it helps heal the vagina; (6) it helps alleviate lower back pain.

Despite the acclaimed preventive benefits of this practice, postpartum baths were not fondly viewed by those who received them. Most of the women noted that the bath, which was usually administered to them by a female relative, was quite painful, due to the extreme heat of the water used. Water was heated over the fire until it became quite hot, after which it was poured into a bucket. The person administering the bath immersed a large cloth in the water, and then pressed it over every part of the new mother's body. Nearly all of the women I interviewed had received a postpartum bath. A woman's mother was mentioned as the person most likely to have given them their postpartum bath. A woman's mother-in-law was the second most mentioned person. The third most cited person was the new mother herself. Three of the 101 younger women who answered this question told me their husbands had performed the task, while one of the older women said that her husband had. Only one woman had not received a hot sponge bath after birth. She had given birth by cesarean section and had been advised by nurses to avoid it because it would interfere with the healing of her surgical scar.

When I asked women if there were any dangers associated with not having this hot sponge bath, they gave a variety of responses. This was an open-ended question, and each women could list up to three possible dangers of not receiving the bath. Although similar, the older and younger women's responses differed slightly, as shown in table 11.1. The four most-cited dangers of not receiving the sponge bath were the same for each group (i.e., blood will coagulate in the body, the woman will be in pain, the woman will die, the woman will have lower back pain). There was a difference, however, in how these consequences were ranked. Although "will die" emerged as the fourth most-cited consequence of not having the hot bath among the younger women, among the older group death emerged as the second most negative consequence of not receiving the bath. The younger women also mentioned more categories of negative consequences than the older women, but this is most likely due to the fact that I interviewed twice as many younger women. Only four women stated that there were no negative health consequences associated with not receiving the hot sponge bath postpartum. All these women were from the younger subset of women. Three of these women had finished the seventh grade; the fourth had attended some years of primary school. Six of the nine younger women who said they didn't know if there were any consequences of not receiving a hot sponge bath postpartum had not attended primary school.

Given that almost every woman I spoke with acknowledged that the postpartum period was fraught with danger and that some of its risks could prove fatal if not prevented, I wanted to know if any of their relatives had died as a result of being pregnant or after giving birth (see table 11.2). A higher proportion of the older women said they had a relative who had died from a pregnancy or birth-related cause than did the younger women: 22.9 percent ($n = 11$) and 16.3 percent ($n = 17$) respectively. This appears to contradict some people's perceptions that in the past, women suffered fewer birth complications as noted already in chapter 7.

When I inquired about the specific causes of death, this subset of women gave a variety of responses (shown in table 11.3). Some women mentioned specific causes of death, such as postpartum hemorrhage (which two women described as "a lot of blood coming out"), infection, placenta problems with blood loss, or symptoms that sounded like eclampsia (the woman's body had swollen up, or she had experienced convulsions). Other causes were less specific, such as the result of sorcery, not receiving the postpartum bath, or the combined result of being promiscuous and looking at the birth blood. Several of the traditional birth attendants I had interviewed the previous year had mentioned this latter behavior as a risk associated with *attending* a woman's birth. Looking at the birth blood, they told me, could harm a person's eyesight. This particular risk could be prevented several ways, one of which required that the birthing woman momentarily place a string of white beads around the neck of the woman who had assisted with her birth.[8]

As suggested by this example, the notion of risk during the postpartum period may also be applied to members of the birthing woman's wider social network. The case study below shows that these risks are multifaceted, involving not only spiritual and physical aspects of risk, but economic factors as well.

Ndalu's Story: Postpartum Hemorrhage
On the afternoon of Friday, June 3, 1994, I returned to Bulangwa, having spent the morning interviewing women at the family planning clinic in Shinyanga town. I was feeling tired and hungry when I arrived, so I

TABLE 11.1. Responses to the Survey Question "What Will Happen If You Are Not Given a Hot Sponge Bath after Giving Birth?" for the Subsets of Older and Younger Women (*N* = 147)[a]

Older Women's Responses (*n* = 46)	*n*	%	Younger Women's Responses (*n* = 101)	*n*	%
Will be in pain	10	20.0	Blood will coagulate inside	18	17.3
Will die	10	20.0	Back/lower back pain	17	16.4
Blood will coagulate inside	7	14.0	Will be in pain	15	14.5
Back/lower back pain	6	12.0	Will die	15	14.5
Blood will rise to the head	6	12.0	Stomach will swell	7	6.7
Embarrassing vaginal noises	5	10.0	Embarrassing vaginal noises	6	5.8
Body will be weak	4	8.0	Will be sick	6	5.8
Stomach will swell	3	6.0	Body will be weak	5	4.8
Will be sick	1	2.0	Blood will rise to the head	5	4.8
Neck problems	1	2.0	General malaise	5	4.8
			Won't stop bleeding	4	3.8
			Body will swell	2	1.9
			Insides will rot	2	1.9
			Neck problems	1	1.0
			Unclean discharge	1	1.0
			Will be unable to sit	1	1.0
			Can't sit if torn	1	1.0
			No consequences	4	1.0
Doesn't know	3	6.0	Doesn't know	9	8.7

[a]Numbers do not add up to 100 percent, because multiple responses were given.

stopped by a friend's house for lunch. While we were eating, she told me that a young woman had stopped by her house looking for me. The woman explained that her relative, who had just given birth at the government clinic, had suffered some type of complication and needed transportation to the mission hospital. Since I wasn't there, my friend suggested she ask one of the Arab shopkeepers for assistance instead.

When I went to look for the woman at the Arab shops, no one had seen her. I then drove to the clinic to find out what the problem was. I learned that the woman in question was Ndalu, the daughter of Mbuke, an older woman who was well-known in the community as an officiant in rituals associated with the birth of twins. The "doctor" on duty, the rural medical aid, told me that Ndalu had given birth in the clinic an hour and a half earlier and had lost a lot of blood, over 500 ml. He added the additional information that he had to remove the placenta manually with his hand, as it had not been expelled after birth.

Since the young woman who had been looking for me had not

TABLE 11.2.   Responses to Survey Question "Have Any of Your Relatives Died because of a Pregnancy or after Giving Birth?" for the Subsets of Older and Younger Women ($N = 152$)

Relative Who Died	Older Women ($n = 48$)		Younger Women ($n = 104$)	
	n	%	n	%
None	37	77.1	87	83.7
Mother	1	2.1	3	2.9
Sister	5	10.4	1	2.9
Daughter	2	4.2	—	—
Paternal aunt	1	2.1	1	1.0
Niece	1	2.1	—	—
Daughter-in-law	1	2.1	—	—
Stepmother	—	—	2	1.9
Cousin[a]	—	—	7	6.7
Sister-in-law	—	—	2	1.9
Other relative	—	—	1	1.0
Total	48	100.0	104	100.0

[a]The category "cousin" represents those women who stated that the relative who died was the child of an aunt or uncle, either paternal or maternal. "Cousin" is my terminology, not theirs. It is also possible that the older women were referring to this category of relative as "sister," a terminology that was often applied to the children of an uncle or aunt.

returned to the clinic, I got in my car and went looking for her again. I found her on the other side of town, walking along the road with a woman who had a small child strapped to her back. Both women were on their way back to the clinic. I learned that the young woman who had been looking for me was Shija, Ndalu's sister-in-law. The woman with the young child was Holo, Ndalu's sister. Mbuke, Ndalu's mother, had apparently already left for the clinic. Both of the women got into my car, and we headed back to the clinic. Along the way, I saw Mbuke on the side of the road and picked her up as well.

When we arrived back at the clinic, Ndalu said she was feeling hungry; she hadn't eaten since the previous day. On hearing this, the "doctor" told one of the nurses to give Ndalu some tea. Another patient at the clinic had some leftover spinach from lunch, which she gave to Ndalu. As Ndalu ate, her three relatives conferred. They decided that Shija and Holo would accompany Ndalu to Kolondoto hospital. Mbuke, the mother, would stay behind to make arrangements to sell a cow, as they would need the money later to cover the costs of Ndalu's hospitalization. It was also decided that

TABLE 11.3.   Responses to Survey Question "What Was the Cause of Her Death?" for the Subsets of Older and Younger Women Who Stated They Had a Relative Who Had Died from a Pregnancy or Birth-Related Cause ($N = 28$)

	Older Women ($n = 11$)		Younger Women ($n = 17$)	
Cause of Death	n	%	n	%
Lost a lot of blood	—	—	2	11.7
Mentioned signs similar to eclampsia	1	9.1	2	11.7
Died after a difficult labor	3	27.3	2	11.7
Placenta problems with blood loss	—	—	2	11.7
At birth, not specified	1	9.1	2	11.7
Miscarriage with hemorrhage	1	9.1	1	5.8
Tightness in chest	—	—	1	5.8
Infection	—	—	1	5.8
Died after a cesarean section	—	—	1	5.8
Had cholera while pregnant	1	9.1	—	—
Died during pregnancy	1	9.1	—	—
Died after giving birth	1	9.1	—	—
Didn't receive a hot sponge bath	1	9.1	—	—
Slept around a lot and then looked at birth blood	—	—	1	5.8
Sorcery	1	9.1	1	5.8
Don't know	—	—	1	5.8
Total	11	100.0	17	100.0

Shija would stay the night at the hospital with Ndalu. Holo would return to Bulangwa with me because she was still nursing a young child. Having settled the matter, we helped Ndalu into the car and drove off. We arrived at the hospital around 4:30, approximately three hours after Ndalu had given birth.

I was impressed by the swiftness of the nurses' response upon our arrival. Two student nurses brought a stretcher and wheeled Ndalu into the ward. Once she was settled onto a bed, another student nurse took her blood pressure, noting aloud that it was quite low.[9] As a nurse set up an IV drip, Ndalu began complaining of a tightness in her chest. Soon afterward, a young man who worked in the hospital laboratory came to take a sample of Ndalu's blood to identify her blood group. He returned within a half an hour to tell us that Ndalu's blood type was O positive and to inform us that the hospital didn't have that particular group currently in stock. Someone would have to donate blood in case Ndalu needed a blood transfusion later on.

One of the nurses then asked Ndalu's relatives why no men had accompanied them to the hospital. Apparently, the hospital didn't like to take blood donations from women because they were usually anemic. They informed us that Holo couldn't donate because she was still breastfeeding. I knew my blood group was A positive, so I wasn't a candidate either. That left Shija. A nurse told her to go to the laboratory and have her blood tested. Shija refused; she did not want her blood drawn. The nurses and I tried to coax her into changing her mind, stressing the fact that Ndalu's life could be in danger, but Shija was steadfast in her refusal. I became frustrated with her and tried to shame her into agreeing to the blood test. "Here I am not even Ndalu's relative," I found myself saying to her, "yet I agreed to drive her to the hospital free of charge. But you, who are a relative of hers, refuse to give blood, even though she might die." One of the nurses again stressed the fact that because no male relatives had accompanied us to the hospital, Shija was the only possibility. Shija didn't say anything, but still looked very determined not to let anyone take a sample of her blood.

Although in retrospect I realize I should have been more understanding about Shija's refusal to give blood, at the time my predominant feeling was irritation rather than empathy. Already starting to feel guilty about my attempts to pressure her, I decided to talk to the lab technician again about the hospital's blood supply. I also wanted to speak about it with the American nurse who lived on the mission compound. On my way out of the maternity ward, I asked two of the nurses if people usually refused to have their blood drawn, even if relatives were quite ill. One told me that many people were indeed leery about having their blood tested. She attributed this to the fact that since blood samples were tested for AIDS (i.e., HIV antibodies), people were afraid they might learn that they had AIDS if they donated blood. She told me this fear was unfounded because a potential donor wouldn't be told if he or she tested positive. Although HIV counseling services were available at the hospital, people weren't usually told they had tested positive unless they specifically asked for the test results. They were simply informed their blood was not compatible.[10]

The other nurse noted that some people refused to give blood because of a widely held belief that blood was a fixed quantity in the body. By donating blood, they decreased their own body's supply of the precious resource.[11] When I later explored the issue of blood donations with a man I knew in the community, he also offered the fear of AIDS or a perception that blood was a fixed quantity as possible explanations for Shija's refusal to donate blood. But he provided an additional explanation. People were also hesitant to donate blood, he told me, because it was "well-known" that instead of giving their blood donation to their family member, hospital personnel might instead sell it to someone else who was willing to pay a high price for it if they or a sick relative needed a transfusion.

When I arrived back at the maternity ward about forty-five minutes later, I learned that Shija had finally consented to have her blood drawn; it was not compatible with Ndalu's. The nurses told us that more relatives would have to come the next day and that this time they should be male. It was now six o'clock in the evening, and I decided to drive back to Bulangwa with Holo. Shija informed me she was coming with us. She was feeling "weak," she said, and couldn't stay at the hospital overnight with Ndalu as originally planned. We finally convinced her to stay by telling her that one of Ndalu's sisters would arrive the next day by bus to take her place. Shija stayed the night and returned to Bulangwa the next day.

Two days later, one of Ndalu's brothers stopped by my house to ask if I would drive him to the mission hospital to bring Ndalu home the following day. When he and I arrived at the hospital the next morning, however, a nurse told us that Ndalu had taken a turn for the worse and couldn't be discharged. Apparently, Ndalu had started hemorrhaging late Friday night, a few hours after our return to Bulangwa. A manual examination of her uterus revealed that pieces of the placenta were still attached to her uterine walls. A doctor at the hospital performed a dilation and curettage to remove the last pieces. An analysis of her blood afterward revealed that her hemoglobin was extremely low: 3.5 (11 to 12 is considered normal). We were informed that she would need a transfusion of blood and monitoring for two days afterward before she could be discharged. A nurse instructed Ndalu's brother to go to the lab to determine if his blood was compatible. When he looked a bit hesitant, she assured him that he had a lot of blood. As with Shija before him, his blood was not compatible. We were told to return the next day with more relatives.

The next morning I returned with another of Ndalu's brothers, a sister, and a female neighbor. The brother's blood was tested but he was excluded as a candidate because his hemoglobin was too low. The sister and neighbor also had their blood tested, but neither proved a suitable match. All three decided to stay overnight in the hope that someone needing a transfusion of blood would have a relative willing to donate their blood to Ndalu in exchange for a blood donation from either woman.[12]

When I returned the next afternoon to pick them up, nothing had been resolved. Ndalu's relatives told me they had remained there the whole day, but had not received much assistance from the nurses. I went again and spoke to the lab technician about the blood supply. It was then that he told me that a male nurse who lived on the mission compound had type O blood and would be willing to donate it for a fee. None of us had any money on us, and so it was decided that Ndalu's brother would return by bus the next morning with cash. Ndalu finally received a blood transfusion on Thursday, June 9, six days after being admitted to the hospital. She was discharged from the hospital two days later. Her total bill for one week's stay came to 15,600 TSH (U.S.$31).

The events that unfolded after Ndalu's postpartum hemorrhage illustrate the complex nature of postpartum risk and the importance of delineating the issues involved in the concept "access to health care." In addition to the very real risk of postpartum hemorrhage and the stark hospital-based reality of a very limited blood supply, her story also highlights the equally important issue of personal perceptions of risk. As her story clearly demonstrates, such perceptions themselves are not static and may change over the course of an emergency. For example, although Shija was quite willing to accompany her sister-in-law Ndalu to the hospital and stay with her throughout her hospitalization, her willingness to do so changed once she was asked to donate blood. The dangers she associated with a withdrawal of her own blood quickly overrode her initial concern with the life-threatening risk of Ndalu's postpartum blood loss. We also saw that although Shija, who was married to Ndalu's brother, didn't want to donate blood, one of Ndalu's neighbors was willing to do so.

Ndalu's story also highlights the variety of costs involved in trying to find a suitable blood donor. In addition to the immediate economic costs of her hospitalization and the cost of paying someone to donate blood, there were costs in terms of time as well. In Ndalu's specific case, these latter costs included the various trips her family members made to the hospital, the hours they spent at the hospital waiting for the problem to be resolved, as well as the time spent away from farming or other everyday activities associated with the maintenance of their households.

CHAPTER 12

Risk and Maternal Health

A reprise:

Mrs. X died in the hospital during labor. The attending physician
certified that the death was from hemorrhage due to placenta previa.
The consulting obstetrician said that the hemorrhage might not have
been fatal if Mrs. X had not been anemic owing to parasitic infection
and malnutrition. There was also concern because Mrs. X had only
received 500 ml of whole blood, and because she died on the operating
table while a caesarean section was being performed by a physician
undergoing specialist training. The hospital administrator noted that
Mrs. X had not arrived at the hospital until four hours after the onset
of severe bleeding, and that she had several episodes of bleeding during
the last month for which she did not seek medical attention. The
sociologist observed that Mrs. X was 39 years old, with seven previous
pregnancies and five living children. She had never used contraceptives
and the last pregnancy was unwanted. In addition, she was poor,
illiterate and lived in a rural area.

—World Health Organization,
"Helping Women off the Road to Death"

I bring this account of women's pregnancy-related experiences to a close
by returning once again to the story of Mrs. X. In light of the other
women's stories we have examined in the preceding pages, how well does
her story capture the complexity of maternal health issues in the community of Bulangwa? Although Anna's miscarriage in the marketplace,
Njile's pregnancy that "turned to the back," the death of Milembe's
"eleven-month-old" fetus, Sayi's prolonged labor, and Ndalu's postpartum hemorrhage all involved risk, in the latter stories we were able to see
the diverse ways the risks those women faced went beyond the individual
women themselves.

One of the things that repeatedly struck me over the course of my
fieldwork in Tanzania was how often the stories women shared with me or

the events I witnessed defied the boundaries laid out in the story of Mrs. X. Sometimes the factors that contributed to women's pregnancy complications were similar to the ones identified in Mrs. X's story. Other times the risks those women encountered were very different. One thing all of their stories had in common, however, was that their experiences would have been misunderstand or misrepresented if put into one small paragraph, consisting of fifteen lines of text. If the details of their experiences are difficult to summarize so as to be relevant for all, what implications does this have for the success of a maternal health initiative that recommended a standard set of solutions be implemented everywhere, irrespective of the context?

Although the accounts of women's pregnancy-related experiences in the preceding pages were diverse and not easily summarized, there are nevertheless some general lessons to be learned from such stories. These lessons can be characterized as suggestions about how to approach the design and implementation of maternal health programs rather than as a blueprint for specific interventions per se.

Delineate the Context of Maternal Health

Although the direct medical causes of poor maternal health outcomes are the same worldwide, beliefs and practices associated with the management of maternal health risk vary considerably between and within societies. We saw examples of this throughout this book. In some cases, local practices surrounding pregnancy and childbirth are directly related to the cultural beliefs or norms shared by those belonging to a specific ethnicity or among people living within a particular setting. In others, people's responses to maternal health risk are a direct result of the socioeconomic status of particular individuals or groups of people, while in still other cases the practices surrounding the management of pregnancy and birth complications may be a reflection of how past and present international recommendations have played out within health facilities at the local level. Given this diversity, delineating the context of maternal health requires gaining an understanding of how risks to maternal health are defined in particular settings and the various strategies that women, men, healers, and health-care workers alike are using to address or counteract them. For example, attention to local practices related to pregnancy and childbirth in Bulangwa revealed that many women were using biomedical and nonbiomedical sources of maternal health care simultaneously. A closer look at the reasons behind this revealed that these two very different systems of maternal care were responding to two very different yet equally important perspectives on maternal health risk: risks *of* motherhood and risks *to* motherhood. Although both have a bearing on maternal health outcomes, attention during the first decade of the Safe Motherhood Initiative was focused exclusively on the former. Women's concerns with unsuccessful fertility, that is, with the very real risk of secondary infertility, did not receive much official attention at all.

Acknowledge the Heterogeneity of Women's Experiences

Delineating the context of maternal health prior to developing interventions also requires that the differences as well as similarities in women's lives be acknowledged. This includes gaining an understanding of the *process* by which certain categories of risk affect different groups of women in different ways, how women perceive their vulnerability to maternal and reproductive risks differently, and the different types of strategies they engage in to counteract them. This type of information is an important first step in helping ensure that maternal health policies and programs remain relevant to the realities of *all* women's lives.

Identify the Unofficial Risks and Unintended Consequences of Policies and Programs

We saw how the beliefs and practices of health-care personnel also had implications for maternal health outcomes. Some of the nurses working in prenatal clinics or in the hospital setting seemed to equate the risk factors illiteracy, poverty, and low status of women with ignorance and inferiority. As a result, they often did not accord their nonliterate clients the same respect as women from a higher socioeconomic status. Thus, as we saw quite vividly in several cases, although illiteracy, poverty, and the low status of women are risks for pregnant women, they are also risks in ways not acknowledged in the Safe Motherhood Initiative. There is, in effect, an unacknowledged flip side to those official risks.

Poverty and the low status of women pose risks to maternal health in other unacknowledged ways as well. Health workers in Tanzania, many of whom are women, earn very low salaries and work in conditions that are often characterized by a lack of the most basic biomedical supplies, such as gloves, medicines, and syringes. The day-to-day frustrations of working in conditions where they receive low pay and are unable to respond appropriately to obstetric emergencies undoubtedly affects health workers' ability to remain motivated at work and, ultimately, the quality of care that pregnant women receive (Bassett et al. 1997; Fonn et al. 1998; Okafor and Rizzuto 1994; Sargent and Rawlins 1991; Sundari 1992).

Some health experts have suggested that the real solution to the problem of maternal mortality is a technical one: women die because they do not have access to emergency obstetric treatment when complications arise (Maine and Rosenfield 1999). Although ensuring access to such emergency care is an important part of addressing the problem of maternal mortality, this solution treats maternal death as an event to be addressed at a particular point in time rather than as part of an ongoing process of care. I would argue that it is precisely because the poor quality of provider-client interactions is a consistent theme in the literature that interventions to improve how women are treated by health-care providers must be accorded equal weight as biomedical interventions. Issues of power between health-care providers and their clients, as well as the broader socioeconomic context of maternal mortality, will continue to be relevant even if emergency obstetric care is physically available.

In 1999, I submitted an article comparing Milembe's pregnancy complication to that of Mrs. X to a women's reproductive health journal for publication. When the editor wrote back, she pointed out (with some exasperation, I suspect) "that Mrs. X's story was always meant to be a simplification." Although my article presented some "relevant and interesting information," she noted, I nevertheless was "mixing up the issues." As she saw it, there were four distinct themes in my paper: (1) the biomedical and social aspects that lead to a maternal death; (2) the quality of treatment that women of different socioeconomic classes receive in the biomedical setting; (3) the disjuncture between allopathic and traditional approaches to care; and (4) a woman's experience of fetal death, what she does about it, what the hospital does about it. "Your woman," she stated quite matter-of-factly, "had a complication, sought care, was taken to the hospital, was admitted, was treated in some form and walked out on her feet. She was never at risk in the same way as was Mrs. X."

The point I was trying to make, I wrote back in response, is that simplifying Mrs. X's story is *precisely* the problem. Given that many who are involved with policy-making at the international level have very little, if any, firsthand experience living in third world settings themselves, simplifications such as Mrs. X's story hinder more than they help. For example, it is only now, more than a decade after the Safe Motherhood Initiative was launched, that rural women's concerns with infertility and miscarriage are starting to receive more explicit attention at the international level. Moreover, despite the place that community participation occupied in the health development discourse in the late 1970s, eliciting input from community members was not identified as one of the essential strategies to "make motherhood safe" when the Initiative was launched in 1987. It was only after the Initiative entered its second decade that community involvement in maternal health programming began to be stressed and officially recognized (Starrs 1998; cf. Pottier 1997; Woost 1997).

Rather than "mixing up" the issues, I continued, I was trying to show that they are connected. The factors that contribute to poor maternal health outcomes do not occur in isolation from each other. For example, given their negative interactions with health-care personnel, how amenable did she think Milembe and her husband would be to returning to that same hospital were she unfortunate enough to experience a life-threatening pregnancy complication in the future? In comparing her story to Mrs. X's, I was raising the possibility that a similar experience might have been the reason behind Mrs. X's delayed arrival at the hospital.

Managing Maternal Health Risk: Future Directions

Tanzania Needs Help to Stem Maternal, Infant Mortality
Dar es Salaam, Tanzania (PANA)—Tanzania Tuesday appealed to the international community to help stymie maternal and child mortality rates in parts of the country. "The appeal to our bilateral partners is to have them continue helping us in rescuing the lives of mothers and children at stake," [according to] a minister of state-in-charge of planning.

It is estimated that between 200 and 400 expectant mothers out of 100,000 die each year during childbirth from preventable complications. Early marriages, uncontrolled pregnancies and harmful practices were the leading causes of death, Vice President Omar Ali said at a function to mark the World Population Day in Dar Es Salaam.

—Pan African News Agency, July 11, 2000

Pregnancy and childbirth continue to pose risks to the health of many Tanzanian women today. It remains to be seen whether or not the "new" definitions of the problem as presented in the excerpt from the Pan African News Agency will be any more effective than their earlier counterparts. Will the solutions proposed be any less generic? Will they take into account perceptions of risk as defined by the people to be targeted?

In his epilogue to *The Anti-Politics Machine,* Ferguson answers the often-asked question "What is to be done?" (to alleviate the poverty, sickness, and hunger seen in many third world countries today), by posing the more specific question "By whom?" Although it is now recognized that "the people" themselves need to be part of the solution, Ferguson adds a cautionary note:

> But, once again, the question is befuddled by a false unity. "The people" are not an undifferentiated mass. Rich and poor, women and men, city dwellers and villagers, workers and dependents, old and young; all confront different problems and devise different strategies for dealing with them. There is not one question—"what is to be done"—but hundreds . . . (1990:281)

In this book, I have tried to show why a false unity of "the people" is problematic even in a small, rural setting with an approximate population of 4,000. In doing so, I have also tried to show how the various discourses surrounding maternal health risk—the colonial and the contemporary, the global and the local, the modern and the traditional—have produced particular kinds of truths about rural Tanzanian women's lives, and how that knowledge, in turn, has had an impact on their pregnancy-related experiences at the local level. I have argued that insufficient attention has been paid to the context in which poor maternal health outcomes occur. This inattention, in turn, has led to the implementation of generic maternal health policies and programs that are not always relevant to the complexities and realities of women's everyday lives. In order to ensure the relevance of maternal health programs in the future, policymakers and program planners must start asking different kinds of questions, ones that highlight the differences as well as similarities in women's experiences. These questions also require that more attention be focused on the process by which access to treatment unfolds, and to the quality of provider-client interactions.

Notes

CHAPTER 1

1. Although the label *developing country* has long been abandoned as problematic by anthropologists and feminist scholars who write critically about development issues in Africa, Latin America, and Asia, it is still commonly used in the literature produced by development organizations and agencies. Therefore, when referring to particular positions adopted by development organizations and agencies, I use the term *developing country*. When taking a position myself, or making an argument that is supported by the anthropological and feminist literature, I use the term *third world*.

2. As we will see in chapter 2, maternal mortality was also raised as an issue of international concern in 1936 by a former member of the Colonial Advisory Medical Committee.

3. The United Nations Children's Fund (UNICEF) and the Population Council also provided support.

4. The more recent 1999 joint WHO/UNFPA/UNICEF/World Bank statement on reducing maternal mortality remarks that the number of annual maternal deaths is now "nearly 600,000" (WHO 1999:1).

5. *Bulangwa* is a Kisukuma word that roughly translated means "learning," an activity that I think best describes the entire period of my fieldwork. In order to protect the privacy of individuals at my fieldsite, I have made the decision to use pseudonyms for the community of study, the names of people who shared their stories with me, as well as those whose work I observed.

6. R. G. Abrahams's (1981) description of his fieldsite in a different community of west central Tanzania during the late 1950s and again in 1974 makes similar references to a fluidity in social relations. He notes, for example, that although the Nyamwezi people, a group that shares cultural and linguistic similarities with the Sukuma (Brandström 1986), made up the largest percentage of the population in the community where he conducted his fieldwork, principles of neighborhood and territorial citizenship rather than ethnic identity were "of greater practical significance in the internal social system of the area's local communities" (Abrahams 1981:5). Abrahams also notes that friendship ties as well as membership in various assistance and ritually based associations (such as those involved with spirit possession and healing) helped to "cut across the boundaries of kinship linkages and even across those of ethnic groups" (1981:12–13; Abrahams 1970).

7. Thaddeus and Maine's (1990) review of the maternal mortality literature is

233

often cited in references to access to treatment. Along with an identification of a delay in the initial decision to seek care, they identify two other types of obstacles: distance to the biomedical facility, along with the related cost of transportation, and the delay in treatment within the institution itself.

8. An extensive review of the critical medical anthropology and political economy of health literature that has informed my approach to this project is beyond the scope of this introduction. But see, for example, Farmer 1992; Frankenberg 1993; Lazarus 1988; Lindenbaum and Lock 1993; Morsy 1990; Scheper-Hughes and Lock 1987; Singer 1995. See also *Medical Anthropology Quarterly* (1986, vol. 17, no. 5) and *Social Science and Medicine* (Baer et al. 1986; Singer et al. 1990) for special issues addressing critical medical anthropology. Other equally influential works include Comaroff 1978; Janzen 1978; Frankenberg 1980; Taussig 1980.

9. Studies of nonbiomedical approaches to illness in the African context, for example, often note that an individual's or family's failure to fulfill obligations to ancestral or nonancestral spirits, or social tensions between family members or even between neighbors, are seen as the source of an individual's health problems (Blakely et al. 1994; Good 1987; du Toit and Abdalla 1985; Evans-Pritchard 1937; Feierman 1984; Feierman and Janzen 1992; Janzen 1992; Ngubane 1977; Sargent 1988; Turner 1967; Yoder 1982).

10. The literature on the impact of development continues to grow. See, for example, the edited collections by Cooper and Packard (1997); Crush (1995); Grillo and Stirrat (1997); Marchand and Parpart (1995); Ram and Jolly (1998); Sachs (1992).

11. These same authors also note that many of these interventions were similar to those targeted at lower- and working-class mothers in Great Britain around the same time (Jolly 1998b; Manderson 1998; Sargent and Rawlins 1992).

12. The anthropologist Judith Justice's (1986) analysis of how foreign aid works in the context of health development programs in Nepal is similar in many ways to Ferguson's analysis of the World Bank's economic development plans for Lesotho. As with Ferguson, Justice's focus is on the structure of development, on the institutions doing the developing (1986:xiii). According to Justice, because of the enormous amounts of capital that they pour into various development projects, international agencies are able to dictate what the country's priorities should be. She notes that "he who pays the piper, calls the tune" (48), while at the same time showing that these tunes are constantly changing. Health-care priorities as defined at the international level are constantly shifting and therefore may be a reflection of current political and economic priorities at the international and national levels rather than a reflection of realities and priorities as expressed by people living at the local level.

CHAPTER 2

1. At the time she wrote the article, Dr. Blacklock was a member of the Colonial Advisory Medical Committee and past member of the Colonial Medical Services in Africa and India.

2. In his cover letter accompanying the copy of Blacklock's article, the British Secretary of State for the Colonies noted that both the Colonial Advisory Medical Committee and the Advisory Committee on Education in the Colonies endorsed the document. He acknowledged that very few funds were currently being spent on the education of women in relation to men and encouraged colonial administrators to "consider ways and means of remedying this defect":

> As the resolution recognizes, greater employment of women in health work may be dependent on an increased supply of women of sufficient general education. It is nowadays generally recognized that for the attainment of social progress in the conditions of most colonial territories the education of women is at least as important as that of men; the increased importance now given to improving nutrition and the large part that women can play in securing that end only emphasizes the need. I fear, however, that the sums spent on the education of women are still small compared with those spent on men's education, and I would ask you to consider ways and means of remedying this defect. (TNA 24840:2)

3. As noted already in chapter 1, when the Safe Motherhood Initiative was launched in 1987, an estimated 500,000 maternal deaths took place each year. Much of the early Safe Motherhood literature also notes that about 99 percent (494,000) of those deaths occur in developing country settings. The corresponding maternal mortality ratio for developing countries as a whole is given as 450/100,000. In other words, 450 women die from pregnancy-related causes for every 100,000 live births that occur in the Third World. The corresponding maternal mortality ratio for developed countries during that same time period is 30/100,000 (Starrs 1987:10). The difference between maternal death ratios and rates will be discussed in more detail in chapter 3.

4. Morsy's (1995) analysis of how the Safe Motherhood Initiative plays out in the Egyptian context is critical of this latter perspective on risk. Taking a skeptical view of the underlying intentions of first world international donors and policymakers who are supporting the Initiative, she suggests that their first and foremost goal is controlling the rate of population growth in third world countries (see also Escobar 1995; Ginsburg and Rapp 1991; Hartman 1987; Kabeer 1994). It is this latter goal, she suggests, rather than improving the survival rate of pregnant and birthing women per se, that drives the Safe Motherhood Initiative.

5. This would mean a maternal mortality ratio of 3,000/100,000—a measurement that is more than six times higher than the ratios referred to as rates in Starrs's 1987 report of the Safe Motherhood Conference (see note 3 above). But Blacklock also acknowledges that widely varying maternal mortality "rates" exist throughout the colonies, noting that some are comparable to England where, according to Loudon 1992, the maternal mortality ratio was around 400/100,000 in the 1930s and early 1940s.

6. Scholarly accounts of demographic trends in East Africa reveal that the population in East Africa actually declined from the 1890s to the 1920s. See Koponen 1996 for a discussion of the environmental and colonial policies that contributed to that decline. See also Feierman and Janzen (1992:25–37) and Turshen

(1984:41–64) for a discussion of related literature. For similar analyses of British concerns with low population levels during the period of colonial rule in Malaysia and Fiji, see Manderson 1998 and Jolly 1998b respectively.

7. Others have noted a similar heterogeneity of opinion among those working on development issues in the contemporary setting. See, for example, Gardner 1997 and Grillo 1997.

8. In terms of colonial development plans for East Africa specifically, Beck (1981) notes that the British government's plan for post–World War I East Africa was the outcome of two main objectives: (1) the upgrading of the European economic sector; and (2) the social improvement of the African population. The social improvement of the natives was to be carried out by a two-pronged approach that included both health and education programs, the content of which was still being debated well into the 1940s. See also Beck 1977.

9. Beck's work reveals similar concerns by medical doctors working during the period of German colonial rule in Tanganyika (1977:33–34). See Little 1991 and Turshen 1984 for a discussion of how British colonial policies negatively affected the health status of local populations in Tanganyika.

10. See Hunt 1990 for a discussion of similar courses in the Belgian Congo that had as their goal the retraining of African mothers.

11. According to an American nurse who had worked at the mission hospital for nearly forty years and whom I interviewed in Shinyanga in 1993, the Maynards were invited by the Church Missionary Society to take over the mission station at Nasa, fifty miles to the north of Mwanza town. They accepted the invitation and arrived in Tanzania in 1912. In 1913 the Maynards decided to leave Nasa to set up a mission station and hospital in the Shinyanga District. The journey on foot from Nasa to Shinyanga took them about one week (today it is an approximately four- to five-hour journey by car). When they arrived, there were no buildings. They pitched their tents under two trees, and Dr. Maynard began treating her first patients under them. The nurse recounting the history of the founding of the mission hospital was the child of American missionaries in Tanzania and had herself been born at the mission hospital. After completing her nursing training in the States, she returned to Tanzania to work as a nurse at the mission hospital from 1955 until she retired in 1994.

12. In addition to the maternity clinic at Kolondoto, there were two other maternity clinics in the Tabora Province: the government clinic, which was located in Tabora town, and a clinic in Kahama town that was built with funds provided by the Native Authorities (TNA 10409:8).

13. In 1920, Britain became the administrator of the Tanganyika territory under a mandate of the League of Nations. Six years later, under the governorship of Sir Donald Cameron, a system of "indirect rule" or Native Authorities was established. Modeled after British colonial policy in Nigeria, the system of Native Authorities in Tanganyika incorporated existing African structures of authority into the colonial administration. See Austen 1967. According to Beck (1981:16), the colonial government's efforts to improve the health of the local population in Tanganyika led to the passage of legislation in 1926 to establish a system of rural health dispensaries that would be maintained by the Native Authorities. She adds

the additional information, however, that debates surrounding just exactly what this system should entail continued until 1946.

14. Archival records for 1934 note that Dr. Maynard's efforts to encourage local women to use the maternity services at Kolondoto Hospital were far more successful than similar services offered through maternity clinics run by the Church Missionary Society (TNA 10721:173). Dr. Maynard's fluency in the local Sukuma language, as well as the fact that (unlike the Church Missionary Society) she did not require conversion to the Christian faith as a prerequisite for treatment at the hospital, were seen as crucial reasons for her success.

15. The policy of disseminating skills in birth management to women who give birth at hospitals is still relevant today in Tanzania and will be discussed in more detail in chapter 7 when we examine contemporary training programs for traditional birth attendants.

16. Under colonialism, hospitals were often segregated along racial lines. See Feierman and Janzen 1992:15 for a discussion of the literature related to this aspect of colonial medical policy.

17. An extract from a letter from the Indian Association of Mwanza to the governor of Lake Province in 1938 provides an example of those anticipated negative reactions:

> This association wish to thank Government for providing a decent maternity home and having thus satisfied a long felt need of Mwanza town. But we regret that the attention given to expectant mothers and babies is most insufficient and inadequate, as it is mostly left to untrained and irresponsible native ayas to execute doctors and nursing sister's instructions. We do not wish to go into details on this subject but your Excellency will appreciate the importance of this and remedy the grievance by removing ayas and substituting qualified Indian nurses to be in superintendence during and after a maternity case. (TNA 12548:75)

18. This informal training of young women has been more formalized in contemporary times in that there is now a school of nursing on the mission compounds. An unregistered nursing school was established at Kolondoto in 1955. It was registered with the government two years later in 1957. As in former times, some of the young women who complete their nurses' training choose to stay on to work as nurses at the hospital. Others seek employment elsewhere after completing their studies.

19. Archival documents make reference to the overwhelming success of the unauthorized maternity and child-care clinics. Apparently this kind of maternity clinic, run by medical officers in the colonial service without authorization or funds from the Colonial Medical Department, began to appear in Tanganyika during the British government's involvement in World War II and was seen as helping to popularize the notion of hospital-based births (TNA 34300:11a).

20. Shangali was a Chagga chief from Machame, an area that is located in what constitutes the present-day Kilimanjaro Region (Illiffe 1979:279; Bates 1965:637).

21. Archival documentation of the subsequent debates and inquiries on maternal and child services for the African population reveals the political tensions

building in the colony during this same period (TNA 34300). For example, an African critique of the government's seeming unwillingness to address the issue of funding maternal and child-care clinics took place during the 1947 Zanzibar Conference of the Tanganyika African Association. In this conference, it was noted that "very little result has been forthcoming," and a request was made that action be taken. Archival documents reveal that "action" was taken two years later in May 1949 in the form of a response by Sneath who suggests that the Africans needed to start helping themselves:

> It is suggested that the reply to the African Association might be that, taking the financial and personnel limitations into account, everything that can be done in the way of health measures, both curative and preventive, is being done. It might therefore be represented to the Association that, physical and practical proof of their intention to help themselves and their fellow-Africans would be by stimulating interest and concrete contributions to the measures mentioned above, and an active role in the attack on disease and the maintenance of a positive attitude to health is to be preferred to vague and loosely worded resolutions which imply criticism of the shortcomings of the government. (50)

See Illiffe (1979:405–35) for a discussion of the African Association. See Beck (1981:11–14) for a discussion of Sneath's tenure as director of medical services.

22. The concern expressed by the director of medical services fifty years ago that certain aspects of Western medicine—such as injections, the dispensing of pharmaceuticals, etc.—can lead to a misplaced faith in the accoutrements of "modern medicine" has been raised in the medical anthropology literature as well. See, for example, Cunningham's (1970) discussion of Thai "injection doctors" and Van der Geest and Whyte's (1988) edited collection on the use and misuse of Western pharmaceuticals in some third world countries.

23. That giving birth far from home is distressful and expensive for Tanzanian women living in rural areas today was a recurring theme in my fieldwork interviews with women in 1994 and will be discussed in more detail in chapter 9.

CHAPTER 3

1. Ester Boserup's (1970) *Women's Role in Economic Development* is considered to be the groundbreaking work in this regard. Her work, which is seen as the catalyst to the formation of the concept "Women in Development," suggested that women's productive role in many third world economies had been largely ignored. A detailed review of the research undertaken during the "UN Decade for Women" is beyond the scope of this present study, but see Escobar 1995:171–92, Kabeer 1994, chap. 1, Parpart 1993, and Sen and Grown 1987 for critical assessments of the "Women in Development" concept.

Feminist debates surrounding the notion of a universal "women's experience" also emerged during this same time period. Much of this latter literature came from feminist scholars of color who expressed the concern that much of the feminist scholarship to date has presented a homogenized view of women's experiences, a view that ignored the experiences of women whose histories are also histories of race and/or class oppression (Amos and Parmar 1984; Carby 1979; Moraga and Anzaldua 1983; see also hooks 1984; Mohanty et al. 1991). For debates within the feminist anthropological literature that explored the question of the universal subordination of women around this same time see Ortner's chapter in Rosaldo and Lamphere's 1974 edited collection *Women, Culture, and Society,* and the corresponding critique in MacCormack and Strathern's (1980) edited collection. See Moore (1988) for a discussion of the various stages of scholarly attention to women within the discipline of anthropology.

2. There are other explanations for this interest in maternal mortality. As noted by Rosenfield and Maine (1985), until the mid-1980s, women's health policy was often couched in terms of the positive effects women's health had on their children's health. One study in Bangladesh, for example, showed that 95 percent of the infants whose mothers died while giving birth or shortly thereafter would also die sometime within their first year of life (Chen et al. 1974, as cited in Winikoff 1988:200). Another earlier justification for the focus on maternal mortality was an economic one. It has been noted that in some agricultural societies women of childbearing age (15 to 49 years old) are responsible for supplying 60 to 90 percent of the labor (WHO 1985). The effects of heavy work loads, poor health, high fertility, and inadequate medical services led some experts at the World Bank to conclude that work output is negatively affected. From their perspective, improving maternal health (which in turn will increase work output) made good economic sense, an argument that is still being put forth by Safe Motherhood advocates today (*Economic and Political Weekly, India* 1987; WHO 1998). Some authors criticized this approach to women's health issues, stating that the focus of development projects should shift away from maternal health to women's health projects because women, in addition to being mothers and wage earners, are dying (WGNRR and ISIS 1988).

3. A review of the extensive Safe Motherhood literature is beyond the scope of this chapter. For examples of studies conducted during the first decade, see Kessel et al. 1995; Maine 1997; MotherCare 1998; WHO 1995a, 1996b.

4. ICD-10 also includes the category of "late maternal death": "The death of a woman from direct or indirect obstetric causes more than 42 days but less than one year after termination of pregnancy."

5. During the first decade of the Safe Motherhood Initiative, maternal mortality ratios where often incorrectly referred to in the literature as maternal mortality rates. The difference between these two measures lies in the denominator used:

> Maternal mortality ratio: Women dying from causes related to pregnancy and childbirth per 100,000 live births. This measure reflects the risk women face of dying once pregnant.

> Maternal mortality rate: Women dying from causes related to pregnancy and childbirth per 100,000 women aged 15–49. This measure reflects both the maternal mortality ratio and the proportion of women who become pregnant within a given year, i.e., the fertility rate.

See Tinker and Koblinsky (1993:2) and Starrs (1998:62) for further clarification.

6. These sources, which are not presented in my adapted version of Ravindran's tables, include statistics from WHO and national government publications, as well as individual research projects. See Ravindran (1988:41) for a listing of these sources.

7. Estimates regarding a woman's risk of dying from a pregnancy-related cause are often presented in different ways in the Safe Motherhood literature. Tinker and Koblinsky (1993:xiii), for example, note that "pregnant women in developing countries face a risk of death that is up to 200 times greater than for women in industrial countries," while another article states that women in developing countries face approximately 440 times the risk of dying from pregnancy in their lifetime than do women who are living in the more developed countries (Winikoff 1988).

8. Feminist critiques of hospital-based births in the West have suggested that some obstetricians may be too quick to diagnose a woman's labor as difficult or obstructed, and as a result many cesarean sections are not medically necessary (Davis-Floyd 1992; Martin 1987). This concern with a rush to perform cesareans is not necessarily a factor in diagnoses of obstructed labor in rural parts of sub-Saharan Africa. Although the numbers of cesarean sections performed in Western countries have been described as abnormally high (25–50 percent of all births) and do not reflect a corresponding rate of obstructed labor, this did not appear to be the case for both of the hospitals near my fieldwork site. As we will see in chapter 6, the number of cesarean sections performed at the government and mission hospitals was quite low: 3 percent of all births. In addition, oftentimes emergency cesareans were delayed either because the woman did not have the economic resources to buy the IV drip, or the electricity in the operating room was cut off due to power failures. The few cases of obstructed labor that I witnessed where cesarean sections were deemed necessary, did, in fact, seem to be literally life-saving rather than the whim of any particular doctor.

9. According to Tietze and Henshaw (Coeytaux 1988:186), Zambia is the only country in sub-Saharan Africa in which abortion is legal on "social or socioeconomic grounds."

10. This particular study is also cited in Winikoff (1988:199) as Wanjala et al. 1985.

11. But see Caplan 1988 for a discussion of her observations of the gender of child malnutrition on Mafia Island, Tanzania.

12. But infertility on the African continent is not limited to those countries south of the Sahara. See Inhorn 1994a for a discussion of infertility among Egyptian women.

CHAPTER 4

1. The Muhimbili Medical Centre is the large government referral hospital, located in Dar es Salaam, the nation's capital.

2. This is the English version of the organization's name. In Kiswahili the organization is known as *Chama Cha Waandishi Wanawake Wa Habari Tanzania*

(CHAWAHATA). Officially registered as a nongovernmental organization in 1987, TAMWA is an organization of female journalists concerned with women's issues in Tanzania.

3. *Sauti ya Siti,* a journal produced in English and Swahili by TAMWA four times a year, focuses on a variety of women's issues.

4. The Women's Global Network for Reproductive Rights, which is based in the Netherlands, is a network of individuals and organizations that campaign for women's reproductive health issues. The network also produces an international newsletter bearing the same name that focuses on women's reproductive health rights around the world.

5. The chairperson identified these conferences as one "on women's issues in [the] SADDAC region" in Arusha and another "on women leaders" that was taking place at the same time in Morogoro.

6. The question of whether people who are engaged in full-time employment can survive on their salaries emerged as a key conversational topic both during my preliminary trip to Tanzania in the summer of 1990 and later during my fieldwork in 1992 through 1994. It seemed as if everyone I spoke with worked more than one job to make ends meet. This fact of everyday life was reinforced by a conversation I had in 1990 with a member of a Tanzanian labor organization who had conducted a study on the cost of living in the capital city. He told me that the study results revealed that although the monthly minimum wage at the time was approximately 3,000 shillings, to actually live at the barest survival level a family needed at least 18,000 to 20,000 shillings per month. Although the size of "family" was not stipulated, the point nevertheless comes across that people's salaries are not sufficient. Even doctors' salaries were quite low, approximately 15,000 shillings per month in 1990. I learned that some doctors took on private patients to make ends meet, a practice that resulted in the neglect of nonpaying patients, as many I spoke with noted. I was also often told that patients wanting scarce medical resources such as medicines, private hospital rooms, beds, blood for transfusions, or attentive treatment had to slip the hospital staff something extra, although the official government policy toward health care until 1993 was that it was free (see Ahmed et al. 1996).

7. TAMWA continued to raise issues regarding women's health during the 1990s, either through their annual Day of Action seminars or in their quarterly journal *Sauti ya Siti.* In 1991, for example, TAMWA chose sexual harassment as their Day of Action theme. Activities focused on bringing the issue of violence against women into the Tanzanian mainstream media. For a summary of that Day of Action, see WGNRR 1991:12–15.

8. Funds for the conference were provided by UNICEF.

9. The term *brideprice* rather than *bridewealth* was used throughout the conference. The advantages of using the term *wealth* versus *price* with regard to marriage negotiations was raised by Evans-Pritchard in his 1931 article "An Alternative Term for Brideprice." Evans-Pritchard (1931:36) suggested "cutting the term [*brideprice*] out of the ethnological literature since . . . it emphasizes only one of the functions of this wealth, an economic one, to the exclusion of other important social functions . . . and since it encourages the layman to think that 'price' used in

this context is synonymous with 'purchase' in common English parlance." This latter use was in fact how the term was used in the context of the conference.

10. Katapa (1994), who conducted a study on the prevalence of arranged marriages in some Tanzanian communities, notes that the Tanzania Law and Marriage Act of 1971 does not apply to Zanzibar, which follows Muslim law. Some of the Zanzibari parents she interviewed stated that they arranged their daughters' marriages so that they "would find a good husband," to "fulfill religious obligations," or to prevent their daughters from engaging in premarital sex. Some of the female parents interviewed had themselves married quite young; four out of fifteen mothers Katapa interviewed had been married before the age of thirteen years, while one woman married at twenty years of age, and the rest were married as teenagers. Of the ten daughters interviewed, none had been married before the age of fourteen, with some marriages occurring when the young girls were in their later teens.

11. But a 1986 article in the *WHO Chronicle* notes that one study found no association between age and maternal deaths in Tanzania (WHO 1986:179).

12. Rwebangira (1994:194) notes that many factions in Tanzania are opposed to abortion as well as to making contraceptives available to unmarried schoolgirls. These factions include some parliament members as well as religious leaders.

13. Several of the chapters in Tumbo-Masabo and Liljeström's 1994 edited collection explore the link between the erosion of initiation rites in Tanzania and the high rates of teenage pregnancy in contemporary times. My article (Allen 2000), in contrast, explores the absence of such rituals among the Sukuma people of west central Tanzania.

14. The issue of harmful practices of traditional midwives will be addressed in chapter 7.

CHAPTER 5

1. Other Africanist scholars have noted the ways in which a community's history of cultural heterogeneity is reflected in its contemporary social and cultural landscape. See, for example, Kopytoff's edited collection (1987) on the reproduction of traditional African societies, in particular Arens's article on the history of the polyethnic community of Mto wa Mbu in Tanzania (Arens 1987). Also important is Cohen and Odhiambo's (1989) work on the historical and anthropological landscape of the Siaya District in western Kenya, Boddy's (1989) discussion of cultural resilience in the Sudan, Janzen's (1992) work that suggests a connection between the emergence of spirit possession cults in certain sub-Saharan African countries and historical patterns of migration and trade routes, and Cohen and Middleton's (1970) edited collection on incorporation and assimilation processes in various African societies. But for a cautionary note on the limits of some historical "data," see Koponen's (1988:23–45) work on late precolonial Tanzania.

2. My attention to Tanzania's colonial past will focus primarily on the period of British presence in Tanganyika from 1916 to 1961. For a discussion of German

colonial rule in northwest Tanganyika from the late nineteenth century to 1916, see Austen 1968 and Illiffe 1979.

3. The son of missionaries, Brandström grew up in west central Tanzania. His scholarly work spans a period of nearly thirty years, from his undergraduate thesis in 1966 on the place of religion in the Sukuma-Nyamwezi context, to his doctoral thesis in 1990 on thought and reality in the Sukuma-Nyamwezi universe, to subsequent publications in the 1990s. See chapter 8 for a discussion of this latter work.

4. I was told a similar version of this by a Nyamwezi friend of mine in 1990. He was more specific, however, noting that the Zaramo people were the ones who asked the Nyamwezi traders and porters where they came from. He also told me that this initial contact with the Zaramo and the "Nyamwezi" people was the major reason that these two groups entered into a joking relationship (*utani*), a relationship that is still considered relevant in the contemporary context, as I will discuss in more detail below. The historian Koponen (1988:71–73, 115), however, cautions that these so-called Nyamwezi may have actually been a much more heterogeneous group than previously thought, including peoples of various ethnicities as well as social status.

5. In 1919 a British colonial officer made a similar observation in his report of the first official tour (by foot) of the Tabora District after the post–World War I transfer of colonial power from the Germans to the British:

> Broadly speaking the collection of tribes inhabiting the Tabora Administrative area are known as Wa-Nyamwezi, Wa-Sumbwa, and Wa-Sukuma, but the former named really embraces the whole area being originally a name given to the natives of the Interior or West by the early Arab travellers and dwellers on the coast. Taking any given point within the district itself, the people to the North, South, East or West are known locally as Wa-Sukuma, Wa-Dakama, Wa-Keya, and Wa-Nyamweli, these being the names of the points of the compass in the local . . . language. (TNA 2551:1–2)

6. This relative "hardness" or "softness" was also jokingly applied by some in the community to the differences in the way these two different peoples prepared *ugali* (*bugali* in Kisukuma). *Ugali,* a mixture of corn flour and water that is boiled until it becomes stiff enough to form into a ball, is a staple of the diet in this area for non-Sukuma and Sukuma peoples alike. Bite-size pieces are then pulled off, formed into a ball, and eaten with sauces, usually at the midday meal. The *ugali* prepared by Sukuma people, I was told, was *ngumu* (hard), a result of less water being used in its preparation, while the *ugali* prepared by Nyamwezi people was softer, like their language (*laini kama lugha yao*). Several people who were used to eating *ugali* prepared in the Sukuma way told me that whenever they ate soft *ugali* (like that prepared by the Nyamwezi of Tabora or the Haya peoples of Bukoba to the north) they never felt full and thus would feel dissatisfied even after finishing their meal.

7. Holmes and Austen (1972:379) note that Roberts (1968b) makes similar observations for the history of migration among the Nyamwezi peoples (see also Roberts 1970; Abrahams 1967, 1970).

8. See, for example, Abrahams 1967, 1981:27–33; Roberts 1968b:117–50; Cory

1951; Holmes and Austen 1972; Itandala 1979; Liebenow 1959; Malcolm 1953:20–33.

9. As part of his job, he occasionally conducted interviews with older community members in order to record their version of local historical events.

10. I also found archival evidence for female chiefs and political intrigue when I visited the Tanzanian National Archives in Dar es Salaam. Two different versions regarding the origin of a ruling clan in southern Sukumaland appear in the colonial record. One source is a 1919 report by a British colonial officer who heard the story while visiting southern Sukumaland soon after the transfer of power from the Germans to the British. In many ways the story presented below is similar to the story told to me by the male healer mentioned above. However, in sharp contrast to the healer's version of the events, in the colonial record we see that the person responsible for intrigue and murder was male rather than female.

> The Wasiha [the people of the Usiha chiefdom that was located in the Shinyanga District] originally came from Negeji in Muanza [Mwanza] District and a daughter of the then reigning chief was installed by her father as Sultan of the Shinyanga—Usiha area. Her name was Giti. Her consort was a man named Mola who made himself unpopular by killing all male relatives of his wife's and all male children born to him apparently in the hopes of himself succeeding to the Sultanship. At length the headmen of Giti took the opportunity of his absence to declare that Zengo a daughter of Giti was to be recognized as the head of the tribe and they divided the district as follows amongst the surviving sisters and one brother of Giti:

Shinyanga	Zengo	(Female)
Ussanda	Malota	(Male)
Mantine	Gigwa	(Female)
Tinde	Nandi	(Female)
Ussule	Chunga	(Female)
Usiha	Kwangu	(Female)

These districts all recognized the Shinyanga Sultan as paramount and do so at the present time. (TNA 2551:13)

Another version of this story was written two years later in 1922 by a different colonial officer:

> When this country was totally uninhabited one Mola a famous hunter who was married to Giti binti Wiga came to these parts in the course of his hunting expeditions and on his return to his home at Negezi he reported so favorably of the country that the then ruling Sultan of Negezi, Wiga, an old man at the time, sent his daughter, who was married to Mola, to found a kingdom in these parts with injunctions that Giti was to rule as Sultan. A small party accompanied the family and they built their first village on the hill of Ikelenga situated in what is now known as the Sultanate of Shinyanga. Mola was jealous of his wife's position and seized the insignia of office and assumed the title of Sultan. Fearing rivals in the form of Giti's two children he murdered them which act incensed and estranged Giti who however continued to live with

him and eventually gave birth to a boy while Mola was away on one of his hunting expeditions. Giti and her followers thereupon plotted to deceive Mola and on his return she informed him of the birth of a daughter and continued the deception by dressing the child as a girl. Mola apparently suspected nothing. When the boy was two years old and able to walk Giti sent word to her father at Negezi and asked for assistance in driving Mola out of her kingdom. Mola was driven out and the son named Izengo ruled in his place. From this time the custom was introduced among this branch of the family that heirs to the Sultanship could only be selected through sisters of the ruling Sultan. So that the law of inheritance in so far as the royal family is concerned is that the eldest son of the eldest sister of the ruling Sultan succeeds him. This was out of respect for the fact that the first Sultan was a woman Giti. This practice was followed until 1905 when the German government ordered that the son of the ruling Sultan should succeed, which is the practice now followed. (TNA 3387)

This latter report also includes a list of the chiefs after the reign of Giti and Izengo; all are male. Although the gender of the chief referred to as Zengo (Izengo) appears to have been transformed from female to male in the two-year interval between these colonial documents, there is, nevertheless a consistent theme that the founding chief of the Usiha clan was female. For other examples in the archival record regarding female chiefs, see Roth 1996:51–52.

11. Indeed, over the course of my fieldwork he often made comments that female power was to be feared. On one occasion, he offered as evidence for women's general untrustworthiness their supposed propensity for sorcery, which in turn was linked to their reproductive powers. We will return to the question of women's propensity for sorcery in later chapters.

12. Beidelman has noted similar (and in his opinion unlikely) myths for the matrilineal Kaguru of Tanzania:

The original group is described as led by a woman because there were no mature men in the group. Like all matrilineal peoples, Kaguru see authority as properly held by men of a matrilineage and any matriarchal tendencies are considered odd: female leadership is here explained away through an abnormal lack of adult males. We are then confronted with the unlikely picture of a band led by a woman and without mature men to protect them as they wander for hundreds of miles over warlike wilds. (1993:78)

Corlien Varkevisser (1971:74–75), who had completed her master's degree in anthropology at the time she conducted research in Mwanza during the latter part of the 1960s, appears to be just as skeptical of the origin story of "wayfaring sisters and one brother" among the Sukuma as Beidelman is about women as leaders in the origin myths for the Kaguru. See, for example, Varkevisser's 1971 article "Sukuma Political History, Reconstructed from Traditions of Prominent Nganda (Clans)." Although the myth of the founding of the Babinza clan (as reported by Itandala) does seem to suggest that Ilembo's sisters founded chiefdoms themselves, it doesn't say that they traveled on their own without men. It could be that there were plenty of mature men in the entourage, but they were insignificant in terms of establishing the chiefdom.

13. Several authors have noted that the conus shell, or *ndeji* in Kisukuma, was one of the important articles of chieftaincy in the past. Cory, for example, notes that it was worn by the chief around the neck or on the wrist (1951). Shorter also mentions the symbolic power of the conus shell in many East and Central African communities:

> One of the most remarkable facts in the history of East and Central Africa is the very ancient and extremely widespread use of the conus-shell as an emblem of authority. The shell originates on the East African coast, but the farther away one goes from the coast the more ritual importance it assumes. (1972:144)

Today the *ndeji* has been transformed into a symbol of the ability to heal people, and thus it was worn by many healers practicing in and around Bulangwa. Other coastal products are also valued for their power by Sukuma and non-Sukuma healers alike in contemporary times. On the three occasions I traveled to Dar es Salaam during my fieldwork, one healer always asked me to bring certain items back for her. One time she asked me to bring a bottle of ocean water and sand. Other times I was asked to bring back certain types of shells that were used as containers for ritual medicines. See the Tabora District Report 1919–1920 (TNA 2551) for a description of other articles of chieftaincy among the Sukuma and Nyamwezi.

14. Boddy (1989:26) has noted a similar central position of ritual as well as political power for women in the Meroë and Christian matrilineal societies of historical Nubia in the Sudan, whereas Lewis's work suggests women's power was peripheral. See also Giles's work (1987, 1989) on women's participation in possession cults on the Swahili coast of East Africa.

15. See also Gray and Birmingham's (1970) edited collection on East African precolonial trading networks.

16. Beidelman, in contrast, notes that *utani* among Kaguru people is tied specifically to notions of pollution and sexuality:

> Kaguru maintain that one cannot entirely respect those with whom one has shared nakedness and sexuality, even though such ties were formalized through marriage. (1993:128)

He notes further that the connections between pollution and sexuality also characterize the *utani* relationship that the Kaguru hold with other peoples. The Kaguru who practice male circumcision stand in *utani* relationship with the uncircumcised Nyamwezi and Hehe peoples "because such men, being uncircumcised and therefore unclean (*sika*), need not be treated politely" (128).

17. A Chagga man who lived in the community told me that a joking relationship also exists between the Chagga and Pare people. He noted that the relationship could, on occasion, become contentious. He gave the example of the funeral he attended for a Chagga man in the Kilimanjaro Region. During the ceremony, the deceased's *mtani,* a Pare man, jumped into the grave and refused to leave it

without a payment from the bereaved family. There was apparently nothing the family could do but pay. In response to my professed sympathy for the bereaved family's predicament, he told me that the joking relationship actually has its own set of rules. The reason the Pare man had jumped into the grave and demanded payment in the first place, he told me, was that the head of the grieving family, who was well-known in the community for his stinginess, hadn't provided much in the way of a funeral feast. The "payment" extracted was subsequently used to buy beer for the funeral guests.

18. Holmes and Austen (1972) also make the point that although the trade in slaves passed through the central regions of Tanzania, slaves were not captured from that area. They were brought primarily from Buganda to the northwest. However, an increase in interethnic warfare that took place in the southern Shinyanga region during the middle of the century may have resulted in prisoners of war being sold into slavery. Roberts (1970:59) makes a related point but also notes that not all slaves were transported out of the interior.

19. See Alpers 1968, Bennett 1971, Holmes and Austen 1972, Kjekshus 1977:124, and Roberts 1968a for more detailed discussion of this period.

20. The impact of this "arms race" was still seen fifty years later, according to evidence provided in the 1926 Annual Report of the Tabora Province:

> During the year special attention was given to the registration of all firearms belonging to natives, and a total of 6,113 muzzle-loading guns are now registered. . . . It is remarkable that of the total number of guns registered in the Province no less than 3,266 are in the Tabora district and 1,930 in Nzega. One can see in that the influence of the past when Tabora was the great interior depot for the Arab ivory hunters and slave traders. (TNA 1733/9/69:17)

21. Kjekshus (1977:2), a political scientist whose scholarly work focuses on the relationship between people and their environment, is highly critical of this latter perspective. He appears skeptical of studies that he characterizes as being overly concerned with political history and that thus tend to portray the situation by the end of the nineteenth century as reflecting a "crisis of authority." He believes that many scholars miss the real reason for the increase in skirmishes during the latter part of the nineteenth century: that the increase in Western goods in the interior via the caravan trade led ultimately to an undermining of the local economies of the interior, resulting in a scarcity of available resources. He also sees the increase in conflict as an indirect result of increases in population, which in turn led to a crisis in the availability of local food products and of land for agriculture and cattle grazing (1977:111–25; cf. Koponen 1988).

22. Gluckman (1963) has noted similar economic and political benefits of village clustering in British Central Africa. See Noble's 1970 doctoral dissertation on the voluntary associations among the Sukuma.

23. Great Britain's usurping of German control over Tanganyika occurred in stages, begun in 1916 in central Tanzania and finalized in 1920 when Tanganyika became a protectorate of Britain through a mandate of the League of Nations (Beck 1977:41; see also Austen 1967; Ingham 1965).

24. Turshen (1984), on the other hand, characterizes the period of colonial rule

under the Germans as quite brutal. She notes, however, that the officials of the central government in charge of the villages were Swahili/Muslim agents (*akidas*) who had been employed by the Arabs and then shifted to German service (31). See also Illiffe's (1979) discussion of the period of German colonial rule.

25. Shinyanga continues to be a site where diamonds and gold are found today.

26. Bakinikana (1974), a Tanzanian whose master's thesis addresses the differential effects of colonialism on precolonial authorities among the Haya and the Sukuma peoples, compares the striking difference in the adherence to Christianity between these two groups. Living among the Haya were many Ganda Christians "who while preaching this alien religion seemed to identify themselves with it as though it was originally a Ganda (African) religion" (1974:146). According to Bakinikana, in contrast to the Haya, the tendency among the Sukuma was to resist conversion to Christianity and to reject it as primarily a European religion. He suggests that this resistance may be a result of "an absence of an influence from African Christians" (146). He notes, however, that conversion to Christianity was much higher among the Sukuma chiefs; 64 percent of the twenty-five chiefs which Liebenow interviewed were Christian (1974:145; see also Liebenow 1959). Bakinikana suggests that chiefs converted more readily to Christianity because of the educational and economic opportunities to be garnered from "pleasing" the European governmental and religious authorities: "Since the government cooperated with the missionaries in different ways, the [chiefs] saw some advantage in becoming Christians" (1974:145). A Kenyan Swahili instructor of mine during my first years of graduate school made a similar comment to me about conversion to Christianity. We had been talking about religion, and he mentioned that he had grown up in Christian boarding schools. When I asked which denomination he was, he chuckled, noting that when he was young, his religious affiliation changed according to which mission school was currently offering free room and board.

CHAPTER 6

1. Hochschild (1999:51) has pointed out that although Stanley marketed *Through the Dark Continent* as excerpts from his journal, those "excerpts" bear little resemblance to the actual journal he kept of his travels.

2. As we saw in the previous chapter, Austen (1968) and Bates (1965) suggest that the government-mandated clearing of brush that characterized the anti–tsetse fly campaigns of the 1920s was responsible for the subsequent soil erosion throughout the area.

3. The fierce competition seen in the Western countries between these two powerful soft drink companies has even reached the rural level in Tanzania. Evidence for this competition takes many forms. In Shinyanga town, for example, Pepsi-Cola distributors provided street signs for virtually every street in the center of town, paved or unpaved, regardless of size. Within a short while, another set of street signs appeared for the same exact set of streets. These new signs carried the Coca-Cola logo and were placed strategically on the opposite side of the street from the street signs displaying the Pepsi-Cola logo. Needless to say, it is almost

impossible to lose one's bearings in Shinyanga town today, since there is not just one set of street markers, but two.

4. Everyone who mentioned this seemed to link the town's gradual economic decline and its accompanying "Asian flight" to the economic policies dating from the mid-1970s, when the Tanzanian government nationalized many privately owned businesses and prosecuted many Arab and Asian members of the community who were suspected of participating in the black market economy. For a more detailed examination of this period see Hedlund and Lundahl 1989; O'Neil and Mustafa 1990; and Yeager 1989. See Campbell 1991 for a review of this and related literature.

5. Children living in the surrounding villages attended primary schools located near their homes.

6. Although persons of mixed Arab and African ethnicity who identify themselves exclusively in terms of their African roots might be referred to by the Kiswahili word *mwarbu,* or Arab, in this specific context it refers to physical rather than cultural characteristics.

7. An example of what can happen if this code is breached occurred during a funeral at the home of an Arab family in the community. One of the Arab guests who had traveled from Shinyanga town arrived at the funeral dressed in a gown that reached approximately two inches below her knees. The "shortness" of her gown and thus her shocking public display of immodesty, especially in the public context of a funeral, was discussed for several days afterward by many of the Arab women over afternoon coffee.

8. There were nevertheless exceptions: two Arab sisters I knew, both in their late thirties, had completed secondary school when they were young.

9. Arab women's low level of involvement with agriculture was the reason some Arabs gave for why Arab women shouldn't marry African men. Arab women shouldn't marry African men, an Arab woman I knew told me, because they would expect their Arab wives to farm the land. Still, there are exceptions even to this generalization. For example, the sister of the Arab woman who provided me with this explanation was married to an African man. Moreover, she was quite a successful business person in her own right, and did no farming herself.

10. Both Beidelman (1963) and Beattie (1963) note similar characteristics of witchcraft beliefs among the Kaguru peoples of Tanzania and the Nyoro peoples of western Uganda. However, although Beidelman states that witchcraft is purchased rather than inherited, he also notes "a taste" for witchcraft can be transmitted as a result of incestuous relationships with matrilineal kin (1963:67–68).

11. Using available Tanzanian government figures on witch killings, Mesaki states that "between 1970 and 1984, 3333 witch-related cases were reported involving the murder of 3692 witch-suspects in 13 regions of mainland Tanzania" (1993:158). These killings are particularly high in Mwanza and Shinyanga:

> Usukuma accounted for 2120 cases and 2246 deaths. Additional figures available for Mwanza and Shinyanga show that between 1984 and 1988 another 827 people were killed. So from 1970 to 1988, 3073 people were killed in the area of Sukumaland after being identified as witches. (189)

12. At the time of my fieldwork from 1992 to 1994, Tanzania's population was estimated at 23.1 million, based on the 1988 census (Bureau of Statistics [Tanzania] and Macro International Inc. 1997).

13. There are actually two main categories of government hospitals: the regional and the district hospital.

14. I also had the opportunity to observe a couple of births at the health center level.

15. User fees were instituted at the government hospital in 1993 (Ahmed et al. 1996). Although women began paying two hundred shillings to give birth at the government hospital (the price equivalent to half a kilo of beef or a kilo of beans), they still were required to bring their own supplies.

16. With the exception of Varkevisser's study, which was part of a larger Dutch project out of the Center for the Study of Education in Changing Societies, the other studies all came out of the Catholic University of America and were designed to study various aspects of social and cultural change among the Sukuma. Two of these studies make particular reference to various aspects of women's reproductive health. Gottfried and Martha Lang (1973) carried out research in the Mwanza Region from July 1961 to December 1962 and in the Shinyanga Region from October 1969 to December 1970. Their primary research interest was on planned social change among the Sukuma. Gottfried Lang notes, however, that the majority of their several thousand survey respondents and informants were male (see Molnos 1973:266). Marlene Reid's research (1969) focused on change in Sukuma health concepts and practices. See also Hatfield 1968; Noble 1970; and Roth 1966. The particular focus of these studies in the early postcolonial years is interesting given that Bakinikana (1974:147) notes that in comparison to the Haya peoples, colonial authorities characterized the Sukuma as being much more resistant to change.

17. One of the women I had listed as having reached menopause had attended primary school until the fifth grade. I originally listed her as having reached menopause because she had told me that she hadn't experienced her menses in over a year, was forty-five years old, had no obvious signs of pregnancy, and had experienced hot flashes. She wasn't sure, however, if she had in fact reached menopause. She thought that perhaps she had a pregnancy that had "turned to the back" (*nda ya gupinda ngongo*). The concept of pregnancies that turn to the back and who experiences them will be discussed in chapter 9. Since she was the only woman in this group who had gone to school, I excluded her from the analysis.

18. In a footnote to his 1990 article (184, n. 8), Brandström notes that there are various forms of conjugal union among what he refers to as the Sukuma-Nyamwezi people (see, for example, Cory's *Sukuma Law and Custom* (1970 [1953]:39–57; see also Bösch 1930). Brandström reduces these various types to three main forms: (1) the union between man and woman resulting from the transfer of bridewealth, (2) widow inheritance, and (3) cohabitation without transfer of bridewealth. It is the first and the third types of unions that emerged as relevant in my interviews with women.

CHAPTER 7

1. The meaning and place of initiation in the contemporary Tanzanian context received a lot of attention from Tanzanian scholars, journalists, and women's health advocates during the late 1980s and early 1990s (Hashim 1989; Kaijage 1989; Shaba and Kituru 1991; Shuma 1994). See my discussion of the absence of puberty initiation rites among the Sukuma (Allen 2000).

2. Various studies of indigenous systems of healing appeared during this same time period and undoubtedly informed health development policy recommendations as they related to primary health care. For examples of cultural practices related to healing in sub-Saharan Africa, see Ademuwagun 1979; Bibeau et al. 1980; Ngubane 1977. See also WHO 1976, 1978b. The literature on indigenous birthing practices is also quite extensive. For examples of anthropological studies of birthing practices that predate the Safe Motherhood Initiative, see Jordan 1978; Kay 1982; Laderman 1983; and MacCormack 1982. See also Jordan's (1990) early critique of TBA training programs and accompanying commentary. For a review of studies of cross-cultural childbirth and related literature, see the introduction to Davis-Floyd and Sargent 1997; Steinberg 1996; and an unpublished WHO report by Edouard and Foo-Gregory (1985).

3. Concerns with the harmful effects of herbs ingested by women during labor has been raised by obstetricians working in other parts of Tanzania as well. Price (1984), for example, estimated that 95 percent of the women in one study of the Southern Highlands of Tanzania were suspected of using herbal medicine during labor. He also notes in addition to causing uterine rupture, herbal remedies, which are taken in various forms, have toxic effects that may lead to liver and renal failure, as well as to serious circulatory problems (1984). He notes that of the 115 maternal deaths he reviewed, two were thought to have been the result of herbal remedies used by the women during their labor.

4. I first heard reference made to a link between adverse pregnancy outcomes and chloroquine use while working as a Peace Corps health volunteer at a maternal and child-care clinic in Gabon in the mid-1980s. Several Gabonese nurses I worked with told me that if I ever heard that a young woman had committed suicide by taking an overdose of chloroquine, I could safely assume she had been pregnant and had actually been trying to abort, not end her life. I heard similar stories during my fieldwork in Tanzania, stories that linked secondary school girls' use of a combination of chloroquine and tetracycline tablets to abortion. See Renne 1996 for a discussion of abortion remedies used by Ekiti Yoruba women in Nigeria.

5. In an unpublished mimeographed document on the Sukuma and Nyamwezi peoples, Hans Cory makes passing reference to midwifery and healing with regard to women's ownership of property. However, as he doesn't provide any further elaboration, I take his use of the word *midwife* to be his own terminology rather than a Sukuma concept per se:

It is characteristic of the relationship between husband and wife that, should the latter acquire property either by inheritance or by her profession (midwifery, medical practice, etc.) she will deposit her property with her brother and not bring it into the house. Undoubtedly the bonds of kinship are stronger than those of matrimony. (n.d.:24)

It is quite possible that he is referring to the general category of female healers, who were called in the cases of retained placenta, or to women who are specialists in fertility medicine. Both of these types of healers, I was told, are simply called *bafumu* (*nfumu* sing.) in the Sukuma language.

6. Sargent (1982) describes a similar practice of giving birth alone among Bariba women in Benin.

7. But as I have already shown in chapter 2, and as the excerpt from the Tanzanian National Archives above reveals, initial attempts to train local women in midwifery skills began during the period of colonial rule in Tanganyika.

8. I heard different opinions on the extent of her midwifery training. Throughout the course of my fieldwork, various people referred to her as a "former nurse at Kolondoto," an occupation that she vehemently denied when I later asked her about it. Yes, she told me, she had lived at Kolondoto for several years, but it was only to take care of her brother who was being treated for leprosy. She even asked me to go and verify the truth of her statements at Kolondoto myself. I eventually did and found that none of the older nurses at the hospital remembered having worked with her, nor did the American nurse who had worked at the mission hospital for almost thirty years. I also spoke with a man who knew her while she lived with her brother in the village for lepers located within the hospital compound. He told me that she arrived around 1958 and left around 1963. Regardless of the source of her training, I spent much time in her village observing her healing practice and learned that she had a vast knowledge of herbal remedies. Specifics of her midwifery and healing practice will be discussed in chapters 8 to 11.

9. In chapter 9 we will revisit this issue of pregnant women being turned away from clinics because they do not have a record of their prenatal care.

10. The idea that births were easier in the past is also a theme in Cory's work (n.d.). I will return to this point again in chapter 11 when I present the results of my interviews with women who had relatives who died from pregnancy or childbirth complications.

11. Despite women's tendency to claim that pregnancy-related taboos were no longer adhered to, some women invoked a general notion of a Sukuma way of doing things as the reason why certain taboos were or were not followed. For example, when I asked women if there were things that they were forbidden to eat or do while they were pregnant, some would respond "We Sukuma don't have any taboos" (*Sisi Wasukuma hatuna mwiko*). This type of comment was also made when comparing Sukuma customs during the postpartum period with those followed by the Arab and some African Muslim women in the community, as will be discussed later in chapter 11. On the other hand, when I asked about the meaning behind certain practices, such as shaving an infant's head within the first month of its life, Sukuma women might respond with the general comment that it was done like that because that was the way the Sukuma people did things (*Sisi Wasukuma,*

tunafanya hivyo), even though this particular practice was common in the community, regardless of a person's ethnicity or religious affiliation.

12. I actually only heard one reference to food taboos during the entire period of my fieldwork, a comment made by a Sukuma woman who was visiting Bulangwa to attend the funeral of a distant relative. I was sitting next to her in the room in which the women attending the funeral had congregated, and we struck up a conversation about why she was there, why I was there, and about my research. I told her that I had been surprised when none of the women in my survey mentioned food taboos. She responded by saying that she herself had heard that a long time ago it was taboo for pregnant women to eat intestines or eggs. The former category of food could result in a birth in which the umbilical cord would be wrapped around the newborn's neck. She couldn't remember the reason why the consumption of eggs was forbidden.

13. One of the manifestations of severe iron-deficiency anemia, according to the sixteenth edition of the *Merck Manual of Diagnosis and Therapy* (Berkow and Fletcher 1992), is that a person with this condition may crave dirt or paint (pica) or ice, as well as suffer from fatigue and loss of stamina.

CHAPTER 8

1. From Fr. George Cotter's (n.d.) collection of Sukuma proverbs.

2. For other studies of African women's fertility-related concerns, see Bledsoe et al. 1998 and Feldman-Savelsberg 1999.

3. An extensive treatment of Brandström's analysis of Sukuma-Nyamwezi cosmology is beyond the scope of this chapter. I am interested in presenting only a brief summary of its core elements in order to discuss their relevance to women's fertility-related experiences in Bulangwa.

4. Unless noted otherwise, the italicized words discussed in this section are in the Sukuma language.

5. The title of Bösch's undated article is not listed in Brandström's 1990 article, so it is not listed in this bibliography either.

6. The historian Iris Berger (1976:161) mentions a similar local proverb for Burundi: "Woman is only the passive earth; it is the man who provides the seed."

7. Brandström situates the symbolic classification regarding left and right in Sukuma-Nyamwezi thought within the context of the anthropological literature on dual classification:

> The Sukuma-Nyamwezi do indeed differ markedly from the pattern recorded from various parts of the African continent of close association of right with male and left with female. The right hand, called "the male hand" among many Bantu-speaking peoples, is generally considered to be "strong" and "good", and it is often associated with patriliny and purity (cf. Werner 1903; Wieschoff 1938; Beidelman 1961; Rigby 1966; Berglund 1976). However, the Sukuma-Nyamwezi have made a different cultural choice. Among them the left hand is symbolically linked to fatherhood and the father's side, and as such the left is the male hand, associated with strength and bravery. As

Granet wrote in his very considerate article on lateral symbolism in China: "The pre-eminence of the right or the left depends always on events, on the occasional circumstances of time and place" (Granet 1973:58). Right and left in Sukuma-Nyamwezi thought is but one example of the "various ways in which different people have used the basic cognitive bricks of dualism to construct edifices of symbolic meaning" (Willis 1985:211). In the cultural "edifice" of the Sukuma-Nyamwezi, the physical weakness of the left has been transformed into "symbolic strength." (1991:123)

As suggested by the passage above, Brandström's analysis provides an interesting exception to other anthropological scholarly writings on dual classification. Due to space limitations, I can not do justice to it here, but wish to direct interested readers to this important aspect of his work.

8. The relevance of the bow to the contemporary setting of Bulangwa merits brief discussion here. Although hunting no longer plays a central role in the everyday life of Sukuma people, the bow does, nevertheless, still have some significance in community life, for example, when a social infraction occurs, such as stealing or not paying debts. The person accused of committing the offense is placed under a form of house arrest and can only leave its premises to buy daily essentials. Only immediate family members are permitted to visit. A person so incarcerated must "turn over his bow" to community authorities until the debt is paid and the sanction of house arrest is lifted. I learned about this use of the bow when a man in Bulangwa was publicly accused and beaten for stealing corn from someone's land. I knew him and believed him to be innocent, and thus I went to visit him to get his version of the story, an action that elicited great concern from a neighbor who cautioned me to be careful or I myself would also be placed under house arrest. The man gave me his version of the story, declaring that he had not, in fact, been placed under house arrest, citing as proof that he still had his bow. Although anyone in the community can be placed under house arrest, I am not sure if Sukuma women and non-Sukuma people are also required to turn over a bow. For a discussion of the history of archery among the Sukuma, see Tanner 1953.

9. See Cory 1944 for a discussion of twin ceremonies among the Sukuma. In Bulangwa, these rituals, known as *ukango,* were also mandated when babies were born in the breech position. One of the perceived dangers of a couple's refusal to carry out this ritual is that it will bring misfortune to the community as whole, such as a failure in the rains. Misfortune could occur at the individual level as well and could have consequences for the health of the parents, their children, or their subsequent descendants. People in Bulangwa acknowledged that these rituals are not as widespread now as they were in the past. They linked this decline to the influence of organized religion. Several people who had twins but had not undergone the *ukango* ritual told me they refused to do so because it was something that pagans (*wapagani*) or people in darkness (*watu wa giza*) did, while they, in contrast, were Christian (*watu wa dini*). See Sargent's (1988) discussion of similar rituals connected to the birth of twins and breech births among the Bariba people of Benin.

10. But "firstborn" can also be contextual. For example, a non-Sukuma friend

of mine, Mama Mary, who was herself a mother of five children, had moved to Bulangwa ten years previously with her three youngest children. Although Mary was her third child, not first, in Bulangwa she became known as Mama Mary, because people in the community knew her in the context of those three children, of whom Mary was the oldest. Even after her daughter Mary moved out of the community several years later, my friend was still referred to as Mama Mary. The way in which a mother and father are addressed can also be temporarily contextual, as in calling a woman or man by the name of one of their other children when that particular child is being stressed in that specific context. Nevertheless, my main point remains the same: parenthood is an important component of a person's social identity, irrespective of their ethnicity.

11. See Beidelman's (1993:92–93) discussion of teknonyms among the Kaguru in Tanzania.

12. This is in sharp contrast to Scheper-Hughes's (1992) observations of children's funerals in a community in northeastern Brazil.

13. In the Sukuma dialect spoken in Bulangwa, the word for diviner was *nfumu*.

14. According to Tanner (1969), the relationship between the living and their ancestors has undergone a transformation over time, a change he linked to the decline in the political power of the chief after the imposition of colonial rule. As discussed in chapter 5, prior to colonial rule, the veneration of ancestors was linked to a chief's ritual and political power. Daily rituals that acknowledged the centrality of ancestral influences in the lives of their living descendants were carried out as preventive measures to ensure adequate rainfall, good harvest, success in warfare, and the general health of the people within the chiefdom. A chief could be replaced if an unusual amount of misfortune occurred within the chiefdom.

Tanner suggested that the attention "now" (i.e., in the late 1960s) paid to ancestors is similar to the role of curative as opposed to preventive medicine. Propitiation of the ancestors, he noted, now takes place only when their living descendants are experiencing misfortune, whether in regard to their health or generally within the context of their daily lives. His reference to the current use of propitiation as a cure rather than as prevention is similar to what I found in Bulangwa, although two people I spoke with (a Sukuma man who was trained as a medical assistant and a woman who took part in my formal interviews) told me they still carried out annual offerings to their ancestors as a form of prevention or insurance against future misfortune.

15. Evidence in the archival records supports Mwana Nyanzanga's reference to drownings resulting from these initiation ceremonies. In 1930 two female initiates into the *Buswezi* society, a spirit possession cult, in Buhungukira, Mwanza, drowned while ritually bathing during the final part of the ceremony. In the official deposition taken during the inquest into the drowning, the father and husband of the two deceased initiates explains how the decision to be initiated was made and how the drowning occurred:

> I am the husband and father of the two deceased. I had two children about seven years ago. My wife was constantly giving birth and the children died after a few days so I went to a doctor of the "Baswezi." He advised me to join

that sect. Since that [time] my wife has born two children who have died and two had done likewise previously. So last month I mentioned the matter to my father who is a disciple of the Kiswezi cult—he advised me to take the old doctor's advice as a cure for my wife's trouble . . .There were four candidates for admission to the sect namely, myself, my wife and my two female children . . .On the sixth day [of the initiation ceremony] we went to a pool of water about breast high and about 10 paces by 10 paces big to wash. When I got in I noticed that the water was "mzito" [heavy] and I fell over. Everyone else did likewise, it was as if an unseen force pushed us over. There was no slime at the bottom of the waterhole. Everyone got out and ran away except myself, my wife and my youngest child. I did not see the latter as I went under and swallowed a lot of water. I cried out and the others came and helped me out but there was no sign of my wife and child. We ran into the water led by the Drs. followed by the candidates, followed by the rest of the sect. As we entered we were surrounded by the older initiates in the water. There were 14 of us . . . My wife and the child who was drowned were holding hands as they went into the water but when their bodies were found they were unclasped. We entered the water to the accompaniment of terrific shouting and yelling. (TNA 19303:3–4)

16. Mwana Nyanzanga names all the babies that she delivers, and almost all are given Christian names, such as James, Mary, John, Moses, etc. She even named one of the newborns "Filipo" after myself and my father because I was known in that particular village as *Mwana Filipo,* "Phillip's child." That children she names may, in turn, be renamed upon returning home is a possibility. Nevertheless, there were several people in that particular village who were known by their Christian names, all of whom she had delivered herself.

17. For the most part here I will limit these to the Kiswahili terms used by both Sukuma and non-Sukuma people.

18. *Mgongo* (*ngongo* in Kisukuma) was also used both in Kiswahili and in Kisukuma to refer to the lower intestinal tract. For example, to describe gas in the lower intestines a person might say that their *mgongo* was "crying" or making noise (*mgongo unalia*). Women also used this phrase to describe the sound made by air pockets in the vaginal tract after giving birth. The prevention of that particularly embarrassing sound was one of the major reasons cited by women for getting postpartum hot sponge baths, a practice that will be discussed in more detail in chapter 11.

19. Even I was not excluded from a scrutiny of my menstrual cycle when a healer conducted a divination of chicken entrails to see if my ancestors agreed I could observe his work. Prior to his arrival (he was with another client about fifty feet away), the man who prepared the chicken for the divination ritual took a cursory look at the entrails and told me that my most recent menstrual flow had been unusually heavy. I actually felt rather disappointed because his "revelation" couldn't have been further from the truth. He also told me that someone had recently stolen a pair of my underwear and was using it in sorcery against me. I must admit feeling genuine relief when the real diviner arrived and started out my divination

by stating that my menses were "normal." Although he didn't say anything about any stolen underwear, he did note that I was currently experiencing some problems with my digestive tract, an observation that was indeed true at the time.

20. An Arab woman who was a good friend of mine told me that a wife would have legitimate grounds for divorce if her husband insisted that they have intercourse during her menses, because she was in a state of ritual uncleanliness.

21. Although this statement is quite similar to statements that some Beng women of the Ivory Coast cite as the reason why husbands and wives might refrain from sexual intercourse during a woman's menses, Gottlieb (1988) acknowledges that in certain contexts (e.g., cooking, entering the forest) menstrual blood is seen as polluting.

22. One of the vendors I interviewed at the herbal market in Shinyanga town told me that a woman who has difficulty conceiving and whose menstrual bleeding begins when the moon is straight above is an example of the most difficult kind of infertility to cure. His treatment of this specific type of infertility occurs in stages. He first gives the woman an herbal remedy to change the timing of her cycle so that the onset of her menses will take place when the moon is either in the west or in the east. Only when this change takes place will he give the woman an herbal remedy to treat her actual infertility.

23. Several women mentioned feelings of embarrassment and fear when they saw their menstrual blood for the first time. One woman told me that when she first saw blood in her underwear, she thought that she had been pierced by a twig while playing outside (*nimechomwa na miti*). Another woman recounted how her brother's wife, who lived in the same compound as she did, noticed that she kept going to the river throughout the day and confronted her about her frequent trips. She replied that she had burst open (*nimepasuka*) and thus kept returning to the river in order to wash the blood away. Her sister-in-law explained to her what was actually happening and how to use a cloth to absorb the menstrual flow.

24. But as results from studies in the Gambia and the United States reveal, confusion about the menstrual cycle is not limited to women living in Tanzanian settings (Bledsoe et al. 1994; Hockenberry-Eaton et al. 1996; Westoff et al. 1969; see also Martin 1987). The study in Gambia, for example, found that only 7 percent of the women in the study who practiced periodic abstinence as a method of birth control identified the middle of the ovulatory cycle as the fertile period (Bledsoe et al. 1994:84). Studies of American women's knowledge about the timing of ovulation also found evidence of misunderstanding. One study in the United States that explored knowledge about ovulation among women who used the pill found that only 58 percent identified the most fertile time as falling between the thirteenth and fifteenth day of a woman's cycle, as opposed to 48 percent of women who used other methods of birth control (Westoff et al. 1969). A more recent United States–based study found that 52 percent of the mothers and 75 percent of the girls who were asked about their knowledge of sexual development were not able to adequately define ovulation (Hockenberry-Eaton et al. 1996:45).

25. As mentioned already in chapter 5, *ugali,* a staple of the midday meal that is eaten with sauces, is a stiff porridge usually made of corn, but occasionally millet, flour.

26. This latter definition belies the complexity of the term. See Reid 1969:68–70 for a discussion of *nzoka* in terms of Sukuma notions of illness in general and with regard to pregnancy and infertility problems specifically (79–80). See Renne's discussion of the connection between menstrual disorders, black blood, and worms among the Ekiti Yoruba of Nigeria (2001).

27. Blood compatibility was a common metaphor used to refer to other aspects of human relations. People, regardless of their ethnicity, who seem to just click or hit it off with one another (to use colloquial English) are said to have "compatible blood" (*damu inapatana*). I first became aware of this concept through a Jaluo friend of mine about six months after arriving in the community. She and I had established a close friendship in a relatively short period of time after I arrived in Bulangwa. Although I had already started meeting a lot of women in the community, for some reason the two of us seemed to get along as if we had been friends for years. I later learned that our friendship was a source of amazement for some people in the community, who supposedly had never seen a friendship between African and white women. After jokingly accusing my friend of using *samba,* a local category of medicine that "caused" me to like her, it was finally agreed that the source of our friendship was the result of the compatibility of our blood.

The characteristics of a person's blood could have other effects. People who have bad luck in finding or keeping a job, or finding a spouse, or those who just seem to have bad luck in general are often diagnosed by healers with a condition known as heavy blood or *damu uzito. Damu uzito* isn't seen as a particularly serious condition, because it is easily treated and cured by washing in a local spiritual medicine over the period of one or two weeks. A person with bad blood (*damu mbaya*), on the other hand, is someone to be avoided at all costs. In trying to explain the meaning of this latter concept to me, Mwana Nyanzanga put it in terms of her own profession: "For example, if I slept with a man who had bad blood, I would start to have bad luck with the births I attend." "Well, what would the cure be?" I asked. "To stop sleeping with him," she replied.

28. Renne (2001) also raises the possibility that the concept of blood incompatibility may reveal something about the character of social relations in general. Her suggestion is useful and relevant to the context of Bulangwa. See discussion of this in the note above.

29. As already noted in chapter 5, there are geographical variations in the Sukuma-Nyamwezi dialect. In Bulangwa and surrounding areas, the hard "k" sound was often replaced by a softer "g." Thus I write *gu ngongo,* rather than the expected *ku ngongo.*

30. Women also spoke about possession by Muslim spirits (*majini* pl., *jini* sing.). *Majini* were not considered ancestors but, rather, outsiders who "came" from faraway places in the Middle East, such as Mecca or Oman (Boddy 1989; Giles 1987; see also Janzen 1992). Although possession by a *jini* was much more common among Muslim women in Bulangwa, both Arab and African, non-Muslims might also experience possession of this sort. Of the 154 women I interviewed, thirty-four women, or 23.2 percent of the sample, told me they had experienced possession at some point in their lives, with one woman stating that she doesn't experience possession because she makes regular offerings to her ancestors. Of these women,

twenty-eight had experienced possession by an ancestral spirit, while six said they had been possessed by a Muslim spirit. When asked whether they had relatives or friends who had experienced possession, the numbers were much larger. Fifty-one percent of the sample (*n* = 80) said they had relatives or friends who had been possessed by an ancestral spirit, while 12 percent (*n* = 19) said that relatives or friends had experienced possession via a Muslim spirit. See Roth 1996:199–220 for additional discussion.

31. My initial insight into fertility-related conditions experienced by men came from informal conversations I had with women. I also gained much insight into male fertility problems from two group interviews I conducted with women who lived in Mwana Nyanzanga's village. After learning something I had never heard before, I checked out this new piece of information with friends and healers in the community. They always verified what the women in the group interviews had told me. I also discussed fertility problems that are common among men with Mwana Nyanzanga, two male healers in Bulangwa, and three male vendors at the herbal market in Shinyanga town.

32. Although Gottlieb (1990:133, n. 7) has noted elsewhere that cold is symbolically associated with fertility in many African societies, this did not appear to be the case in Bulangwa. See de Heusch 1987 for an analysis of the connection between heat and gestation among the Thonga of southern Africa.

33. Varkevisser (1973:102–3) also makes reference to local methods of birth control used by Sukuma women in Mwanza, as well as to the fact that some women acknowledged "willfully" breaking taboos in order to prevent conception.

CHAPTER 9

1. At the lay midwifery clinic in El Paso, we measured the fundus with a tape measure from the upper edge of the pubic bone to the top of the uterus while the pregnant woman lay flat on her back. See Davis 1987:16 for a description of the fundal measurement.

2. Cory (1970 [1953]:91) provides a slightly different account than either Varkevisser's or mine. He invokes the term *kulela nda* only in terms of the pregnancies of unmarried women. He mentions the practice of *kutwalilwa nda* whereby the woman's father or nearest paternal relative would send two of the pregnant women's relatives to the home of the woman's lover to announce that he has been named as the father. This announcement took place once the woman's pregnancy became obvious (92). *Kulela nda,* according to Cory, is a version of *kutwalilwa nda.* In some areas of Sukumaland (he doesn't specify which) the lover of the unmarried pregnant woman moved in with the woman's family, leaving only after the woman gave birth. Cory's data on the effects of a man's promiscuity during his wife's (or lover's) pregnancy are also different from both Varkevisser's and mine:

> For the father exists no taboo [limiting sexual intercourse] but during the pregnancy of his wife and even after the birth for a number of months he uses a medicine called *makile* which annihilates the evil influences of his extra-mat-

rimonial connections for the child. This is an almost obligatory medicine, and for instance, in Sumbwa, it is used by both parents. (n.d.:26)

As we can see, Cory makes no mention of the husband "watching the womb" in the above passage. We learn instead that a husband's extramarital relations are a possibility during his wife's pregnancy and in fact a "risk" to his unborn child. A man can nullify the effects of his actions by taking local medicine.

3. Short stature, more than five previous pregnancies, and pregnancies occurring before the age of fifteen or over the age of thirty-five were some of the factors included in this calculation of being "at risk." See Hayes's (1991) critique of the risk approach and accompanying commentaries.

4. All of the rural medical aids and medical assistants (a higher category of health-care personnel) I met throughout the course of my fieldwork were male.

5. Although the control may be subtle, the result of it, that is, the humiliation of being talked about, is not. I became aware of just how devastating the consequences of this subtle control through gossip can be when an Arab woman in Shinyanga committed suicide after her husband accused her of infidelity. Various versions of the tragedy were recounted afterward, but they all centered around the misinformation one of the husband's relatives had given him. It appears that while the husband was out of town, his best friend, an Indian man, happened to stop by his home to inquire about his whereabouts and to greet the wife. She offered him coffee, which he stayed to drink, and he then left. A relative of the husband (an unreliable young man, as he was later described to me) happened to see the Indian man leaving the house and jumped to the conclusion that he was having an affair with his relative's wife. Upon the husband's return, his relative took him aside to tell him of his wife's supposed illicit affair. That evening the husband went to his parents' home, sent for his wife, and when she arrived, confronted her in front of his parents with the "proof" of her infidelity. He immediately declared three *talaka,* divorcing her on the spot. I was later told that this giving of the *talaka* all at once is actually a drastic measure and rarely done. Instead, a husband's uttering of *talaka* is usually done in stages, with much involvement and negotiation. A man may give his wife one or two and then may never give her a third. Although the giving of the first and second *talaka* also means that the couple is divorced, it is once the third is given that there is no possibility of reconciliation in the future. Thus, the man's own family members were quite shocked at his drastic measure and pleaded with him to change his mind. He refused and told his wife to pack up her belongings and return to her parents that same evening. As she was packing to leave, she took an overdose of chloroquine and died several hours later. All in the Arab community were quite shocked at the suicide, as was the husband; he threatened to commit suicide himself. When I later spoke to an Arab friend about it, she told me that the woman's decision to take her own life was largely a result of the public humiliation that such an accusation would cause her. Although not everyone would have necessarily believed that she had committed adultery, she would never have been able to live that accusation down, and people would have talked about it for a long time to come.

6. It is important to note here that Arab women's embarrassment regarding

issues of sexuality is itself contextual. For example, many of the conversations I had with Arab women, either alone or in groups, could, on occasion, get rather bawdy. Making overt references to sex in mixed company, however, just wasn't done. That does not mean that issues of sexuality were not of public interest. In fact, the Arab community seemed to pay a lot of attention to various aspects of people's sexual lives. Young Arab brides, for example, are expected to be virgins. Evidence of a bride's virginity was demonstrated on the wedding night in the form of the bloodstained sheets from the bed on which the marriage was consummated. Although the evidence of her virginity is displayed only to certain family members, it would be discussed among members of the Arab community afterward, as public proof of the young woman's virginity brings honor to her family. Apparent interest in others' sexuality can also be seen in the significance attached to the preparation of the Arab specialty known as *boku-boku,* a rice and goat meat dish that was always eaten in the community on Muslim holidays. The preparation of this dish is time-consuming; the rice is boiled together with the meat until it is very soft. It is then worked by a combination of stirring and beating with a large wooden ladle, about three feet long, until it gains the consistency of soft Play-Doh. It is arduous work, and this final stage of preparation is often done by several Arab women together, or by male African workers. There is also a lot of uncertainty surrounding its preparation; rather than turning to Play-Doh, it can, on occasion, turn into an inedible watery substance similar to porridge. This latter failure is believed to be the result of a person's sexual uncleanliness. It was general knowledge among the Muslim members of the community familiar with Arab customs that *boku-boku* will turn into porridge if it is prepared in a household where someone is sexually unclean, meaning that someone in the household had recently engaged in sexual intercourse but had not bathed afterward. This failure, in turn, brings considerable shame and humiliation to the household that prepared the dish. I learned about this during the first year of my fieldwork, when it occurred at a neighbor's home on the first day of the Muslim holiday of Id el Fitr. The family in question had invited several other Arab families to eat with them. At the last minute of preparation, after the guests had already arrived and were waiting to eat, the *boku-boku* turned into porridge. This family's public humiliation was talked about for several days afterward over coffee in several of the Arab households I visited. Some speculated that the husband and wife had sex the previous night, but that one of them had not washed afterward. Others told me that the family placed the blame for the failed *boku-boku* on the sexual uncleanliness of the African worker involved in the preparation.

7. Although neither of the two men who owned private clinics in Bulangwa provided maternity care, pregnant women who experienced complications sometimes showed up at their doors.

8. Before leaving for the field I had purchased several disposable birthing kits from a supply company for lay midwives. Whenever I traveled to the villages I always carried one of these kits in my car, in case of emergencies.

9. The *khanga,* a piece of cloth worn by African and Arab women alike, has many functions. Women might use a *khanga* as a sling to carry a child on their back, or wear it wrapped around their waists to protect their clothes from dust, or

on their heads at funerals as a sign of respect. In Anna's case, the women's *khanga* functioned as walls to protect her modesty.

10. That he was overworked was an accurate self-assessment. Despite the fact that there was a government clinic in town, people rarely went there as a first choice because it was often out of medicine. When he opened the doors to this particular private clinic every morning at around eight o'clock, he sometimes found as many as thirty people waiting to be seen. He didn't close them again until six in the evening.

11. In their study of the reported use of herbal remedies during pregnancy among women attending urban and rural prenatal clinics in Tanga, Tanzania, Mbura et al. (1985) found a reported prevalence of 43.3 percent and 40.2 percent respectively. See also Mabina et al. 1997 and Varga and Veale 1997 for herbal use during pregnancy among South African women.

12. Stomach (*tumbo* in Swahili; *nda* in Sukuma) is the word many women used to refer to the abdominal area. *Nda* is also the Sukuma word for pregnancy (*mimba* in Swahili).

13. The phenomenon of pregnancies simply "disappearing" or "turning to the back" is known in other parts of Tanzania as well. A Tanzanian female journalist I spoke with in Dar es Salaam told me it had happened to a woman she knew casually. The woman had even worn a maternity dress for over a year. Although she looked pregnant, she never gave birth. The journalist told me that she later learned secondhand that the woman's pregnancy had "disappeared" and so she never asked the woman about it directly.

14. People often made the distinction between healers who used medicines to cure people (*waganga*) and healers, or sorcerers, who used medicines with the intent of causing harm (*wachawi*). But, as was pointed out to me on several occasions, even benevolent healers knew how to concoct harmful medicines, as it was only by knowing the ingredients of those harmful medicines that they were able to counteract them with more powerful medicines of their own.

15. As her research was in Mwanza, Varkevisser uses the word *kupindya,* whereas *gupinda* is how this condition was referred to in Shinyanga.

16. Kleiner-Bossaller describes a similar category of pregnancy known as *kwantacce* among Muslim Hausa-Fulani women in northern Nigeria (1993; see also Feldman-Savelsberg 1999 for Cameroon). *Kwantacce* is referred to as a "sleeping" or "lying down" pregnancy, a condition that can be experienced by young and old women alike—even among women who have already reached the age of menopause. These pregnancies apparently start out as normal, but then cease to grow after the fourth or fifth month. The pregnancy remains in this suspended state until the woman uses a medicine to return the pregnancy to its starting point. If successful, she will give birth nine months later (Kleiner-Bossaller 1993:19). Pregnancies that were "returned" to their proper place in Bulangwa, however, were often said to continue from the gestational age they were when they initially turned to the back. Although Kleiner-Bossaller's description of this condition in Nigeria shares many similarities to pregnancies that "turn to the back" in Bulangwa—for example, both are seen as being caused by jealous persons using sorcery, or unintentionally by women who were actually trying to abort—there are

also some differences. In the Nigerian case, it is the "pregnant" woman herself who makes the diagnosis, whereas in Bulangwa, the diagnosis was often made by a local healer, a diagnosis that the woman may or may not agree with.

17. One of the nurses told me that a sister of a nurse she knew had experienced this condition twice during her first pregnancy. The pregnancy disappeared for the first time when she was five months pregnant. She had all the signs of pregnancy: missed menses, growing abdomen, and the presence of fetal heartbeats when nurses listened for them at the clinic. She woke up one morning and the pregnancy was simply gone, without any signs of miscarriage. The nurse recounting this story told me that the young woman took local medicine and the pregnancy returned. At seven months, it disappeared again. She eventually learned that she had been bewitched by her cowife. Another nurse told me about one of her clients who had been five months pregnant. The woman had definitely been pregnant, the nurse told me, because she had measured the fundal height herself. One day the woman woke up and the pregnancy was gone; there were no signs of blood. The woman told her that she had felt it when it turned to the back.

18. Although several other non-Sukuma people I spoke with also described *nda ya gudpinda ngongo* as a Sukuma phenomenon, one of the Arab women I interviewed in Bulangwa told me that her first pregnancy had "turned to the back."

19. When I asked women whether they had relatives or friends whose pregnancies had "turned to the back," the numbers were much larger, with 34 percent of the women stating that they knew of relatives or neighbors who had suffered from this condition. Of these fifty-three women, twenty-one said the women with this condition had been neighbors, two said they had been friends, while the remaining thirty women said that they had been relatives.

20. Although Mwana Nyanzanga knew I was neither a nurse nor a doctor, she knew that I had received some training in lay midwifery prior to arriving in Tanzania, and so from time to time she asked me for my opinion about specific cases.

21. She listened for heartbeats using a hollowed-out gourd. She placed the smaller end next to her ear and the wider end on the pregnant woman's abdomen.

22. As she had already been scolded by the nurses on the maternity ward for not having a card, it is likely that in the time it took us to walk to the MCH clinic on the opposite end of the hospital, Milembe had come up with an explanation as to why she didn't have a card.

CHAPTER 10

1. From Fr. George Cotter's (n.d) collection of Sukuma proverbs.

2. But male health personnel didn't always enter with business directly related to birth. Once, as I was observing on the labor ward in Shinyanga's regional hospital, a man came in during a woman's labor to make sure that members of the nursing staff were up to date on their political party membership cards. As he sat and chatted with them at a nearby table, the woman in labor, who was lying naked on the birthing table a few feet away, used a corner of the cloth she was lying on to cover her vagina.

A Tanzanian freelance journalist writing on the conditions pregnant women encounter on the labor wards in some Tanzanian hospitals has made similar observations:

> What is shocking I have discovered . . . is that some women working in hospitals find it exciting to pop in the "labor ward" to see who is next in the production line. Her job is not related to midwifery, yet she stands and gapes at another woman who can barely feign modesty with her most private parts exposed to make way for the event of the moment. Within a few moments she cables the message on, how so and so was positioned, attributes of the unfortunate's anatomy and the expressions . . . which were uttered in agony. . . . All this along with the fact that most labor wards throughout the various hospitals position their beds or stretchers with the feet of the patient facing the door or entrance of said ward. Only in a few are there any screens, and seldom if ever is the screen to maintain an element of privacy. Thus one can see clerical staffs, ward orderlies, even the odd porter popping a head around a door. (Cushnie-Mnyanga 1989:19)

3. One day, when I mentioned to the nursing staff on duty that in America husbands often stayed with their wives throughout labor and childbirth, most didn't think it was a very good idea. If the husband was present during a wife's labor, one of them told me, the woman would "act" as if she were in more pain than she actually was because her husband was watching. One of the younger nurse assistants, who was not married and had not yet given birth, proclaimed she would want her husband with her during labor, a comment that elicited chuckles from her coworkers.

4. Tensions and power struggles were also present in the female-centered birthing clinic in El Paso, although there they had more to do with conflicts between health-care providers themselves than between providers and clients as in Tanzania. During the first week of my training in El Paso, for example, I often heard comments by trainees and staff that the "energy" at the clinic could, on occasion, become quite "weird." This weird energy, I gradually learned, was an outcome of several factors. Sometimes it seemed to be merely a result of sleep deprivation; the shifts at the clinic were twenty-four hours, and depending on the number of births that took place on a particular day, trainees and staff alike might not get an opportunity to sleep. Another source of tension was the result of interactions between midwifery trainees themselves. Some had prior experience attending births before coming to the El Paso clinic. Others, like myself, had not. In fact, soon after my arrival, I realized that I was the source of some of the tension between students. I was perceived as a wimp because initially I was more comfortable observing births rather than actually taking part in them. This hesitancy on my part was met with a lot of resentment on the part of students and staff alike. Everyone else had started by doing, I was informed, so I shouldn't receive any special treatment. Part of my hesitation was due to my training as an anthropologist in which observation is a key element in the fieldwork experience. But to a greater extent my hesitation was due to the fact I didn't like the idea of learning the ropes of midwifery by practicing on women's bodies. See Davis-Floyd 1992 for a discussion of similar aspects of medical training in U.S. training hospitals.

5. Although *wazungu* (*mzungu,* sg.)was the Kiswahili word generally applied to white people, Europeans and Americans alike, its meaning often depends on the context in which it is used. Fabian (1995), for example, cites an example of how he mistranslated the word while going over transcripts of his interviews with an informant from the Shaba Region of Zaire (i.e., the Democratic Republic of Congo). Initially he translated *muzungu* (from the Kiswahili dialect spoken in the Shaba Region) as "an American white man." He later made the connection that the American referred to in the interview was actually Bennetta Jules-Rosette, an American woman whose dissertation Fabian had reviewed in 1977. As Fabian notes:

> I do not remember exactly when I made the connection, but eventually it became clear to me that she must have been the person I had taken to be a white man. That revealed a first misunderstanding: the person was a woman, not a man. But there is another twist to this story: Bennetta Jules-Rosette is an African-American. That signals the problems with translating the Swahili term *muzungu.* It distinguishes one class of non-Africans (there are others) on the bases of origin, socioeconomic status, and political position, but not of color. (1995:43)

Fabian's observations about the complexity of the term were also relevant in the context of my fieldwork in Shinyanga and Bulangwa. A West African man, who was the director of a UN-funded development project in Bulangwa, lived with his wife and children in a big house far from the center of town. People often referred to him as the *mzungu mweusi,* a term that can be translated either as "the black white man" or the "black European," because many in the community felt he put on airs and thought himself to be superior.

6. As a guest, I also received special treatment. One day, after observing a birth in which the woman had not received much assistance from nurses sitting nearby, one of them turned to me and offered me a frozen ice treat. Not wanting to appear rude, I took it, but found the whole incident ironic—here were several nurses and myself sitting around eating frozen ices while the woman who had just given birth received nothing at all. At the time, I found myself comparing this to my experiences at the clinic in El Paso, where women were given juices and a yogurt shake to drink immediately after giving birth.

7. Retractions, a condition whereby the newborn infant has difficulty breathing, can often be diagnosed by a visual inspection (the baby's rib cage flares and belly collapses in a seesaw fashion). Retractions in the newborn infant may indicate several things about the newborn's lungs: they are either damaged, immature, or obstructed (Davis 1987:88). When these occurred at the birthing clinic in El Paso, an ambulance was called, and the newborn was rushed to the nearby hospital.

8. Checking to make sure a placenta is complete is quite important, because any pieces left attached to the uterus could cause the woman to hemorrhage.

9. Although she didn't specify which type of skin, Brandström notes that the skin on which Sukuma-Nyamwezi women gave birth was a cowhide "originating from the herd that made its mother its father's wife" (1991:122). This symbolically established the newborn child as "a two-sided child, a child of both the left and right side" (122).

10. As noted already in chapter 6, Mwana Nyanzanga's "hospital" was a three-room structure consisting of an examining room/postpartum room, a room for dispensing medicines, and a birthing room. The instruments she boiled were part of the birthing kit she had been given during the first training seminar for traditional birth attendants in 1986. The kit included scissors and pieces of string she had cut from the ball of string included in her birth kit. She would use the string to tie the umbilical cord in three places and the scissors to cut it.

11. As this was the first time I had observed a birth in a remote setting, I wanted to be sure the labor was progressing normally, and so I checked her dilation. In the subsequent births I observed at her home, I only did this on a few occasions.

12. Although some women may dilate more quickly than others and differently for each birth, from my experience attending births in El Paso, I had come to expect that birth was imminent (meaning it could take place within the next two to four hours) once a woman's cervix had dilated to seven or eight centimeters.

CHAPTER 11

1. Some Muslim women made further distinctions within this forty-day period. The first seven days of an infant's life, for example, were seen as a particularly dangerous time. Because of the heightened sense of danger during this first week, an infant was not supposed to leave its mother's bedroom or be left alone, even for a moment. This first week was dangerous, an Arab neighbor explained to me, because it was the period of time in which evil spirits (*mapepo mabaya*) could harm the newborn child by switching or changing its soul (*kubadilisha roho yake*). She gave me the example of an Arab woman she knew who left her newborn child alone for a moment during the first week of its life. During that brief moment, the evil spirit present in the room changed the child into an imbecile. Apparently, he was never quite right in the head again, even as an adult (*Sasa, akili zake siyo sawa*).

2. But Riesman notes that the knife is also used by Muslim Fulani women of Burkina Faso as a means of protection during the postpartum period, both for themselves and for their newborn:

> Another form of protection that is never omitted is a piece of iron, usually a knife. For the first weeks, and sometimes much longer, the baby will always have a knife, or at least a scrap of a knife blade, lying nearby. . . . The mother, too, carries the same protection. Whenever she goes out of the house, to wash or urinate, for instance, she carries her *garjaahi* (straw-cutting knife) tucked into her skirt at all times. And she is never allowed to be alone at all during the first seven days after giving birth. A companion goes with her to the bush when she needs to relieve herself. (1992:109)

3. Similar to what I had found in my interviews with women who had participated in the UN-sponsored seminars for traditional birth attendants, she told me that many of the women who attended the training seminars she conducted had never actually delivered a baby themselves, although they may have sat with women during their labor and then cut the cord once the placenta had come out.

She stressed this latter point. Many of the women she spoke with told her that they wouldn't touch the baby until after the placenta had been totally expelled from the woman's body.

4. In her book on Kuru sorcery, Lindenbaum (1979:67) mentions a similar perception of the benefits of pit latrines in communities of Fore peoples in the Eastern Highlands of Papua New Guinea. In addition to preventing the spread of diseases linked to fecal contamination, the building of latrines in this particular community had unintended benefits as well, in that latrines provided a safe place in which community members could dispose of their hair and nail clippings, food scraps and feces, and thus prevent sorcerers from gaining access to materials they needed in order to bewitch people and cause their ill health.

5. These dance competitions are usually held in a large open field with two dance groups occupying separate corners of the field. The winning group was determined by which group of dancers drew the biggest crowd. A variety of medicines were used by each of the competing dance groups, either to enhance the group's own ability to draw spectators to their corner of the field or to sabotage the other group's ability to do so. For an earlier description of these dance societies see Hall 1936. See Bessire 2001 for a more contemporary description on the Internet, complete with color photos.

6. One of the traditional birth attendants I had interviewed during the first year of my fieldwork also told me that some nurses sold placentas as ingredients for local medicines.

7. Cory (1944), who described how this particular ritual was performed in different parts of Sukumaland in the past, notes that in one locale the placenta was placed in a pot and buried at the doorway of the parents' house, while in another locale the preferable place was near water, sometimes near a watering hole for cattle.

8. When I mentioned this to a man I knew, he told me that the same thing was also said about the occupational hazards of being a butcher: it caused poor eyesight. In other words, the blood of humans and animals had the capacity to damage the eyesight of a person who looked at it too much.

9. She initially told me that Ndalu's blood pressure had registered 20/0. She later clarified this statement by stating that they had been having problems with that particular blood pressure cuff, and that she couldn't read the bottom number.

10. Although I didn't spend much time speaking with hospital personnel about the specific policies regarding HIV counseling, I did speak informally about it with friends. One man I knew told me that he been tested for the virus at the government hospital in Shinyanga town during the last month of his wife's second pregnancy. She had experienced complications during a previous birth and had needed a blood transfusion. Doctors were anticipating similar complications with her second pregnancy, so her husband was asked to donate blood prior to the onset of her labor. His blood was tested, and he was told it was virus-free.

11. Some of the nurses I spoke with during my first trip to Tanzania in 1990 gave similar interpretations of people's refusal to give blood. They attributed the "current" blood shortage to the fact that "these days" fewer people were donating blood. According to them, most people refused to donate blood because they were

afraid they would contract AIDS in the process or because of their belief that donating blood would decrease their own body's supply of it. They also noted that people weren't always informed they had the virus if health-care personnel believed that the person might decide to commit suicide upon learning they had the virus. Despite the fact that some HIV counseling services were available in 1990 in Dar es Salaam, those services were relatively new and not very widespread.

12. I later learned that this was a common practice. Although the blood of the potential donor might be found incompatible with the person for whom they had agreed to donate, a suitable donor might be found among relatives of other patients waiting for transfusions. If that proved to be the case, each could donate their blood in exchange for the other.

References

Abrahams, R. G.
  1967   The peoples of greater Unyamwezi, Tanzania. In Daryll Forde, ed.,
          Ethnographic Survey of Africa, vol. 17. London: International African
          Institute.
  1970   The political incorporation of non-Nyamwezi immigrants in Tanza-
          nia. In Ronald Cohen and John Middleton, eds., *From Tribe to Nation
          in Africa: Studies in Incorporation Processes,* 93–113. Scranton, PA:
          Chandler.
  1981   *The Nyamwezi Today: A Tanzanian People in the 1970s.* Cambridge:
          Cambridge University Press.
Abu-Lughod, Lila
  1993   *Writing Women's Worlds: Bedouin Stories.* Berkeley: University of
          California Press.
Ademuwagun, Z. A.
  1979   *African Therapeutic Systems.* Waltham, MA: Crossroads.
Aggarwal, V. P., and J. K. G. Mati
  1982   Epidemiology of induced abortion in Nairobi, Kenya. *Journal of
          Obstetrics and Gynecology East Central Africa* 1:54–57.
Ahmed, A. M., D. P. Urassa, E. Gherardi, and N. Y. Game
  1996   Patients' perception of public, voluntary and private dispensaries in
          rural areas of Tanzania. *East African Medical Journal* 73 (6): 370–74.
Allen, Denise Roth
  2000   Learning the facts of life: Past and present experiences in a rural Tan-
          zanian community. Special issue of *Africa Today.* Sexuality and Gen-
          erational Identities in Sub-Saharan Africa. Elisha P. Renne and Kears-
          ley A. Stewart, eds., 47 (3/4): 3–27.
Alloo, Fatma
  1988   Report on the Meeting on Maternal Mortality. Tanzania Media
          Women Association, Dar es Salaam, Tanzania. Mimeograph.
Alpers, Edward.A.
  1968   The nineteenth century: Prelude to colonialism. In B. A. Ogot and J.
          A. Kieran, eds., *Zamani: A Survey of East African History,* 238–54.
          Nairobi: East African Publishing House.
Amos, Valerie, and Pratibha Parmar
  1984   Challenging imperial feminism. *Feminist Review* 17:3–19.

Appadurai, Arjun
    1996   *Modernity at Large: Cultural Dimensions of Globalization.* Minneapolis: University of Minnesota Press.
Appell, Laura W. R.
    1988   Menstruation among the Rungus of Borneo: An Unmarked Category. In Thomas Buckley and Alma Gottlieb, eds., *Blood Magic: The Anthropology of Menstruation,* 94–112. Berkeley: University of California Press.
Arens, W.
    1978   Changing patterns of ethnic identity and prestige in East Africa. In R. E. Holloman and S. A. Arutiunov, eds., *Perspectives on Identity,* 211–20. The Hague: Mouton.
    1987   Taxonomy and dynamics revisited: The interpretation of misfortune in a polyethnic community. In Ivan Karp and Charles S. Bird, eds., *Explorations in African Systems of Thought,* 165–80. Washington, DC: Smithsonian Institution.
    1989   Mto wa Mbu: A rural polyethnic community in Tanzania. In Igor Kopytoff, ed., *The African Frontier: The Reproduction of Traditional African Societies,* 242–54. Bloomington: Indiana University Press.
Austen, Ralph A.
    1967   The official mind of indirect rule: British Policy in Tanganyika, 1916–1939. In Prosser Gifford and Wm. Roger Louis, eds., *Britain and Germany in Africa: Imperial and Colonial Rule,* 577–606. New Haven: Yale University Press.
    1968   *Northwest Tanzania under German and British Rule: Colonial Policy and Tribal Politics, 1889–1939.* New Haven: Yale University Press.
Backett, E. M., A. M. Davies, and A. Petros-Barvazian
    1984   The risk approach in health care. With special reference to maternal and child health, including family planning. *WHO Public Health Papers* 76:1–113.
Baer, Hans A., Merrill Singer, and John Johnson, eds.
    1986   Towards a Critical Medical Anthropology. Special issue of *Social Science and Medicine* 23 (2).
Bakinikana, Isaya Kaitaba Mugala
    1974   The Effects of Colonialism on Pre-Colonial Authorities among the Haya and the Sukuma of Tanzania. M.A. thesis, University of Minnesota.
Bassett, Mary Travis, Leon Bijlmakers, and David M. Sanders
    1997   Professionalism, patient satisfaction and quality of health care: Experience during Zimbabwe's structural adjustment programme. *Social Science and Medicine* 45 (12): 1845–52.
Bates, Margaret
    1965   Tanganyika: Changes in African life, 1918–45. In Vincent Harlow and E. M. Chilvers, eds., *History of East Africa,* 625–38. Oxford: Clarendon.

Beattie, John
    1963   Sorcery in Bunyoro. In John Middleton and E. H. Winter, eds., *Witch-craft and Sorcery in East Africa,* 27–55. New York: Praeger.

Beck, Ann
    1977   Medicine and society in Tanganyika, 1890–1930: A historical inquiry. *Transactions of the American Philosophical Society* 67 (3): 3–59.
    1981   *Medicine, Tradition, and Development in Kenya and Tanzania, 1920–1970.* Waltham, MA: Crossroads.

Beidelman, T. O.
    1961   Right and left among the Kaguru: A note on symbolic classification. *Africa* 31:250–57.
    1963   Witchcraft in Ukaguru. In John Middleton and E. H. Winter, eds., *Witchcraft and Sorcery in East Africa,* 57–98. New York: Praeger.
    1993   *Moral Imagination in Kaguru Modes of Thought.* Washington: Smithsonian Institution Press.

Belsey, M. A.
    1976   The epidemiology of infertility. *WHO Bulletin* 54:319.

Bennett, Norman R.
    1968   The Arab impact. In B. A. Ogot and J. A. Kieran, eds., *Zamani: A Survey of East African History,* 216–37. Nairobi: East African Publishing House.
    1971   *Mirambo of Tanzania ca. 1840–1884.* London: Oxford University Press.

Berger, Iris
    1976   Rebels or status seekers? Women as spirit mediums in East Africa. In Nancy J. Hafkin and Edna G. Bay, eds., *Women in Africa: Studies in Social and Economic Change,* 157–81. Stanford: Stanford University Press.

Berglund, Axel-Ivar
    1976   *Zulu Thought-Patterns and Symbolism.* London: Hurst.

Berkow, Robert, and Andrew J. Fletcher, eds.
    1992   *The Merck Manual of Diagnosis and Therapy.* Rathway, NJ: Merck Research Laboratories.

Bessire, Aime H. C.
    2001   The Bagula and Bagika Dance Societies. http://www.photo .net/sukuma/dance.html. (Access date July 1, 2001.)

Bibeau, Giles, Ellen Corin, Mulinda, Mabiala, Matumona, Kukana, and Nsiala
    1980   *Traditional Medicine in Zaire: Present and Potential Contributions to the Health Services.* Ottawa: International Development Research Centre.

Blacklock, Mary
    1936   Certain aspects of the welfare of women and children in the colonies. *Annals of Tropical Medicines and Parasitology* 30:221–64.

Blakely, Thomas D., Walter E. A. van Beek, and Dennis L. Thompson, eds.
    1994   *Religion in Africa.* London: James Currey.

Bledsoe, Caroline, Fatoumatta Baja, and Alan G. Hill
    1998   Reproductive mishaps and Western contraception: An African challenge to fertility theory. *Population and Development Review* 24 (1):
            15–57.
Bledsoe, Caroline H., Alan G. Hill, Umberto D'Alessandro, and Patricia Langerock
    1994   Constructing natural fertility: The use of Western contraceptive technologies in rural Gambia. *Population and Development Review* 20 (1):
            81–113.
Blohm, W.
    1933   *Die Nyamwezi, Gesellschaft und Weltbid.* Hamburg: Friedericksen, De
            Gruyter.
Boahen, A. Adu
    1987   *African Perspectives on Colonialism: The Johns Hopkins Symposia in
            Comparative History.* Baltimore: Johns Hopkins University Press.
Boddy, Janice
    1989   *Wombs and Alien Spirits: Women, Men, and the Zar Cult in Northern
            Sudan.* Madison: University of Wisconsin Press.
Boerma, Ties
    1987   The magnitude of the maternal mortality problem in sub-Saharan
            Africa. *Social Science and Medicine* 24 (6): 551–58.
Boerma, Ties, Mark Urassa, and Raphel Isingo
    1996   Female infertility and its association with sexual behavior, STD, and
            HIV infection in Tanzania. TANESA Working Paper, No. 14.
            Mwanza, Tanzania.
Bösch, F.
    1930   *Les Banyamwezi, Peuple de l'Afrique Orientale.* Münster: Bibliotheca
            Anthropos.
Boserup, Ester
    1970   *Women's Role in Economic Development.* New York: St. Martin's.
Brandström, Per
    1986   Who is a Sukuma and who is a Nyamwezi: Ethnic identity in west-central Tanzania. Vol. 27, Working Papers in African Studies. Uppsala:
            African Studies Programme, Department of Anthropology, University of Uppsala.
    1990   Seeds and soil: The quest for life and the domestication of fertility in
            Sukuma-Nyamwezi thought and reality. In Anita Jacobson-Widding
            and Walter van Beek, eds., *The Creative Communion: African Folk
            Models of Fertility and the Regeneration of Life,* 167–86. Stockholm:
            Almqvist and Wiksell International.
    1991   Left-hand father and right-hand mother: Unity and diversity in
            Sukuma-Nyamwezi thought. In Anita Jacobson-Widding, ed., *Body
            and Space: Symbolic Models of Unity and Division in African Cosmology and Experience,* 119–41. Stockholm: Almqvist and Wiksell International.

Browner, Carole H., and Carolyn F. Sargent
  1990 Anthropology and studies of human reproduction. In Thomas M. Johnson and Carolyn F. Sargent, eds., *Medical Anthropology: Contemporary Method,* 215–29. New York: Praeger.
Bureau of Statistics [Tanzania] and Macro International, Inc.
  1997 *Tanzania Demographic and Health Survey 1996.* Calverton, MD: Bureau of Statistics and Macro International.
Burton, R. F.
  1860 *The Lake Regions of Central Africa.* London: Longmans.
Campbell, John
  1991 The unmaking of Tanzania and the march towards capitalism? *Africa* 61 (2): 265–77.
Caplan, Pat
  1988 Engendering knowledge: The politics of anthropology. *Anthropology Today* 4 (5): 8–12.
  1989 Perceptions of gender stratification. *Africa* 59 (2): 196–208.
Carby, Hazel V.
  1979 White women listen! Black feminism and the boundaries of sisterhood. In Centre for Contemporary Cultural Studies, University of Birmingham, ed., *The Empire Strikes Back: Race and Racism in 70s Britain,* 212–35. Birmingham: Hutchinson.
Chen, L. C., M. C. Gesche, S. Ahmed, A. I. Chowdhury, and W. H. Mosley
  1974 Maternal mortality in rural Bangladesh. *Studies in Family Planning* 5 (11): 334–41.
Coeytaux, Francine M.
  1988 Induced abortion in sub-Saharan Africa: What we do and do not know. *Studies in Family Planning* 19 (2): 186–90.
Cohen, David, and E. S. Atieno Odhiambo
  1989 *Siaya: The Historical Anthropology of an African Landscape.* London: James Currey.
Cohen, Ronald, and John Middleton, eds.
  1970 *From Tribe to Nation in Africa: Studies in Incorporation Processes.* Scranton, PA: Chandler.
Collier, Jane F., and Sylvia J. Yanagisako
  1989 Theory in anthropology since feminist practice. *Critique of Anthropology* 9 (2): 27–37.
Comaroff, Jean
  1978 Medicine and culture: Some anthropological perspectives. *Social Science and Medicine* 12 (4): 247–54.
  1993 The diseased heart of Africa. In Shirley Lindenbaum and Margaret Lock, eds., *Knowledge, Power, and Practice,* 305–29. Berkeley: University of California Press.
Comaroff, Jean, and John Comaroff, eds.
  1993 *Modernity and Its Malcontents: Ritual and Power in Postcolonial Africa.* Chicago: University of Chicago Press.

Cooper, F., and R. Packard, eds.
    1997   *International Development and the Social Sciences: Essays on the History and Politics of Knowledge.* Berkeley: University of California Press.
Cory, Hans
    1944   Sukuma twin ceremonies—Mabasa. *Tanganyika Notes and Records* 17:34–43.
    1949   The ingredients of magic medicines. *Africa* 19 (1): 13–32.
    1951   *The Ntemi: The Traditional Rites in Connection with the Burial, Election, Enthronement and Magic Powers of a Sukuma Chief. Custom and Tradition in East Africa.* London: Macmillan.
    1952   The people of the Lake Victoria region. *Tanganyika Notes and Records* 33:22–29.
    1960   Religious beliefs and practices of the Sukuma/Nyamwezi tribal group. *Tanganyika Notes and Records* 54:13–26.
    1970   [1953] *Sukuma Law and Custom.* Westport, CT: Negro Universities Press.
    n.d.   The Sukuma and Nyamwezi. Mimeograph.
Cotter, Fr. G.
    n.d.   *Sukuma Proverbs.* Nairobi: BeeZee Secretarial Services.
Crush, J., ed.
    1995   *Power of Development.* London: Routledge.
Cunningham, Clark
    1970   The "injection doctors." Antibiotic mediators. *Social Science and Medicine* 4:1–24.
Cushnie-Mnyanga, Jamila
    1989   We have an issue. *Sauti ya Siti* (5) (March): 19.
Daily News (Tanzania)
    1988   MMC records more maternal deaths. *Daily News,* May 6, 1988.
Davis, Elizabeth
    1987   *Heart and Hands: A Midwife's Guide to Pregnancy and Birth.* 2d ed. Berkeley, CA: Celestial Arts.
Davis-Floyd, Robbie
    1987   The technological model of birth. *Journal of American Folklore* 100 (398): 479–495.
    1992   *Birth as an American Rite of Passage.* Berkeley: University of California Press.
Davis-Floyd, Robbie E., and Carolyn F. Sargent, eds.
    1997   *Childbirth and Authoritative Knowledge: Cross-Cultural Perspectives.* Los Angeles: University of California Press.
de Certeau, Michel
    1984   *The Practice of Everyday Life.* Berkeley: University of California Press.
de Groot, A. N. J. A., W. Slort, and J. van Roosmalen
    1993   Assessment of the risk approach to maternity care in a district hospital in rural Tanzania. *International Journal of Gynecology and Obstetrics* 40:33–37.

de Heusch, Luc
    1987   Heat, physiology, and cosmogony: *Rites de passage* among the
        Thonga. In Ivan Karp and Charles S. Bird, eds., *Explorations in
        African Systems of Thought*, 27–43. Washington, DC: Smithsonian
        Institution.
Delaney, Carol
    1988   Mortal flow: Menstruation in Turkish village society. In Thomas
        Buckley and Alma Gottlieb, eds., *Blood Magic: The Anthropology of
        Menstruation*, 75–93. Berkeley: University of California Press.
DiGiacomo, Susan M.
    1987   Biomedicine as a cultural system: An anthropologist in the kingdom of
        the sick. In Hans A. Baer, ed., *Encounters with Biomedicine: Case Stud-
        ies in Medical Anthropology*, 315–46. New York: Gordon and Breach
        Science Publishers.
Dixon-Mueller, Ruth
    1993   *Population Policy and Women's Rights: Transforming Reproductive
        Choice.* Westport, CT: Praeger.
Dixon-Mueller, Ruth, and Judith Wasserheit
    1991   *The Culture of Silence: Reproductive Tract Infections among Women in
        the Third World.* New York: International Women's Health Coalition.
Douglas, Mary
    1969   Is Matriliny Doomed in Africa? In Mary Douglas and Phyllis M. Kay-
        berry, eds., *Man in Africa*, 121–35. London: Tavistock.
    1985   *Risk Acceptability according to the Social Sciences.* New York: Russell
        Sage.
    1992   *Risk and Blame: Essays in Cultural Theory.* London: Routledge.
Duden, Barbara
    1992   Population. In Wolfgang Sachs, ed., *The Development Dictionary: A
        Guide to Knowledge as Power*, 146–57. London: Zed.
du Toit, Brian M., and Ismail H. Abdalla, eds.
    1985   *African Healing Strategies.* New York: Trado-Medic.
Eastman, Carol M.
    1971   Who are the Waswahili? *Africa* 41:228–36.
Economic and Political Weekly
    1987   Editorial. Safe motherhood: World Bank's discovery. *Economic and
        Political Weekly, India* 22 (10): 388.
Edouard, Lindsay, and Cecile Li Hoi Foo-Gregory
    1985   *Traditional Birth Practices: An Annotated Bibliography.* Geneva:
        World Health Organization.
Escobar, Arturo
    1985   Discourse and power in development: Michel Foucault and the rele-
        vance of his work to the Third World. *Alternatives* 10:377–400.
    1995   *Encountering Development: The Making and Unmaking of the Third
        World.* Princeton: Princeton University Press.
Evans-Pritchard, E. E.
    1931   An alternative term for brideprice. *Man* (42) (March): 36.

1937   *Witchcraft Oracles and Magic among the Azande.* Oxford: Clarendon.

Fabian, Johannes
1995   Ethnographic misunderstanding and the perils of context. *American Anthropologist* 97 (1): 41–50.

Farmer, Paul
1992   *AIDS and Accusations: Haiti and the Geography of Blame.* Berkeley: University of California Press.

Feierman, Steven
1984   The social roots of health and healing in modern Africa. *African Studies Review* 28 (2/3): 73–145.

Feierman, Steven, and John M. Janzen
1992   *The Social Basis of Health and Healing in Africa.* Berkeley: University of California Press.

Feldman-Savelsberg, Pamela
1999   *Plundered Kitchens, Empty Wombs: Threatened Reproduction and Identity in the Cameroon Grassfields.* Ann Arbor: University of Michigan Press.

Ferguson, James
1990   *The Anti-Politics Machine: "Development," Depoliticization, and Bureaucratic Power in Lesotho.* Cambridge: Cambridge University Press.

Fonn, S., M. Xaba, K. Tint, et al.
1998   Maternal health services in South Africa. *South African Journal of Medicine* 88 (6): 697–702.

Fortney, Judith
1997   Ensuring skilled attendance at delivery: The role of TBAs. Presentation at the Safe Motherhood Technical Consultation, Colombo, Sri Lanka.

Foster, Stanley O.
1996   Malaria in the pregnant African woman: Epidemiology, practice, research and policy. *American Journal of Tropical Medicine and Hygiene* 55 (1): 1.

Foucault, Michel
1979   *Discipline and Punish: The Birth of the Prison.* Translated by Alan Sheridan. New York: Vintage.
1980   Truth and Power. In *Power/Knowledge: Selected Interviews and Other Writings, 1972–1977.* New York: Pantheon.

Frankenberg, Ronald
1980   Medical anthropology and development: A theoretical perspective. *Social Science and Medicine* 14b:197–207.
1993   Risk: Anthropological and epidemiological narratives of prevention. In Shirley Lindenbaum and Margaret Lock, eds., *Knowledge, Power and Practice,* 219–42. Berkeley: University of California Press.

Gabba, Anna
1989   Old women victims of witch hunt. *Sauti ya Siti* (5) (March): 31.
1990   Old Women Accused As Witches in Tanzania's North-Western

Regions. Tanzania Media Women's Association, Dar es Salaam. Mimeograph.

Galaty, John G.
1993   Maasai expansion and the new East African pastoralism. In Thomas Spear and Richard Waller, eds., *Being Maasai: Ethnicity and Identity in East Africa,* 61–86. London: James Currey.

Gardner, Katy
1997   Mixed messages: Contested "development" and the "Plantation Rehabilitation Project." In R. D. Grillo and R. L. Stirrat, eds., *Discourses of Development: Anthropological Perspectives,* 133–56. Oxford: Berg.

Giles, Linda
1987   Possession cults on the Swahili coast: A re-examination of theories of marginality. *Africa* 57 (2): 234–58.
1989   Spirit Possession on the Swahili Coast: Peripheral Cults or Primary Texts? Ph.D. diss., Dept. of Anthropology, University of Texas at Austin.

Ginsburg, Faye D., and Rayna Rapp
1991   The politics of reproduction. *Annual Review of Anthropology* 20:311–43.

Ginsburg, Faye D., and Rayna Rapp, eds.
1995   *Conceiving the New World Order: The Global Politics of Reproduction.* Berkeley: University of California Press.

Gluckman, Max
1963   *Order and Rebellion in Tribal Africa.* New York: Free Press of Glencoe.

Gluckman, Max, V. C. Mitchell, and J. A. Barnes
1949   The village headman in British Central Africa. *Africa* 19 (2): 89–106.

Good, C. M.
1987   *Ethnomedical Systems in Africa.* New York: Guilford.

Good, Mary-Jo Delvecchio
1980   Of blood and babies: The relationship of popular Islamic physiology to fertility. *Social Science and Medicine* 14B:147–56.
1995   Cultural studies of biomedicine: An agenda for research. *Social Science and Medicine* 41 (4): 461–73.

Gottlieb, Alma
1988   Menstrual cosmology among the Beng of Ivory Coast. In Thomas Buckley and Alma Gottlieb, eds., *Blood Magic: The Anthropology of Menstruation,* 55–74. Berkeley: University of California Press.
1990   Rethinking female pollution: The Beng case (Cote d'Ivoire). In Peggy Reeves Sanday and Ruth Goodenough Gallagher, eds., *Beyond the Second Sex: New Directions in the Anthropology of Gender,* 65–79. Philadelphia: University of Pennsylvania Press.

Granet, M.
1973   Right and left in China. In R. Needham, ed., *Right and Left: Essays on Dual Classification,* 43–58. Chicago: University of Chicago Press.

Gray, Richard, and David Birmingham, eds.
  1970   *Pre-Colonial African Trade: Essays on Trade in Central and Eastern Africa before 1900.* London: Oxford University Press.
Greenhalgh, Susan, ed.
  1995   *Situating Fertility: Anthropology and Demographic Inquiry.* Cambridge: Cambridge University Press.
Grillo, R. D.
  1997   Discourses of development: The view from anthropology. In R. D. Grillo and R. L. Stirrat, eds., *Discourses of Development: Anthropological Perspectives,* 1–33. Oxford: Berg.
Grillo, R. D., and R. L. Stirrat, eds.
  1997   *Discourses of Development: Anthropological Perspectives.* Oxford: Berg.
Hall, R. de Z.
  1936   The dance societies of the Wasukuma, as seen in the Maswa District. *Tanganyika Notes and Records* 1:94–96.
Hamilton, S., B. Popkin, and D. Spicer
  1984   *Women and Nutrition in Third World Countries.* New York: Bergin and Garvey.
Harrison, Kelsey A.
  1996   Macroeconomics and the African mother. *Journal of the Royal Society of Medicine* 89 (7): 361–62.
  1997   Maternal mortality in Nigeria: The real issues. *African Journal of Reproductive Health* 1 (1): 7–13.
Hartman, Betsy
  1987   *Reproductive Rights and Wrongs: The Global Politics of Population Control and Contraceptive Choice.* New York: Harper and Row.
Hartwig, Gerald W.
  1970   The Victoria Nyanza as a trade route in the nineteenth century. *Journal of African History* 11:535–52.
Hashim, Leila Sheikh
  1989   Unyago: Traditional family-life education among the Digo, Bondei, Muslims, Sambaa, Segeuju and Zigua of Tanga Region. Paper presented at the Day of Action on Maternal Mortality Workshop, Tanzanian Media Women's Association, Dar es Salaam.
Hatfield, Colby
  1968   The Nfumu in Tradition and Change: A Study of the Position of Religious Practitioners among the Sukuma of Tanzania. Ph.D. thesis, Catholic University, Washington, DC.
Haub, C., M. M. Kent, and M. Yanagishita
  1991   *1991 World Population Data Sheet.* Washington, DC: Population Reference Bureau, Inc.
Hayes, M. V.
  1991   The risk approach: Unassailable logic? *Social Science and Medicine* 3:64–70.

Hedlund, Stefan, and Mats Lundahl
 1989   *Ideology as a Determinant of Economic Systems: Nyerere and Ujaama in Tanzania.* Research Report, no. 84. Uppsala: Scandinavian Institute of African Studies.
Hepburn, Sharon J.
 1988   Western minds, foreign bodies. *Medical Anthropology Quarterly* 2 (1): 59–74.
Herz, B., and A. R. Measham
 1987   *The Safe Motherhood Initiative: Proposal for Action.* Washington, DC: World Bank.
Hochschild, Adam
 1999   *King Leopold's Ghost: A Story of Greed, Terror, and Heroism in Colonial Africa.* Boston: Mariner.
Hockenberry-Eaton, Marilyn, Mary Jane Richman, Colleen DiIorio, et al.
 1996   Mother and adolescent knowledge of sexual development: The effects of gender, age, and sexual experience. *Adolescence* 31 (121): 35–47.
Holmes, C. F.
 1969   A History of the Bakwimba of Usukuma, Tanzania from Earliest Times to 1945. Ph.D. thesis, Boston University.
 1971   Zanzabari influence at the southern end of Lake Victoria: The lake route. *African Historical Studies* 4 (3): 477–507.
Holmes, C. F., and R. A. Austen
 1972   The pre-colonial Sukuma. *Journal of World History* 14 (2): 377–405.
Hone, E. D.
 1936   Raid! *Tanganyika Notes and Records* 1 (2): 98–100.
hooks, bell
 1984   *Feminist Theory: From Margin to Center.* Boston: South End Press.
Hunt, Nancy Rose
 1990   Domesticity and colonialism in Belgian Africa. *Signs* 15 (3): 447–73.
 1999   *A Colonial Lexicon of Birth Ritual, Medicalization, and Mobility in the Congo.* Durham: Duke University Press.
ICD-10
 1992   *International Classification of Disease and Related Health Problems.* 10th rev. Geneva: World Health Organization.
Illiffe, John
 1979   *A Modern History of Tanganyika.* Cambridge: Cambridge University Press.
Ingham, Kenneth
 1965   Tanganyika: The mandate and Cameron, 1919–1931. In Vincent Harlow and E. M. Chilver, eds., *History of East Africa,* 543–93. Oxford: Clarendon.
Inhorn, Marcia C.
 1994a *Quest for Conception: Gender, Infertility, and Egyptian Medical Traditions.* Philadelphia: University of Pennsylvania Press.
 1994b Interpreting fertility: Medical anthropological perspectives. *Social Science and Medicine* 39 (4): 459–61.

Inhorn, Marcia, and Kimberly A. Buss
     1994   Ethnography, epidemiology and infertility in Egypt. *Social Science and Medicine* 39 (5): 671–86.
Itandala, Buluda
     1979   Ilembo, Nkanda and the girls: Establishing a chronology of the Babinza. In J. B. Webster, ed., *Chronology, Migration, and Drought in Interlacustrine Africa,* 145–73. New York: Africana.
Jacobs, Alan H.
     1967   A chronology of the pastoral Maasai. In Bethwell Ogot, ed., *Hadithi I. Proceedings of the annual conference of the Historical Association of Kenya in Nairobi, Kenya, 1967,* 10–31S. Nairobi: East African Publishing House.
Janzen, John
     1978   *The Quest for Therapy in Lower Zaire.* Berkeley: University of California Press.
     1992   *Ngoma: Discourses of Healing in Central and Southern Africa.* Berkeley: University of California Press.
Jolly, Margaret
     1998a   Introduction: Colonial and postcolonial plots in histories of maternities and modernities. In Kalpana Ram and Margaret Jolly, eds., *Maternities and Modernities: Colonial and Postcolonial Experiences in Asia and the Pacific,* 1–25. Cambridge: Cambridge University Press.
     1998b   Other mothers: Maternal 'insouciance' and the depopulation debate in Fiji and Vanuatu, 1890–1930. In Kalpana Ram and Margaret Jolly, eds., *Maternities and Modernities: Colonial and Postcolonial Experiences in Asia and the Pacific,* 177–212. Cambridge: Cambridge University Press.
Jordan, Brigitte
     1978   *Birth in Four Cultures: A Crosscultural Investigation of Childbirth in Yucatan, Holland, Sweden, and the United States.* London: Eden.
     1990   Cosmopolitical obstetrics: Some insights from the training of traditional midwives. *Social Science and Medicine* 28 (9): 925–44.
Justesen, Aafke
     1988   The tip of the iceberg: Maternal mortality. Paper presented at the Tanzania Media Women's Association Seminar on Maternal Mortality. Goethe Institut. Dar es Salaam, Tanzania.
Justice, Judith
     1986   *Policies, Plans, and People: Foreign Aid and Health Development.* Berkeley: University of California Press.
Kabeer, Naila
     1994   *Reversed Realities: Gender Hierarchies in Development Thought.* London: Verso.
Kaijage, Theresa J.
     1989   A strategy for family health promotion at household and community level. Paper presented at the Day of Action on Maternal Mortality, Tanzanian Media Women's Association, Dar es Salaam.

Kaisi, M.
  1988 The rest of the iceberg. Paper presented at the Tanzania Media Women's Association's Seminar on Maternal Mortality in Goethe Institute, Dar es Salaam, Tanzania.
  1989 *The Safe Motherhood Initiative in Tanzania: Role of the Health Sector.* Dar es Salaam: Ministry of Health.
Kasonde, J. M., and I. Kamal
  1998 Safe motherhood: The message from Colombo. *International Journal of Gynecology and Obstetrics* 63 (Supplement1): S103–S105.
Katapa, Rosalia S.
  1994 Arranged marriages. In Zubeida Tumbo-Masabo and Rita Liljeström, eds., *Chelewa, Chelewa: The Dilemma of Teenage Girls,* 76–95. Uppsala: Scandinavian Institute of African Studies.
Kaufert, Patricia A., and John O'Neil
  1993 Analysis of a dialogue on risks in childbirth: Clinicians, epidemiologists, and Inuit women. In Shirley Lindenbaum and Margaret Lock, eds., *Knowledge, Power and Practice: The Anthropology of Everyday Life,* 32–54. Berkeley: University of California Press.
Kay, Margarita, ed.
  1982 *Anthropology of Human Birth.* Philadelphia: F. A. Davis.
Keesing, Roger M.
  1987 Anthropology as interpretive quest. *Current Anthropology* 28:161–76.
Kessel, E., R. Cook, and I. Rosenfield, eds.
  1995 Practical issues in safe motherhood. *International Journal of Gynaecology and Obstetrics.* Supplement 50 (2).
Kilbride, Phillip Leroy, and Janet Capriotti Kilbride
  1990 *Changing Family Life in East Africa: Women and Children at Risk.* University Park: Penn State University Press.
Kisseka, M.
  1973 Heterosexual Relations in Uganda. Ph.D. thesis, University of Missouri.
Kjekshus, Helge
  1977 *Ecology Control and Economic Development in East African History.* London: Heinemann.
Kleiner-Bossaller, Anke
  1993 Kwantacce, the 'sleeping pregnancy,' A Hausa concept. In Gudrun Ludwar-Ene and Mechthild Reh, eds., *Gros-Plan Sur Les Femmes en Afrique (Afrikanische Frauen Im Blick; Focus on Women in Africa),* 17–30. Bayreuth African Studies Series 26.
Kleinman, Arthur, and Joan Kleinman
  1996 The appeal of experience; the dismay of images: Cultural appropriations of suffering in our times. *Daedalus* 125 (1): 1–23.
Koponen, Juhani
  1988 *People and Production in Late Pre-Colonial Tanzania: History and Structures.* Uppsala: Scandinavian Institute of Development Studies.
  1996 Population: A dependent variable. In Gregory Maddox, James L. Gib-

lin, and Isaria N. Kimambo, eds., *Custodians of the Land: Ecology and Culture in the History of Tanzania*, 19–42. London: James Currey.

Kopytoff, Igor, ed.
1987   *The African Frontier*. Bloomington: Indiana University Press.

Kortmann, M.
1972   *Malaria and Pregnancy*. Utrecht: Drukkeriji, Elinkwijk.

Laakso, Annette, and Ingvor Agnarsson
1997   *How Rural Women in Tanzania Raise Money to Finance Their Delivery Care*. Uppsala, Sweden: Unit for International Child Health, Uppsala University.

Laderman, Carol
1983   *Wives and Midwives: Childbirth and Nutrition in Rural Malaysia*. Berkeley: University of California Press.

Lang, G. O., and M. B. Lang
1973   The Sukuma of Northern Tanzania. In Angela Molnos, ed., *Cultural Source Materials for Population Planning in East Africa*, vol. 3: 224–33. Nairobi: East African Publishing House.

Larsen, Ulla
2001   Primary and secondary infertility in Tanzania. Submitted for publication.

Lazarus, Ellen
1988   Theoretical considerations for the study of the doctor-patient relationship: Implications of a perinatal study. *Medical Anthropology Quarterly* 2:34–59.

Lesthaeghe, R., P. O. Ohadike, J. Kocher, et al.
1981   Child-spacing and fertility in sub-Saharan Africa: An overview. In Hilary J. Page and Ron Lesthaeghe, eds., *Child-Spacing in Tropical Africa: Traditions and Change*, 3–23. London: Academic.

Lewis, I. M.
1971   *Ecstatic Religion: An Anthropological Study of Spirit Possession and Shamanism*. Baltimore: Penguin.

Liebenow, J. G.
1959   The Sukuma. In Audrey Richards, ed., *East African Chiefs: A Study of Political Development in Some Uganda and Tanganyika Tribes*, 229–59. New York: Praeger.

Lindenbaum, Shirley
1979   *Kuru Sorcery: Disease and Danger in the New Guinea Highlands*. Mountain View, CA: Mayfield.

Lindenbaum, Shirley, and Margaret Lock, eds.
1993   *Knowledge, Power, and Practice: The Anthropology of Medicine and Everyday Life*. Berkeley: University of California Press.

Little, Marilyn
1991   Imperialism, colonialism and the new science of nutrition: The Tanganyika experience, 1925–1945. *Social Science and Medicine* 32 (1): 11–14.

Lock, Margaret, and Deborah Gordon, eds.
   1988   *Biomedicine Examined: Culture, Illness, and Healing.* Dordrecht: Kluwer Academic.
Loudon, Irvine
   1992   *Death in Childbirth: An International Study of Maternal Care and Maternal Mortality, 1800–1950.* Oxford: Clarendon.
Mabina, M. H., J. Moodley, and S. B. Pitsoe
   1997   The use of traditional herbal medication during pregnancy. *Tropical Doctor* 27:84–86.
MacCormack, Carol P., ed.
   1982   *Ethnography of Fertility and Birth.* Prospect Heights, IL: Waveland.
MacCormack, Carol P., and Marilyn Strathern, eds.
   1980   *Nature, Culture, and Gender.* Cambridge: Cambridge University Press.
Maglacas, A. Mangay, and John Simons, eds.
   1986   The potential of the traditional birth attendant. *WHO Offset Publication* No. 95.
Maguire, G. Andrew
   1969   *Towards "Uhuru" in Tanzania: The Politics of Participation.* London: Cambridge University Press.
Mahler, Halfdan
   1987   The Safe Motherhood Initiative: A call to action. *Lancet* 1 (8533): 668–71.
Maine, D., ed.
   1997   Prevention of Maternal Mortality Network. *International Journal of Gynaecology and Obstetrics* Supplement 59 (2).
Maine, Deborah, and Allan Rosenfield
   1999   The Safe Motherhood Initiative: Why has it stalled? *American Journal of Public Health* 89 (4): 480–82.
Malcolm, D. W.
   1953   *Sukumaland: An African People and Their Country.* London: Oxford University Press.
Mandara, M. P., and G. I. Msamanga
   1988   Maternal mortality in Tanzania. Paper presented at the Annual Conference of the Tanzanian Public Health Association, Arusha, Tanzania.
Manderson, Lenore
   1998   Shaping reproduction: Maternity in early twentieth century Malaya. In Kalapana Ram and Margaret Jolly, eds., *Maternities and Modernities: Colonial and Post Colonial Experiences in Asia and the Pacific,* 26–49. Cambridge: Cambridge University Press.
Marchand, Marianne H., and Jane L. Parpart
   1995   *Feminism/Postmodernism/Development.* London: Routledge.
Martin, Emily
   1987   *The Woman in the Body: A Cultural Analysis of Reproduction.* Boston: Beacon.

1988   Premenstrual syndrome: Discipline, work, and anger in late industrial societies. In Thomas Buckley and Alma Gottlieb, eds., *Blood Magic: The Anthropology of Menstruation,* 161–81. Berkeley: University of California Press.

Martinez, Renee, Ingrid Johnston-Robledo, Heather M. Ulsh, et al.

2000   Singing "the baby blues": A content analysis of popular press articles about postpartum affective disturbances. *Women and Health* 31 (2/3): 37–56.

Mauldin, W. Parker

1994   Maternal mortality in developing countries: A comparison of rates from two international compendia. *Population and Development Review* 20 (2): 413–21.

Mbura, J. S. I., H. N. Mgaya, and H. K. Heggenhougen

1985   The use of herbal medicine by women attending antenatal clinics in urban and rural Tanga district in Tanzania. *East African Medical Journal* 62 (8): 540–50.

Mesaki, Simon

1993   Witchcraft and Witch-Killings in Tanzania: Paradox and Dilemma. Ph.D. diss., University of Minnesota.

1995   The preponderance of women as victims in Sukuma witch killings. In Peter G. Forster and Sam Maghimbi, eds., *The Tanzanian Peasantry: Further Studies,* 279–90. Brookfield, USA: Avebury, VT.

Middleton, John, and E. H. Winter, eds.

1963   *Witchcraft and Sorcery in East Africa.* New York: Praeger.

Mohanty, Chandra Talpade

1991   Under western eyes: Feminist scholarship and colonialist discourse. In Chandra Talade Mohanty, Ann Russo, and Lourdes Torres, eds., *Third World Women and the Politics of Feminism,* 52–79. Bloomington: Indiana University Press.

Mohanty, Chandra Talade, Ann Russo, and Lourdes Torres, eds.

1991   *Third World Women and the Politics of Feminism.* Bloomington: Indiana University Press.

Molnos, Angela, ed.

1973   *Cultural Source Materials for Population Planning in East Africa,* vols. 1–3. Nairobi: East African Publishing House.

Moore, Henrietta L.

1988   *Feminism and Anthropology.* Minneapolis: University of Minnesota Press.

Moraga, Cherrie, and Gloria Anzaldua

1983   *This Bridge Called My Back: Writings by Radical Women of Color.* New York: Kitchen Table.

Morsy, Soheir A.

1990   Political economy in medical anthropology. In Thomas Johnson and Carolyn F. Sargent, eds., *Medical Anthropology: Contemporary Theory and Method,* 26–46. New York: Praeger.

1995   Deadly reproduction among Egyptian women: Maternal mortality and the medicalization of population control. In Faye D. Ginsburg and Raya Rapp, eds., *Conceiving the New World Order: The Global Politics of Reproduction,* 162–76. Berkeley: University of California Press.

MotherCare
1998   *Mother Care Matters. Five Years of Learning and Action. A Compendium of Quarterly Newsletters and Literature Reviews on Maternal and Neonatal Health and Nutrition.* Arlington, VA: John Snow.

Nachtigal, G.
1988   The role of unwanted pregnancy. Case studies. Paper presented at the Tanzania Media Women's Association's Seminar on Maternal Mortality in Goethe Institute, Dar es Salaam, Tanzania.

Needham, R., ed.
1960   *Right and Left: Essays on Dual Classification.* Chicago: University of Chicago Press.
1981   *Circumstantial Deliveries.* Berkeley: University of California Press.

Ngubane, Harriet
1977   *Body and Mind in Zulu Medicine: An Ethnography of Health and Disease in Nywuswa-Zulu Thought and Practice.* London: Academic.

Noble, Charles
1970   Voluntary Associations of the Basukuma of Northern Mainland Tanzania. Ph.D. thesis, Catholic University of America.

Nowak, R.
1995   New push to reduce maternal mortality in poor countries. *Science* 269:780–82.

Ntukula, Mary
1994   The initiation rite. In Zubeida Tumbo-Masabo and Rita Liljeström, eds., *Chelewa, Chelewa: The Dilemma of Teenage Girls,* 96–119. Uppsala: Scandinavian Institute for African Studies.

Okafor, Chinyelu B., and Rahna R. Rizzuto
1994   Women's and health care providers' views of maternal practices and services in rural Nigeria. *Studies in Family Planning* 25 (6): 353–61.

Omolulu, O.
1974   L' importance de l'allaitement maternelle. *Afrique Médicale* 120:485–87.

O'Neil, Norman, and Kemal Mustafa, eds.
1990   *Capitalism, Socialism, and the Development Crisis in Tanzania.* Aldershot: Avebury and Gower.

Ong, Aiwha
1988   Colonialism and modernity: Feminist re-representations of women in non-Western societies. *Inscriptions* 3/4:39–104.

Pala, Achola O.
1977   Definitions of women in development: An African perspective. *Signs* 3 (1): 9–13.

Pan African News Agency
2000   Tanzania Needs Help to Stem Maternal, Infant Mortality. July 11. http://allafrica.com/stories/200007180303.html.

Parpart, Jane L.
    1993   Who is the "other"?: A postmodern feminist critique of women and development theory and practice. *Development and Change* 24 (3): 439–64.
Pigg, Stacy Leigh
    1993   Unintended consequences: The ideological impact of development in Nepal. *South Asian Bulletin* 8 (1): 45–58.
    1995   Acronyms and effacement: Traditional medical practitioners (TMP) in international health development. *Social Science and Medicine* 41 (1): 47–68.
Pottier, Johan
    1997   Towards an ethnography of participatory appraisal and research. In R. D. Grillo and R. L. Stirrat, eds., *Discourses of Development: Anthropological Perspectives,* 203–27. Oxford: Berg.
Price, T. G.
    1984   Preliminary report on maternal deaths in the Southern Highlands of Tanzania in 1983. Paper presented at the Conference of the Association of Gynaecologists and Obstetrics of Tanzania, August 1984, Dar es Salaam.
Puja, Grace Khwaya, and Tuja Kassimoto
    1994   Girls in education—and pregnancy at school. In Zubeida Tumbo-Masabo and Rita Liljeström, eds., *Chelewa, Chelewa: The Dilemma of Teenage Girls,* 54–75. Uppsala: Scandinavian Institute of African Studies.
Ram, Kalpana, and Margaret Jolly, eds.
    1998   *Maternities and Modernities: Colonial and Postcolonial Experiences in Asia and the Pacific.* Cambridge: Cambridge University Press.
Ravindran, Sundari
    1988   Maternal mortality rates for selected countries. *Maternal Mortality: A Call to Women for Action.* Special issue: International Day of Action for Women's Health, May 28. A Joint Publication of the Women's Global Network on Reproductive Rights and the Latin American and Caribbean Women's Health Network 40.
Ravindran, Sundari, and Marge Berer
    1988   Maternal mortality statistics: What's in a number? *Maternal Mortality: A Call to Women for Action.* Special issue: International Day of Action for Women's Health, May 28. A Joint Publication of the Women's Global Network on Reproductive Rights and the Latin American and Caribbean Women's Health Network 5–6.
Reid, Marlene
    1969   Persistence and Change in the Health Concepts and Practices of the Sukuma of Tanzania, East Africa. Ph.D. thesis, Catholic University of America.
Renne, Elisha
    1996   The pregnancy that doesn't stay: The practice and perception of abortion by Ekiti Yoruba women. *Social Science and Medicine* 42 (4): 483–94.

2001   "Cleaning the inside" and the regulation of menstruation in South-western Nigeria. In Etienne van de Walle and Elisha Renne, eds., *Regulating Menstruation: Beliefs, Practices, Interpretations.* Chicago: University of Chicago Press.

Riesman, Paul
1992   *First Find Your Child a Good Mother: The Construction of Self in Two African Communities.* New Brunswick: Rutgers University Press.

Rigby, P.
1966   Dual symbolic classification. *Africa* 36:1–16.

Roberts, Andrew, ed.
1968a   *Tanzania before 1900.* Nairobi: East African Publishing House.

Roberts, Andrew
1968b   The Nyamwezi. In Andrew Roberts, ed., *Tanzania before 1900,* 117–50. Nairobi: East African Publishing House.

1970   Nyamwezi trade. In Richard Gray and David Birmingham, eds., *Pre-Colonial African Trade: Essays on Trade in Central and Eastern Africa before 1900,* 39–74. London: Oxford University Press.

Rosaldo, Michelle Zimbalist, and Louis Lamphere, eds.
1974   *Woman, Culture, and Society.* Stanford: Stanford University Press.

Rosenfield, Allan, and Deborah Maine
1985   Maternal mortality—A neglected tragedy. Where is the M in MCH? *Lancet* 2:83–85.

Roth, Denise M.
1996   Bodily Risks, Spiritual Risks: Contrasting Discourses on Pregnancy in a Rural Tanzanian Community. Ph.D. diss., Department of Anthropology, University of Illinois at Urbana-Champaign.

Roth, Warren
1966   Three Cooperatives and a Credit Union as an Example of Culture Change among the Sukuma. Ph.D. thesis, Catholic University of America.

Royston, Erica, and Sue Armstrong
1989   *Preventing Maternal Deaths.* Geneva: World Health Organization.

Ruck, N.
1996   Work motivation in African medical services. *Africa Health* (May): 23–27.

Rwebangira, Magdalena Kamugisha
1994   What has the law got to do with it? In Zubeida Tumbo-Masabo and Rita Liljeström, eds., *Chelewa, Chelewa: The Dilemma of Teenage Girls,* 187–215. Uppsala: Scandinavian Institute of African Studies.

Rwebangira, Magdalena K., and Rita Liljeström
1998   *Haraka, Haraka . . . Look before You Leap: Youth at the Crossroad of Custom and Modernity.* Stockholm: Nordiska Afrikainstitutet.

Sachs, Wolfgang, ed.
1992   *The Development Dictionary: A Guide to Knowledge As Power.* London: Zed.

Sargent, Carolyn F.
1982   *The Cultural Context of Therapeutic Choice: Obstetrical Care Decisions among the Bariba of Benin.* Dordrecht: D. Reidel.

1988   Born to die: Witchcraft and infanticide in Bariba culture. *Ethnology* 27 (1): 79–95.

1989   *Maternity, Medicine, and Power.* Los Angeles: University of California Press.

Sargent, Caroline, and Joan Rawlins

1991   Factors influencing prenatal care among low-income Jamaican women. *Human Organization* 50 (2): 179–87.

1992   Transformations in maternity services in Jamaica. *Social Science and Medicine* 35 (10): 1225–32.

Scheper-Hughes, Nancy

1992   *Death without Weeping: The Violence of Everyday Life in Brazil.* Berkeley: University of California Press.

Scheper-Hughes, Nancy, and Margaret Lock

1987   The mindful body: A prolegomenon. *Medical Anthropological Quarterly* 1 (1): 6–41.

Sen, Gita, and Caren Grown

1987   *Development, Crises, and Alternative Visions.* New York: Monthly Review.

Shaba, Marie, and Davie Kituru

1991   Unyago. *Sauti ya Siti* 14:24–26.

Shoka, John Luhende

1972   Ideology and Nation-Building in Tanzania: A Micro-Study of Shinyanga District, 1961–1970. Ph.D. thesis, University of Washington.

Shorter, Aylward

1972   Symbolism, ritual and history: An examination of the work of Victor Turner. In T. O. Ranger and I. N. Kimambo, eds., *The Historical Study of African Religion,* 139–49. Berkeley and Los Angeles: University of California Press.

Shuma, Mary

1994   The case of the matrilineal Mwera of Lindi. In Zubeida Tumbo-Masabo and Rita Liljeström, eds., *Chelewa, Chelewa: The Dilemma of Teenage Girls,* 120–32. Uppsala: Scandinavian Institute for African Studies.

Singer, Merrill

1995   Beyond the ivory tower: Critical praxis in medical anthropology. *Medical Anthropology Quarterly* 9 (1): 80–106.

Singer, Merrill, Hans Baer, and Ellen Lazurus

1990   Critical medical anthropology: Theory and research. Special issue of *Social Science and Medicine* 30 (2).

Smith, Dorothy

1987   *The Everyday World as Problematic.* Boston: Northeastern University Press.

Stanley, Henry M.

1969   [1878] *Through the Dark Continent.* New York: Greenwood.

Starrs, Ann
  1987 *Preventing the Tragedy of Maternal Deaths. Report of the Safe Motherhood Conference held in Nairobi, Kenya, February 1987.* New York: Family Care International.
  1998 *The Safe Motherhood Action Agenda: Priorities for the Next Decade.* Report of the Safe Motherhood Technical Consultation held in Sri Lanka, October 1997. New York: Family Care International.
Steinberg, Susanne
  1996 Childbearing research: A transcultural review. *Social Science and Medicine* 43 (12): 1765–84.
Stoler, Ann Laura
  1992 Rethinking colonial categories: European communities and the boundaries of rule. In Nicholas B. Dirk, ed., *Colonialism and Culture,* 319–52. Ann Arbor: University of Michigan Press.
Sundari, T. K.
  1992 The untold story: How the health care systems in developing countries contribute to maternal mortality. *International Journal of Health Services* 22 (3): 513–28.
Sutton, J. E. G.
  1968 The settlement of East Africa. In B. A. Ogot and J. A. Kieran, eds., *Zamani: A Survey of East African History,* 69–99. Nairobi: East African Publishing House.
Swantz, Marja-Liisa
  1969 The Religious and Magical Rites Connected with the Life Cycle of the Woman in Some Bantu Ethnic Groups of Tanzania. Thesis, University of Dar es Salaam.
Tanner, R. E. S.
  1953 Archery amongst the Sukuma. *Tanganyika Notes and Records* 35:63–67.
  1955 Maturity and marriage among the Northern Basukuma of Tanganyika. *African Studies* 13 (3): 123–33.
  1957 The magician in Northern Sukumaland, Tanganyika. *Southwestern Journal of Anthropology* 13 (4): 344–51.
  1958 Sukuma ancestor worship and its relationship to social structure. *Tanganyika Notes and Records* 50:52–62.
  1969 The theory and practice of Sukuma spirit mediumship. In John Beattie and John Middleton, eds., *Spirit Mediumship and Society in Africa,* 273–89. New York: Africana.
  1970 The witch murders in Sukumaland: A sociological commentary. *Crime in East Africa,* 4. Uppsala: Scandinavian Institute of African Studies.
Taussig, Michael
  1980 Reification and the consciousness of the patient. *Social Science and Medicine* 14B:3–13.
Tesfaye, Wolde-Medhin
  2002 Cultural Spaces, Habitats of Power: Smallholders, Local Community

and the "Modernizing" State in Warahimanu, Wollo, Ethiopia. Ph.D. diss., Department of Anthropology, University of Illinois at Urbana-Champaign.

Thaddeus, Sereen, and Deborah Maine

1990   *Too Far to Walk: Maternal Mortality in Context. Findings from a Multidisciplinary Literature Review.* Prevention of Maternal Mortality Program, Center for Population and Family Health, Columbia University.

Tietze, C., and S. Henshaw

1986   *Induced Abortion: A World Review 1986.* New York: Alan Guttmacher Institute.

Tinker, Anne, and Marjorie A. Koblinsky

1993   Making motherhood safe. World Bank Discussion Papers, No. 202. Washington, DC: World Bank.

TNA (Tanzania National Archives). Regional Files

2551	Tabora District Report. 1919–1920
3387	Local Tribe Particulars. 1922.
1733/14	Annual Report. Tabora District. 1923.
1733/4	Annual Report. Tabora District. 1925.
1733/20	Annual Report. Shinyanga Sub-District. 1925.
1733/9	Annual Report. Tabora Province. 1926.
12548	Medical and Sanitary. Lake Province. 1938.

TNA. Secretariat Files

1072	Missions: Subsidy to Medical. Vol. 1. 1927.
10409	Training of Native Midwives and Welfare Workers. 1927–1929.
19303	Baswezi. 1930.
23384	Native Authorities. 1936–37.
24840	Certain Aspects of the Welfare of Women and Children in the Colonies. 1937.
24840/1	Certain Aspects of the Welfare of Women and Children in the Colonies. 1937–1938.
34300	Maternity and Welfare Clinics and Financial Assistance to Expectant Mothers. 1946.

Treichler, Paula

1989   What definitions do: Childbirth, cultural crisis and the challenge to medical discourse. In B. Dervin and L. Grossberg, eds., *Rethinking Communication,* 424–53. Beverly Hills, CA: Sage.

Tumbo-Masabo, Zubeida, and Rita Liljeström, eds.

1994   *Chelewa, Chelewa: The Dilemma of Teenage Girls.* Uppsala: Scandinavian Institute for African Studies.

Turner, Victor

1967   *Forest of Symbols: Aspects of Ndembu Ritual.* Ithaca: Cornell University Press.

Turshen, Meredith

1984   *The Political Ecology of Disease in Tanzania.* New Brunswick: Rutgers University Press.

1999 *Privatizing Health Services in Africa.* New Brunswick: Rutgers University Press.

UNDP (United Nations Development Programme)
1993 *Human Development Report 1993.* New York: Oxford University Press.

United Republic of Tanzania
1992 *Safe Motherhood Strategy for Tanzania.* Dar es Salaam: Ministry of Health.

Van der Geest, Sjaak, and Susan R. Whyte, eds.
1988 *The Context of Medicines in Developing Countries: Studies in Pharmaceutical Anthropology.* Dordrecht: Kluwer.

Varga, C. A., and D. J. H. Veale
1997 *Isihlambezo:* Utilization patterns and potential health effects of pregnancy-related traditional herbal medicine. *Social Science and Medicine* 44 (7): 911–24.

Varkevisser, Corlien M.
1971 Sukuma political history, reconstructed from traditions of prominent nganda (clans). *Tropical Man* 4:67–91.
1973 *Socialization in a Changing Society: Sukuma Childhood in Rural and Urban Mwanza, Tanzania.* Translated by Donald A. Bloch. The Hague: Centre for the Study of Education in Changing Societies.

Vaughan, Megan
1991 *Curing Their Ills: Colonial Power and African Illness.* Stanford: Stanford University Press.

Verderese, Maria de Lourdes, and Lily M. Turnbull
1975 The traditional birth attendant in maternal and child health and family planning: A guide to her training and utilization. *WHO Offset Publication* No. 18.

Walraven, G. E. L.
1996 Primary reproductive health care in Tanzania. *International Journal of Obstetrics and Gynecology and Reproductive Biology* 69:41–45.

Wanjala, S., N. Murugu, and J. Mati
1985 Mortality due to abortion at Kenyatta National Hospital, 1974–1983. In Ruth Porter and Malol O'Connor, eds., *Abortion: Medical Progress and Social Implications,* 41–52. London: Pimtman (Ciba Foundation).

Wasserheit, Judith N.
1989 The significance and scope of reproductive tract infections among Third World women. *International Journal of Gynecology and Obstetrics* Supplement 3: S145–S168.

Were, Gideon S.
1968 The Western Bantu peoples from A.D. 1300 to 1800. In B. A. Ogot and J. A. Kiernan, eds., *Zamani: A Survey of East African History,* 177–97. Nairobi: East African Publishing House.

Werner, A.
1973 [1903] Note on the terms used for "right hand" and "left hand" in the Bantu languages. *Journal of African Society* 13:112–16. Reprinted in

R. Needham, ed., *Right and Left: Essays on Dual Symbolic Classification.* Chicago: University of Chicago Press.

Westoff, Charles

2000   Personal communication, May 2, Princeton, NJ.

Westoff, Charles F., Larry Bumpass, and Norman B. Ryder

1969   Oral contraception, coital frequency, and the time required to conceive. *Social Biology* 16 (1): 1–10.

WGNRR (Women's Global Network on Reproductive Rights)

1991   Maternal mortality and morbidity report 1991. *Women's Global Network on Reproductive Rights.*

WGNRR and ISIS

1988   Maternal mortality: A call to women for action. International day of action for women's health, May 28. Special issue produced by the Women's Global Network on Reproductive Rights and the Latin and Caribbean Women's Health Network/ISIS International.

WHO (World Health Organization)

1976   African traditional medicine: A report of an expert group. *AFRO Technical Report Series,* No. 11. Brazzaville: WHO Regional Office for Africa.

1977   Something for all and more for those in greater need. A "risk approach" for integrated maternal and child health care. *WHO Chronicle* 31:150–51.

1978a The Alma Ata conference on primary health care. *WHO Chronicle* 32 (11): 432–38.

1978b The promotion and development of traditional medicine: Report of a WHO meeting. *WHO Technical Report Series,* No. 622. Geneva: World Health Organization.

1979   Traditional birth attendants: A field guide to their training, evaluation, and articulation with health services. *WHO Offset Publication No. 44.*

1981   Global strategy for health for all by the year 2000. *Health for All Series, Vol. 3.* Geneva: World Health Organization.

1985   Women, health and development: A report by the Director-General. *WHO Offset Publication* No. 90.

1986   Maternal mortality: Helping women off the road to death. *WHO Chronicle* 40 (5): 175–83.

1991a *Maternal Mortality: A Global Factbook.* Compiled by Carla AbouZahr and Erica Royston. Geneva: World Health Organization.

1991b *Midwifery Education: Action for Safe Motherhood.* WHO/MCH/91.3. Geneva: World Health Organization.

1992   *Traditional Birth Attendants. A Joint WHO/UNFPA/UNICEF Statement.* Geneva: World Health Organization.

1995a Maternal health and Safe Motherhood: Findings from concluded research studies. *World Health Statistical Quarterly* 48:2–3.

1995b *Natural Family Planning: What Health Workers Need to Know.* Geneva: World Health Organization.

1996a *Safe Motherhood. Foundation Module: The Midwife in the Community. Education Material for Teachers of Midwifery.* Geneva: World Health Organization.

1996b *Mother-Baby Package: Implementing Safe Motherhood in Countries.* Geneva: World Health Organization.

1998 Safe motherhood as a vital social and economic investment. *World Health Day Fact Sheets* WHD98.2. Geneva: World Health Organization.

1999 *Reduction of Maternal Mortality. A Joint WHO/UNFPA/UNICEF/ World Bank Statement.* Geneva: World Health Organization.

WHO and UNICEF

1996 *Revised 1990 Estimates of Maternal Mortality: A New Approach by WHO and UNICEF.* Geneva: World Health Organization.

Wieschhoff, H. A.

1973 [1938] Concepts of right and left in African cultures. *Journal of the American Oriental Society* 58:202–17. Reprinted in R. Needham, ed., *Right and Left: Essays on Dual Symbolic Classification.* Chicago: University of Chicago Press.

Willis, R. G.

1985 Do the Fipa have a word for it? In D. Parkin, ed., *The Anthropology of Evil,* 209–23. New York: Basil Blackwell.

Winikoff, Beverly

1988 Women's health: An alternative perspective for choosing interventions. *Studies in Family Planning* 19 (4): 197–214.

Wood, Geof

1985 The politics of development policy labelling. *Development and Change* 16 (3): 347–73.

Woost, Michael D.

1997 Alternative vocabularies of development? "Community" and "participation" in development discourse in Sri Lanka. In R. D. Grillo and R. L. Stirrat, eds., *Discourses of Development: Anthropological Perspectives,* 229–53. Oxford: Berg.

World Bank

1993 *World Development Report 1993: Investing in Health.* New York: Oxford University Press.

Yeager, Roger

1989 *Tanzania: An African Experiment.* Boulder: Westview.

Yoder, P. Stanley, ed.

1982 *Issues in the Study of Ethnomedical Systems in Africa.* Los Angeles: Crossroads Press.

Young, Allan

1982 The anthropologies of illness and sickness. *Annual Review of Anthropology* 11:257–85.

Zimbwe, Moma

1988 Training of traditional birth attendants at Pangani Village Health Project. Paper presented at the Tanzanian Women Media Association's Seminar on Maternal Mortality in Goethe Institute, Dar es Salaam, Tanzania.

Index

Abortion, 20, 37, 43, 44, 46, 47–48, 57, 58, 61, 62, 148, 177, 251
Abrahams, R. G., 9, 76–77, 233, 246–47
Abu-Lughod, L., 5–6
Access to care, 11, 15, 19, 22, 45, 54, 63, 98, 148, 160, 186, 233
  during British colonial rule in Tanganyika, 22, 25, 31, 32
  references to, in the Safe Motherhood literature, 11, 45, 229, 233–34
  and social distance, 11
African Inland Mission, 25–29, 238
Age, 44, 99–100, 242
Alloo, F., 57, 58, 59
Alma Ata Conference, 109
Ancestors, 10, 65, 69, 91, 104, 121, 131, 138–39, 164, 255
  ethnicity of, 138
  gender of, 138
  and healing in the African context, 234
  and influence on fertility, 125–27, 138
  Maasai, 138
  Taturu, 138
Anemia, 20, 46, 49, 54, 64, 118, 158, 222, 224, 252
Anna's story, 170–72, 226
Appadurai, A., 12–13, 65, 75
Arabs, in nineteenth-century Tanzania, 9, 76–78, 243, 247
Arab women in Bulangwa, 10, 91, 249
  and discussions on sexual matters, 260–61

and farming, 249
and interactions with health-care providers, 185, 196–97
and menstrual taboos, 129, 257
and postpartum rituals, 212–13, 252
and public codes of modesty, 164–65, 249, 261
social control of, 88, 165, 260
See also Bulangwa
Austen, R., 9, 69, 70, 71, 79, 236, 243, 244, 247

Bakinikana, I., 82, 248
Bariba (Benin), 254
Bassett, M., 197
Bates, M., 81
Beck, A., 24, 236, 238, 247
Beidelman, T. O., 245, 246
Berger, I., 74, 252
Biomedicine, approaches to healing, xvi, 12, 120, 227–28
  and colonial discourse, 13–14
  comparison to nonbiomedical approaches to health, xvi, 12, 227–28
  and maternal health care in Bulangwa, 91–96
  "performance" of, 16
Birth control. *See* Contraceptives; Family planning
Blacklock, M., 19–25, 33, 234, 235
Bledsoe, C., 132, 257
Blood
  bad blood, 258